Teaching and Assessing in Clinical Practice

A Reader

edited and introduced by

CAROL M. DOWNIE MSc RGN RM RNT

PRINCIPAL LECTURER, SCHOOL OF HEALTH
FACULTY OF HUMAN SCIENCES
UNIVERSITY OF GREENWICH

and

PHILIP BASFORD RGN RNT ARRC

PRINCIPAL LECTURER, SCHOOL OF HEALTH
FACULTY OF HUMAN SCIENCES
UNIVERSITY OF GREENWICH

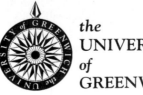

the
UNIVERSITY
of
GREENWICH

First published in 1997 for internal University use.

Second edition published in 1998 by Greenwich University Press and prepared for publication by

Procurement and Business Services Department
University of Greenwich
Woolwich Campus
Wellington Street
London
SE18 6PF

ISBN 1 86166 108 8

Designed and produced for the Procurement and Business Services Department by Angela Allwright.

Te**aching** and **ssessing** i**n** **ractice**

Contents

Foreword

Some years ago concern developed among commercial airlines that military trained pilots were too macho in the cockpit. On encountering a crisis they would take control, tell people what to do and centre the resolution of the problem entirely on their own mental resources. This was not considered the best approach. For each crisis is unique and dealing with it is therefore a learning process. And two heads are better than one.

Most times when I am in need of professional health care I am having my own little crisis and in both psychological and physiological terms my crisis is unique, just as much as for those aeroplane passengers. The solutions to my situation are most reliably developed and delivered by an expert team who are inclined to learn from each other and learn about me. Learning must pervade the clinical area.

The achievement of this ideal, however, depends on the expertise of experienced health care workers and the extent to which they are inclined to create such learning environments and induct trainees into it. Carol Downie and Philip Basford have assembled a collection of works which will help with both.

From these well-selected readings students and experienced practitioners alike will get direct access to a multiplicity of authors whose contributions range from fundamental insights into learning for practice, through to down-to-earth guidance on helping oneself and others to learn in the clinical environment.

While indispensable for nurses, midwives and health visitors, I do hope doctors and care assistants will use it too — and of course, airline pilots.

John Humphreys
Professor of Professional & Vocational Education
Pro Vice-Chancellor
University of Greenwich
September 1988

Introduction

"As a registered nurse, midwife or health visitor, you are personally accountable for your practice and, in the exercise of your professional accountability, must:

14.   *Assist professional colleagues, in the context of your own knowledge, experience and sphere of responsibility, to develop their professional competence and assist others in the care team, including informal carers, to contribute safely and to a degree appropriate to their role."*

(UKCC Code of Professional Conduct, 1992)

The Nurses and Midwives Act (1983), Rule 18, refers to a number of competencies that a trained practitioner needs to develop. The overall aim of these competencies is to develop a nurse or midwife who is proficient in care management, care collaboration, resource management, health promotion and *facilitation of learning*.

In the role of facilitator some of the skills practitioners are expected to display are those of teaching, assessing and evaluation. They also have to act as effective guides, mentors, supervisors and role models. In order to fulfil these roles and demonstrate the required skills, practitioners must also be able to plan effectively, be organised, be able to motivate and perhaps most importantly be able to demonstrate competent communication skills. From this it is clear that the teaching and assessing role of the registered nurse or midwife is by no means a simple one and requires the development of a wide range of sometimes quite complex skills to enable him/her to be able to carry out the roles effectively.

Teaching and assessing and the accompanying responsibilities are not something that a registered nurse or midwife can easily avoid if he/she is to fulfil the requirements laid down within the UKCC *Code of Professional Conduct* (1992). The purposes of the units of study in teaching and assessing are to provide assistance in the development of theoretical knowledge and to allow an exploration of how this knowledge can be applied in practice. All such units taught within the School of Health at the University of Greenwich are substantially based on the English National Board's *Teaching and Assessing in Clinical Practice* (ENB 997, 998) outline curricula.

This Reader is divided into five discreet sections which reflect the main content areas of teaching and assessing units. The first section provides materials related to The Concept of the Adult Learner and an attempt has been made to provide a range of sources on this topic which will complement the formal theoretical input received. As nursing and midwifery students are by definition adults, it would seem logical to explore this concept and gain a clearer understanding of the adult in a learning situation.

The second section follows logically from the first in that it looks at How Adults Learn. In this section the materials provided are designed to help in the exploration of a range of theories of learning and factors which influence the learning process such as individual differences in learning styles, learning skills and experience.

Facilitating Clinical Learning is covered in the third section and the materials here were specifically chosen to illustrate how theoretical concepts and ideas can actually be applied in a practical setting. Very often students find theoretical concepts rather abstract and obscure and have great difficulty in identifying any meaningful relationship between the two. The extracts and articles provided will hopefully help in making this relationship clearer.

Reflective Practice is becoming increasingly relevant and essential in modern nursing and midwifery. The fourth section focuses on this topic and provides a range of materials which give a broad overview of the concept and its application to modern nursing and midwifery practice.

The final section covers Evaluation and Assessment, two key skills required of any registered practitioner. Again a range of materials is provided to help demystify the theories of assessment and evaluation and allow an exploration of the roles of assessor and evaluator.

It would be unwise to consider that the contents of this book provide a definitive collection of articles and extracts, negating the need for further reading and investigation. It would be expected that it will merely provide a fairly secure foundation and that further investigation will be required to make your knowledge base more secure.

Carol Downie and Philip Basford
July 1997

Publisher's note

The contents of the readings in this anthology have been reproduced as they appear in the publications from which they are taken. In the majority of cases footnotes and bibliographic material are included, the exceptions being where they are of excessive length.

The Concept of the Adult Learner

The extracts and articles reproduced in this section are designed to give a reasonably balanced view of andragogy and experiential learning. Linked to the formal theoretical input that will be provided as part of your unit of study, you should find these of value in developing your understanding of adult learning and the role you have to play in facilitating the process. Much has been written about adult learning theory in relation to nursing and midwifery education, and to gain a more in-depth understanding of this aspect of teaching and assessing further reading and investigation will be necessary.

Malcolm Knowles (1990) is possibly one of the best known theorists in relation to adult learning and adult learners; it was he who developed the concept of andragogy. Andragogy is based on the assumption that adults differ in a range of ways from children in their approach to learning. As all the students in nursing and midwifery education are adults, it would seem reasonable for anyone facilitating their learning to be familiar with Knowles' work and to have explored the concept of the adult learner.

In the past, traditionally, nursing and midwifery education was delivered using a predominantly pedagogical approach. That is to say that strategies used to teach were, in the main, teacher-led and teacher-centred with the students playing a very passive, childlike role in the learning process. This has not entirely changed, nor perhaps is it entirely appropriate that a pedagogical model is never used, but there are significant advances in ensuring facilitation strategies are suitable for the students involved in the learning process.

Milligan (1995) very concisely summarises the key elements of andragogy by stating that it is:

> 'facilitation of adult learning that can best be achieved through a student centred approach that . . . . enhances student's self concept, promotes autonomy, self direction and critical thinking, reflects on experience and involves the learner in the diagnosis, planning, enacting and evaluation of their own learning needs.'

If one accepts that these elements are essential in nursing and midwifery education, then it is incumbent on anyone involved in this process to develop their knowledge and skills of adult learning strategies in order for them to be able to facilitate learners in the most appropriate and beneficial manner.

Those using this Reader will almost entirely be involved in the facilitation of learning in the clinical environment where the vast amount of learning is experiential in nature. Experiential learning is viewed by Kolb (1984) as knowledge emerging through the transformation of experience. Kolb sees learning as a core process in human development and this development is gained through experience. Many of the elements of andragogy can be demonstrated within Kolb's (1984) *Experiential Learning Cycle*, and it becomes clear that these two combined can offer those involved with nurse education a very useful means of assisting those in a learning situation to develop a range of skills which will equip them to function more effectively as qualified practitioners.

References

Knowles M (1984) *Andragogy in action: Applying modern principles of adult learning.* Jossey-Bass, San Francisco.

Kolb D (1984) *Experiential learning cycle.* Prentice Hall, New Jersey.

Milligan F (1995) In defence of andragogy. *Nurse Education Today* 15: 22–27.

1.   Adult Students

Who are they . . . ?

Alan Rogers

A profile

Much attention has been given in recent writings on adult education to the adult learner. Whole books have been devoted to the topic, and most general studies of adult education, based on the premise that all forms of teaching adults ought to be student-centred rather than teacher-centred, contain sections dealing with the way adults learn.

Drawing a profile

One feature of this discussion has been the compilation of lists of general characteristics of the adult student. Their aim is to help teachers of adults to become more conscious of what they are doing when they draw up a profile of their students, to test out the items specified to see which do not apply to their particular group and to identify other characteristics specific to their teaching context. One of the more helpful of these lists is that compiled by Harold Wiltshire (1977), but like so many it is limited in its application in that it is directed more towards the traditional student in non-vocational liberal adult education of an academic orientation than to basic education, practical skill-based courses or professional development programmes.

In many of these descriptions there are a number of myths about the adult student participant. Large generalisations are frequently made. It has been suggested at various times that adult students are people well beyond schooldays, full of a mixture of regret, determination, guilt and ambition, but dogged by lack of confidence and self-belief, harrassed by noise and diversions, facing problems of time and space to study, tiredness and opposition and mockery from spouses and friends. (These descriptions have all come from a number of recent writings purporting to describe the general principles on which adult education is predicated.) But clearly these do not describe all (or even perhaps many) adult students. Each such description needs to be drawn up with a proper regard to the individual group in question.

We all draw some picture of who our student participants are going to be. We do this as an integral part of the process of planning the programme and the course. Most of us can rely on past experience to help us, but new teachers of adults cannot do this; they may turn to other more experienced teachers to assist them, but even this is not always possible.

The process of compiling such a profile is often unconscious. We rarely make explicit the views we hold about the prospective learners, their abilities and motivations, what we can and cannot expect from them. Even in those programmes where the goals are

Alan Rogers: 'Adult Students: Who are they . . .?' from *TEACHING ADULTS* (Open University Press, 1996; 2nd edn), pp. 51–73.

negotiated with the potential learners, the teacher-planner still makes several assumptions: for example, that the participants want to join in, that they are willing to entertain the notion of change and that they are capable of engaging in the processes put before them.

We thus fall into unquestioned and possibly false presuppositions about our prospective student participants. We may on occasion assume that the learners are at the opposite extreme from our goals: that they possess no skills at all, if our goals relate to the acquisition of skills; that they are completely ignorant of the subject in hand, if our goals are knowledge-related; that they hold negative attitudes, if our goals are attitude change; that they have not yet begun to comprehend, if our goals are concerned with understanding; that they lack all forms of confidence, if our goal is confidence-building. None of this may be true. Indeed, it is most unlikely to be true. Those who come on a bird-watching course are already more likely than not to know something about the subject; those who attend car-maintenance classes will invariably have had some experience of a car; those who wish to learn about women in literature are most likely to have done some reading in this field already and will have views on the subject; those who come to family planning classes often know more than their teachers allow for. Unless we make conscious what we believe about our potential student participants, we are in danger of presupposing falsehoods.

Testing the profile

Having compiled a list of apparent characteristics of our potential learners, it is necessary to test these assumptions at the earliest possible moment. In some forms of teaching adults — correspondence courses, for example, or the educational programmes offered by the media, and the self-directed learning materials prepared by many agencies — the teacher-planners never meet the learners, so that the assumptions made cannot easily be assessed to see whether they are right or wrong. But in most other cases it will quickly become apparent whether we have judged correctly what the prospective student participants are able to do, what they are willing to do and what they want to do. Sometimes we will get it all wrong, so that there is nothing to be done after the first meeting with the participants other than to redesign the whole learning package. As with most skills of teaching, however, we can improve with practice; but even after long experience, because every group of adult learners is different, we must still test whether the presuppositions we have made about our student participants are correct or not, so that the programme of work can be revised or amplified as necessary.

Teachers are sometimes reluctant to do this in their first encounter with the student participants. It may be that they are hesitant to expose themselves from the start of their relationship with the learners, to give the impression that they are in any way uncertain. Or, having prepared something for the first meeting, they may be anxious to go ahead and give it. These teachers sometimes justify this on the grounds that the participants who have turned up want to have something 'meaty' at the first session so as to judge better the content, level and pace of learning involved in the course, that some prospective participants would find a first meeting devoted to a general discussion about the course an unsatisfying experience. Or the teacher accepts at face value the student participants' assessment of their own ignorance of the subject, their inability to contribute anything useful towards setting the goals and constructing the programme of work. There are many reasons for not opening up the assumptions we have made about the participants to challenge.

Despite all of this, it might be better to spend at least part of the first meeting with any group of adult student participants listening rather than talking, assessing whether the assumptions we have made about their interests and abilities are right or not. Even if we do not do this at the first meeting, the task will have to be done at some stage during the course. It should be done as early as possible so that there is no lengthy gap between bringing together their expectations as learners and our expectations as teachers.

The range is wide

In order to test out these presuppositions, we need to undertake the process consciously rather than subconsciously. It is useful to write down our description of the potential student participants, and here we run into the biggest problem of all. Most of us teach in groups, and the wide range of those who join such groups, even small groups, may hinder us from making realistic judgements about what we can in general expect from our student-learners.

Let us take one example as illustration. It is now thought that intelligence is not a fixed inherent ability that cannot be improved after the end of formal schooling, or a range of abilities that grow and decline along mathematical curves. Rather it is seen as being 'plastic'; it rises to peaks or falls into troughs throughout adulthood, largely governed by whether the activities engaged in and the environmental factors are stimulating and encouraging or whether they are damaging and inhibiting. Particularly the development of intelligence seems to be dependent as much on the amount of educational experience one has received and on the subsequent use of learning skills in one's occupations as it is on the basic learning ability developed when young. People who have had a good deal of education and who have been engaged in tasks calling for considerable and regular amounts of new learning will be 'more intelligent' at 50 than they were at 25; conversely, those who have been employed in occupations that have not required them to engage in new learning are likely not to have developed their intelligence to the same extent. Thus in any group of adults engaged in a learning programme, the range of learning ability, even among people of roughly the same age and same initial education, is likely to be considerably wider than in a comparable group of children.

Lifespan studies

It may be useful at this point to outline the general conclusions of what have been called 'lifespan studies' in relation to adult learning; for if learning is a process of personal changes made in adapting to changed situations and experiences, the study of different patterns of life is likely to throw light on such learning.

In the 1970s and 1980s, a general view of lifespan development emerged based on ideas about the major points of meaningful change that occur during adulthood. This was thought to give teachers a useful basis for this process of drawing a profile of their student participants. Although it is given less credence today, it is still worth reviewing this field. What follows is not intended to be a comprehensive guide to this area of study but an introduction. Teachers who want to pursue the subject further are referred to the books listed at the end of the chapter.

The terms 'growth', 'change' and 'development' are used in a variety of senses. Some educational writers see 'change' as quantitative accumulations to the content of thought, and 'development' as a qualitative transformation of one's thinking structures; but these distinctions omit any reference to intention and purpose. A more satisfactory definition sees 'change' as value-free, indicating an undirected process, whereas 'development' implies purposeful change, directed towards the achievement of some goal.

A number of writers see adult progression as growth, the gradual and natural increase of maturity. Others see it as development, i.e. goal achievement. For writers like Piaget and Kohlberg, the goal is one of 'rational autonomy'; for others there is the increasing sense of perspective as well. Viewed in goal-achievement terms, it is possible to determine stages of progress. On the other hand, some writers have rejected the concept of 'development' and replaced it with a more or less value-free view of change throughout adult life.

General considerations

It seems to be accepted that there are, for the adult, few (if any) age-related changes. Unlike the child and the adolescent, whose different stages are recognised (even if not universally agreed), adults change and develop more by experience and by the exercise of abilities than by mere age. There are physical changes that occur with increasing age, but none of these is related to any specific age, and the changes that take place differ for each individual.

Additionally there is in the West a strong emphasis on the physical elements in human make-up. Thus ageing is seen as a phenomenon to be resisted, something to be overcome rather than welcomed and valued for the wisdom and status it brings.

Adult development has several other dimensions. On the one hand, there are the changes that occur within each person as the years advance. On the other hand, there are those changes within the social and cultural context of the individual which call for new responses. We are dealing with a changing person in a changing world. Change, not stability, is the norm.

Among those many changes are variations in perspectives, including the view of the ageing process itself. Traditionally in Western societies, youth has been seen in positive terms while ageing has been regarded more negatively. But in recent years, views in relation to older persons have shown significant changes, with growing positive attitudes towards older age groups and rather more negative attitudes towards younger people, perhaps a result of the increasing number of older persons in society as a whole. In many developing countries on the other hand, influenced by Western cultural patterns, the reverse would seem to be happening, despite the increasing number of older persons in various forms of adult education. Society is not only imposing roles on individuals but is constantly reinterpreting those roles — and all these changes will call for learning on the part of every adult.

Ages of man and woman

Most of us are acquainted with Shakespeare's 'seven ages of man': the infant, the schoolboy, the lover, the soldier, the justice, the 'lean and slipper'd pantaloon', and finally second childhood. Since Shakespeare's time there have been many attempts to better this description of adult changes. Some are very general: Whitehead's successive phases of romance, precision and rationalizatlon, or Egan's romantic stage, philosophic stage and eirenic or fulfilled stage. Some still display the so-called 'plateau effect' of Shakespeare: growth, maturity and decline. The very title of the University of the Third Age perpetuates the outdated concept of a three-stage life consisting of growth, performance and 'completion'.

Recently it has been recognised that some of the earlier schemata relating to adult development were too closely tied to successive stages, and attempts have been made to break away from this. There is however still a tendency to see adults in too great an isolation from the social and physical environment in which they are located, to see society as static while the individual changes, to underestimate the effect of changes in social structures and values on the adult. Equally there is an underestimate of the effect that different educational and cultural backgrounds and different experiences can have on adults.

Dominant concerns

The most influential group of lifespan theories are those that see changes during the adult phase of life in terms of dominant concerns. Havighurst (1952) suggested that the individual passes through eight main stages; after the two periods of childhood and adolescence comes adulthood, a 'developmental period in about as complete a sense as childhood and adolescence are developmental periods'. From 18 to 30, adults are focusing their life; there is a concern for self-image. Self is a major preoccupation, not society (voting and civic duties are less frequent at this period). This is a period of experimentation, of settling into jobs and love affairs. Education tends to be turned to by some as an instrument for occupational advancement. From 30 to 40, adults are collecting their energies; this is a period of stability and relatively less introspection, less self-doubt. The job is now most important, with child-rearing a close second. Involvement in education now tends towards the expressive rather than the instrumental. The decade from 40 to 50 is a period of self-exertion and assertion. This is the peak of the life cycle. Public and civic activities are more prominent, whereas participation in educational programmes tends to decline. This stage is characterised by a turning out towards society from oneself, the family and the job. 'Action' is the means of dealing with the world, and this emphasis on action brings about the first consciousness of physical deterioration.

From 50 to 60, adults maintain their position and at the same time change roles; educational involvement is for expressive rather than instrumental purposes. There is increasing evidence of physical deterioration (sight and hearing), and larger amounts of energy have to be exerted to avoid losing ground. Often it is asserted that the adult is more passive and deferential, with a sagging sense of self-assurance. 'Thought' rather than 'action' is the means of dealing with the world, and there is more concentration on short-term rather than long-term achievements. The adult spends the years between 60 and 70 deciding whether and how to disengage. This is often the period of the death of friends and relatives, of less social concern, of less active preoccupations and more short-term gratifications. From 70 onwards is the period of making the most of disengagement. Healthy adults are not too preoccupied with the past, are self-accepting and relatively content with the outcomes of their life, but often the period is characterised by poor health, reduced means and dependence on others.

Havighurst's views, as set out above, are frequently cited by adult educators. They are almost the only ones that relate such changes directly to educational activities. But they are too simplistic, too rigidly tied to ages, and they are based on Western male-dominated concepts of a successful work career. Major changes in social structure have rendered such a neat analysis suspect.

These considerations have led to a more sequential approach without tying each stage too closely to ages. Neugarten (1977) speaks of adulthood as representing a 'movement from an active, combative, outer-world orientation to . . . an adaptive, conforming inner-world orientation'. Three stages are identified: a period of expressiveness, expansiveness and extroversion, of autonomy and competence (up to about the age of 30); an intermediate period of reorientation; and a third stage of change from active to passive modes of relating to the environment with greater introversion.

Tensions

Erikson (1965) sees the stages of human development in terms of different tensions. There is the general and continuing tension between 'the inner wishes . . . and the demands to conform to other people's standards and requirements', which all people experience and which leads to compromises if the adult is 'to maintain the integrity of his [sic] personality'. In addition there are a series of developmental tensions; in puberty and adolescence, there is the tension between identity and role confusion; in young adulthood, intimacy versus isolation; in adulthood, generativity versus stagnation; and in 'maturity', the integrity of the self versus despair. The educational implications of each stage are delineated: initial education for the child and adolescent, vocational education for the young adult, social and community education for the adult, and philosophical and creative education for the mature. Boshier (1989) similarly speaks of tensions (incongruence); he draws upon the work of Carl Rogers (1974) to depict the individual as having

> 'two problems; maintaining inner harmony with himself [sic] and with the environment. Incongruence is developed within the person (intra-self) and between the person and other-than-self experiences (self/other) . . . . The research of life-cycle psychologists supports the notion that younger [adults] manifest more intra-self and self/other incongruence than older, more mature [people].'

> (Boshier 1989: 147–50)

Time perspectives

Lifespan changes may be seen in terms of how time is viewed. Some writers have suggested that the child sees the future as far away; for the adolescent, the future is rosy; for the adult, time is finite, while the mature adult feels that time is running out. Friedman elaborated this version of the 'plateau' theory of lifespan changes, being particularly conscious that successive stages do not correlate with ages. He thus overlapped some stages:

- The *entry stage* (say 18–25): orientation is to the future — the future will be better than the present; change is good.

- *Career development* (say, 20–50): orientation is increasingly more to the present than to the future; away from interest in promotion towards an interest in the intrinsic value of work, together with participation and achievement in non-work areas.

- *Plateau* (say, 35–55): the main time-focus moves from the present to a feeling that time is running out; there is increasing neuroticism, especially among the lower socio-economic groups, who cope less well than professionals and managers (!).

After 55 comes a period of decline.

Sex and class factors

As these examples show, there is considerable sex and class bias in such analyses. This indicates the origin of most of the studies — amongst American white professional males, those who on the whole predominate in continuing education programmes in the United States. The sexual bias is surprising; all of these theories relate to male careers despite the fact that women predominate in most forms of non-vocational adult education. The women's movement has been seeking to redress the balance, exploring the cycle of adulthood for women. Similarly, it is likely that the lifespan stages and expectations of blacks are different from those listed above.

The class bias has received less attention. Almost all the above descriptions rely upon doubtful assumptions concerning the social and educational background of the participants; they relate to the educated, the professionally employed and the ambitious. One attempt to redress this balance towards the working class (by Guy Hunter, quoted in Stephens and Roderick, 1971) suggests that

> 'there is a rough sequence in a working life which the intellectual is too apt to forget. After the first period of school and pure technical training, the worker, for the ten years from 15 to 25, is pitchforked into practical life — finding and holding a job after marriage and founding a home on small resources . . . between 25 and 35, as the worker approaches a more responsible job, education should broaden his ideas of the nature of authority, of the social and human implications of any new job, of the deeper purposes of society. Once this broadening process has been started, it may well lead on into history, literature and art. It means at 21 bread

and butter and the wage packet. At 30 it may include ideas of status, leisure, civic responsibility; and at 40 and thereafter it may deepen into a concept of the good life.'

(p. 195)

Roles and crisis points

This attempt to draw up an alternative lifespan sequence to that of the male professional still assumes a working life. Long-term unemployment on a large scale and changes in attitudes to work and retirement have thrown doubt on much of the existing research. These changes and the patronising air that surrounds such efforts to define working-class life stages have led to a number of different approaches, some of which concentrate on the pattern of family life and/or lifestyles. Others seek not so much for the variations between separate groups of adults but for a comprehensive view of development common to all adults. A way forward is found in concentrating on the changing *roles* of the adult or on the crisis points that occur in the life of most adults of a particular generation, whether male or female, working class or middle class, black or white — although reactions to these new roles and crisis points vary considerably according to experience and the culture of the individual.

The most common roles and crisis points identified (Sheehy, 1976) usually relate to the first job, marriage, parenthood, the departure of children from the home, bereavement (especially the loss of parents and spouse), separation and divorce, loss of a job or other role, retirement and (less sequential and more occasional) moving house (a major period of stress in the lives of many people). Amongst these writers, a common crisis point is seen to occur somewhere about the age of 40 in both males and females.

Summary

The search for the stages of man or woman is still under way. From our point of view as teachers, it is wise to remember that adults age; and that, with ageing,

- physical changes occur, to a greater extent for some people than for others and in different ways;

- roles change, all calling for new learning, and there may on occasion be difficulties in adapting to new roles or to new perceptions of roles;

- various crisis points are passed, sometimes easily, sometimes with difficulty.

The mixed group that most teachers of adults face will not only possess a wide range of ability; they will also be at different ages and at different stages of development, and will in any case react in different ways to the very varied changes each one is experiencing in their own life.

General characteristics of adult student-learners

Despite the wide variations that exist between the members of our learning group, however, it is still possible to identify some of the common characteristics of adult student participants. What follows is my list; you may find it helpful to decide for yourself how far each of the categories is appropriate in your own circumstances. I have selected seven characteristics that seem to me to be true of the large majority of adult learners, whatever their situation or stage of development, although cultural settings may modify these to some extent:

- The student participants are adult by definition.
- They are in a continuing process of growth, not at the start of a process.
- They bring with them a package of experience and values.
- They come to education with intentions.
- They bring expectations about the learning process.
- They have competing interests.
- They already have their own set of patterns of learning.

1. They all are adults by definition

We have seen that adulthood is an ideal, never fully achieved. The concept implies movement, progress towards the fulfilment of the individual's potential, the development of balanced judgements about themselves and others, and increasing independence. Our student participants are people who are becoming more mature, and the way we teach adults should encourage this development in self-fulfilment, perspective and autonomy.

The most visible way in which the adult learners exercise their adulthood in relation to our programme of work is by voluntarily choosing to come to our classes. Adult student participants are not dependent in the way children are. Malcolm Knowles, who has written one of the more perceptive accounts of the subject (*The Adult Learner*, 1990), suggests that adulthood is attained at the point at which individuals perceive themselves to be essentially self-directing (although this may not be for many persons a single point). He points out that there is a natural process of maturation leading organically towards autonomy, but that this is limited by what the social culture permits. In many societies the culture does not encourage the development in some groups of people (women, for instance, especially married women, in many parts of the world) of those abilities needed for self-direction. Self-directedness then is often partial; it may not extend to all parts of life (including to education). Knowles points to the gap or tension that exists in these cases between the drive and the ability to be self-directing.

Some people will feel more strongly than others this compulsion, this urge to take control of their own lives, to be involved increasingly in the decision-making processes affecting their life choices. But it is there in virtually all adults nonetheless. The educational process for adults, to be effective, should coincide with this process of maturation. A situation that reverses the trend, treating the developing adult as a child, will find itself faced on most occasions with major blocks to learning. Our programme must adapt itself to this increasing sense of self-determination if it is to maximise learning.

Against this must be set the fact that some adults, re-entering education after some time away from school, expect to be treated as children. The expectations of 'being taught' are sometimes strong, and if these expectations are not met in some way or other, once again learning is hindered. Experience suggests however that even the most docile group of adult students, happy for much of the time to be passive learners as if they were back in school again, will at the right time rebel against their teachers when the affront to their adulthood becomes too great. It can be a great help to provoke such a situation when we feel the time has come to break up the more formal atmosphere and secure greater participation by the students in their own learning process.

2. *They are all engaged in a continuing process of growth*

Contrary to some assumptions, adult student participants have not stopped growing or developing. They are not at a static period in their lives, a plateau between the growth stages of youth and the declining stage of old age; they are still people on the move. Whatever our view about the way adults develop, the key issue is that growth and change are occurring in all aspects of our student participant's life — in the physical arena, in the intellectual sphere, in the emotions, in the world of relationships, in the patterns of cultural interests. This is true of all participants in all types of adult learning. The pace and direction of these changes vary from person to person; but that it is happening cannot be called into question.

The teacher should take this pattern of change seriously. The people we are trying to help to learn are not passive individuals; they are actively engaged in a dynamic process. And they are in the middle of this process, not at the start. They may be at the start of a new stage of the process, but this stage will draw upon past changes and will in turn contribute to the whole programme of development and growth. It is a process that, although continual, is not continuous; it usually proceeds in spurts, triggered off by new experiences (such as the adult class itself) or new perceptions.

We are normally aware of this process of change within ourselves; indeed, coping with teaching adults itself forms part of the changing pattern of our lives. But we are sometimes reluctant to accept that such a process occurs within the student participants, that they are in the midst of a series of changes when they come to us. It is not practical for us to know all our student participants intimately enough to assess accurately the position each of them has reached and the way by which they have got there. But we can be aware that the process is in every case still continuing. Sensitivity to this fact, and to the fact that the educational experience we offer forms part of this ongoing change process, helps a great deal in creating our responses to the varying demands the students make upon us.

3. *They all bring a package of experience and values*

Each of the learners brings a range of experience and knowledge more or less relevant to the task in hand. New students are not new people; they possess a set of values, established prejudices and attitudes in which they have a great deal of emotional investment. These are based on their past experience. Knowles (1990) suggests that, for children, experience is something that happens to them; for adults, experience serves to determine who they are, to create their sense of self-identity. When this experience is devalued or ignored by the teacher, this implies a rejection of the person, not just the experience.

This is true in all fields of teaching adults, even in the formal technical and higher educational programmes, but it becomes particularly important for the adult teacher in those contexts where personal growth forms the major objective of the educational programme. The tensions and concerns of both the learner and the teacher in these contexts have been particularly well described by John Wood in his 'Poem for Everyman' (1974).

Poem for Everyman[1]

I will present you
parts
of
my
self
slowly
if you are patient and tender.
I will open drawers
that mostly stay closed
and bring out places and people and things
sounds and smells, loves and frustrations, hopes and sadnesses,
bits and pieces of three decades of life
that have been grabbed off
in chunks
and found lying in my hands
they have eaten
their way into my memory
carved their way into my
heart
altogether — you or I will never see them —
they are me.
if you regard them lightly
deny that they are important
or worse, judge them
I will quietly, slowly
begin to wrap them up,
in small pieces of velvet,
like worn silver and gold jewelry,
tuck them away
in a small wooden chest of drawers

and close.

Such sentiments are not characteristic of all adult student participants. Far from being reticent, some are confident, and a few positively push their views and experiences at the group and at the teacher. But it is perhaps true of more adults in learning situations than we are aware of. The teacher of adults needs to be sensitive to the situation whenever it arises, and it often occurs in the most unlikely of settings and in every class, whether it is a closed group brought together for a specific training purpose, an open-recruitment general-interest course, a highly structured formal class or a community education or development group.

What are the implications of students' prior experience, knowledge and values for our approach to teaching?

First this 'package' determines what messages are received by the learner. The student participants see all new material they encounter through the lens of their existing experience and knowledge (just as the teacher does), and this may distort the messages. Constant feedback from the participants is essential if the teacher is to remain alive to exactly what the student is learning.

Secondly, in those cases where the student participants do not believe that they possess any relevant experience or knowledge, where they insist that they 'know nothing at all about the subject', it is possible to help them to become aware that they do in fact possess relevant material. For unless the new learning is related to this existing reservoir of experience and knowledge, it cannot be fully absorbed into the person; it will sit uneasily with the rest of the individual's make-up, it will be compartmentalised from the rest of their being and will thus not fully affect their attitudes and behaviour. It is not a difficult skill for the teacher to acquire to explore with the participants something of what they already know about the matter in hand: words and phrases relating to the subject of the course, collected from the participants and listed on a blackboard or otherwise, can demonstrate to them that they are able to contribute towards the programme of learning. It is usually necessary only for the teacher to make a beginning; once the process has begun, the participants will normally be able to continue the exploration for themselves and find new ways of relating the content of the course to different parts of their own experience and knowledge. The start of the process is the most difficult step for some of the student participants to take, but it is an essential one before deep and permanent learning can take place.

Thirdly, not all of this set of values, experience and knowledge is correct or helpful to the required learning. What is correct and helpful needs to be confirmed and reinforced; what is not correct needs unlearning. Experience of teaching adults reveals that there is often as much unlearning to be done as new learning, and because of the emotional investment in the existing patterns of experience and knowledge, the unlearning process is one of the more difficult tasks facing the teachers of adults.

Fourthly, this experience and knowledge (some of it unique to the individual participant and therefore new to the teacher) is a major resource for learning and can be harnessed into the work of the class to the enrichment of the whole group. Much new material can be drawn out from the student participants rather than be presented by the teacher to the taught. Theoretically, we should all start from where the student participants themselves are; but since we usually teach in groups this is not often possible except where the contract to learn has ensured that a more or less homogeneous group has been created. But the utilisation of the varied experience and knowledge of all the members of the group is essential not only to ensure effective learning at a personal level; it will help to bind together the group and make all of its members richer.

4. *They usually come to education with set intentions*

It is often argued that adult students come to adult education because of a sense of need. We shall look at this area of needs in adult education [in more detail later], but here we must note one or two points. First, it is not always strictly true that the members of our classes are motivated by needs; some job-related programmes, for instance, contain participants who have little or no sense of need. Perhaps it is more useful to talk of all adult student participants as having a set of 'intentions', which for many of them can imply the meeting of a felt need.

Secondly, for those who do come out of a want or need, it is on occasion a confused area. Sometimes the participant is imbued with a vague sense of unease and dissatisfaction. The reason for attending that they give to others and even on occasion to themselves is not the true reason; sometimes the reason is not related to learning at all but more towards social contact or getting out of the house or to please some third person (some research suggests that there is a high correlation between attending some forms of adult education and problems within the marriage relationship, to take but one example). Even when this sense of need is related to learning, there is at times an uncertainty as to what it is that they should be learning. R. D. Laing has expressed something of this in his poem 'Knots' (from the 1972 book of the same title):

> *Knots*[2]
>
> There is something I don't know
>   that I am supposed to know.
> I don't know *what* it is I don't know
>   and yet am supposed to know,
> and I feel I look stupid
>   if I seem both not to know it
>   and not know *what* it is I don't know.
> Therefore I pretend I know it.
>   This is nerve-racking
>   since I don't know what I must pretend to know.
> Therefore I pretend to know everything.
>
> I feel you know what I am supposed to know
> but you can't tell me what it is
> because you don't know that I don't know what it is.
>
> You may know what I don't know, but not
>   that I don't know it,
> and I can't tell you. So you will have to tell me everything.

At one end of the spectrum of student intentions then is the satisfying of some vague and ill-articulated sense of need. At the other end are those who are present out of a desire to solve a clearly identified problem or to undertake a particular learning task which they feel is required for the performance of their social or vocational roles — for example, to learn a language for their next holiday; to acquire mastery over a computer for job or leisure fulfilment; to understand the development processes of very young children to help them cope at home; or to come to a knowledge of one of the systems of government to enable them to play a more effective role in their local community. In the course of their own continuing development, these people find that they need a specific skill or knowledge or understanding to enable them to fit more easily into some existing or new situation. Even those who come to adult education classes in search of 'a piece of paper', a qualification, rather than new learning may be there for different motives. For some, it is the necessary preliminary to securing promotion or access to more education; for others, it is part of their pursuit of self-affirmation, a need to achieve a goal for themselves. A number come to seek reassurance, confirmation of their ability to achieve the goal. There is a wide range of such wants and intentions. These purposes, often perceived clearly, are almost always concrete and meaningful to their immediate concerns, though on occasion the learning is intended for longer-term future application.

These are the two extremes to this spectrum of adult intentions: those who come to achieve a particular piece of learning related to their present pattern of life, and those who come for social and/or personal reasons or out of some general indeterminate sense of urgency. In the middle are the many who come to learn a 'subject'. Here are those who wish to learn history or cooking or painting or bird-watching, material that is specific enough but not directly related to the solution of an immediate problem. For them it is a matter of interest, of adding to the richness of their present way of life.

Often no clear-cut distinction may be drawn between these three groups. Nevertheless, they may be more or less equated with what C. O. Houle, in his classic work *The Inquiring Mind* (1961), has identified as the three main orientations of the adult learner. In any adult learning situation, he claims, some of the student participants are *goal-oriented*. They wish to use education to achieve some external objective such as a certificate or promotion or to solve an immediate problem facing them. For them the learning experience tends to come to an end once the objective (often separate from the learning process) has been achieved.

A second group is described as *activity-oriented*. They like the atmosphere of the adult class, they find in the circumstances of the learning a meaning for themselves independent of the content or of the announced purpose of the activity. They attend because they get something out of the group apart from the subject-matter involved; it meets a range of needs that are mainly personal and/or social. These people frequently seek the continuance of the activity even though the content of the learning may well change; they may pass from one class to another, searching for satisfaction in the activity itself.

The third group is described as *learning-oriented*. They desire the knowledge or skill for its own sake. They pursue the subject out of interest and will continue to pursue it even without the assistance of a formal programme of adult learning (see Figure 1).

The implications for the teacher of the different intentions of each of these three groups (and of the many who occupy places on the spectrum between these three positions) are considerable. The responses of each group to the demands of the learning programme will vary. Those participants who are motivated to attend courses out of some sense of internal need may on occasion exhibit anxiety, sometimes mixed with hesitation and uncertainty; for the concept of need is threatening, demeaning both to oneself and to others. Such anxiety can be a useful thing — it can promote learning provided it is not too great. A gentle encouragement of the sense of need and particularly an attempt to focus it upon particular learning objectives that may help towards meeting the needs often bring about greater readiness to learn. The development of a clearer conception of the nature of the learning task and of the relevance of the material to the immediate concerns of the participant is an essential preliminary to the use of the learning programme to satisfy such needs. On the other hand, those whose motivation is to achieve some external goal (to pass an examination, for instance) will often reveal a great keenness. Here too, the clearer the awareness of purpose and of the relevance of the task to meet this purpose, the greater the motivation to learn.

Figure 1   Orientations of learning

Orientation	Intentions	Learning process	Continuation at end of programme?
Goal-oriented; end product	Achievement; problem-solving/ attainment	Learning most in certain specific areas	Process ceases on 'successful' completion of course
Learning-oriented	Interest in subject	Learning in all parts of subject-matter	Continued learning in same or related subject area
Activity-oriented	Social or personal growth needs; often indeterminate	Find in activities satisfactions to needs	A new situation or activity is sought

5. They bring certain expectations about education itself

Adult student participants come to their learning programmes with a range of expectations about the learning process, a series of attitudes towards education in general. These are usually based on their experience of schooling and of education since leaving school (if any). The conception of what education is and what it is for varies widely. Some people enjoyed their years in school; others did not. A number of our student participants assume that adult education will be like school. They expect to be taught everything by a teacher who 'knows everything'; they expect to be put back *in statu pupillari*, which is what education and learning imply for them. On the other hand, some are more confident, willing to engage for themselves directly with the material being handled. For some of them the joy of the adult class is that it is unlike school. Even for many of those who enjoyed their schooldays, the value of adult education is often that the contents and the methods employed are different from those experienced in the formal education system (Figure 2).

These expectations have different results on the attitudes of the participants towards the work of the group. Some tend more towards conformism, while others seek for a measure of independent learning. Some see, in the formal structure of an adult education class, support for themselves, feeling more at home with 'being taught' —

though they may still be anxious as to whether their skills of learning are adequate for the purpose or not. They may feel that their ability to learn has declined since they were last in education (and this may be true; on occasion we may have to spend some time with our student participants boosting their confidence and, even in some advanced courses, strengthening their skills of formal learning). Some of those who have had experience of education over a longer time may look for a less formal structure or become impatient, wishing to push on faster; they feel able to deal with the material easily.

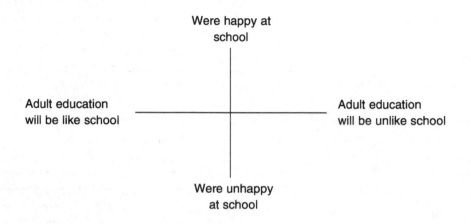

Figure 2   Orientations of learning

In particular, both kinds of student participant bring with them a set of *self-horizons* relating to the sort of material they can or cannot master. Most of us believe that there is some subject or other that we can never learn, that is just not compatible with our range of inherent abilities and interests. It is odd that so many voluntary adult students still find themselves in classes containing a good deal of material that from the start they are adamant they will never be able to learn. Students attend courses in religion and yet say they cannot cope with 'theology'; students join art classes with a firm belief that they can never learn to draw. Learning in parts of these fields is not for them; they confine themselves to the role of 'looker-on', as presumably they were at times in school. They may plead age, using this as an excuse to avoid causes of failing for other reasons. By contrast there will be those who see the entering of new areas as a challenge, difficult but not beyond the learning resources they can call upon.

We need to explore these views, about schooling, learning and what is expected in education, from an early stage in the learning programme. The worst thing we can do is treat all the participants alike, teaching one course to them all. The problem of the teacher of adults faced with a mixed group of student participants, encouraging those with low self-horizons and keeping the more self-reliant satisfied with their own progress, is one of constantly making choices between alternatives, of balancing between the needs of one sub-group and those of another while maintaining loyalty to the subject-matter of the course and the group as a whole.

6. *They all have competing interests*

Apart from those adults, still too few, who are for a relatively short period engaged in full-time courses, adult students are part-time. Education for them is a matter of secondary interest; it is not their prime concern. It is constantly overshadowed by the 'realities' of life: their job or lack of job, their family situation, their social life, other competing issues.

The adults who come to join us in the learning enterprise come from a complete social environment. They all have relationships such as parents, partners, workmates and friends, as well as being students. Adult learners should not be divorced from their background if their learning is to be relevant and thus effective. We need to take seriously the whole of the context within which our student participants live and where they use the new learning they have acquired. Students in other parts of the educational world may be taken out of their life situation to concentrate on their learning, but part-time adult learners continue to live within their world and to apply what they learn in that world.

Within that background there are factors supporting the learning endeavours as well as some militating against these same endeavours. Not all of the competing concerns that the participants bring with them to our programmes are hindrances. Some are supportive. Indeed, periods of intensive study can hardly be carried through without the identification of the support networks existing all around the adult learner, and it is to the advantage of both teacher and student participant to encourage the full exploitation of these supporting factors. This is particularly true where the class is a one-off episode, not backed up by other studies as it is at school or college. A short course, taken part-time and on its own, assumes in the life of many student participants rather less significance than it has for the teacher we must not be surprised if our students' attention is at times distracted towards the more urgent problems of the family's health, or the omission to fulfil some promised errand, or problems at work.

7. *They all possess set patterns of learning*

Adults are engaged in a continuing process of lifelong learning, and they have already acquired ways of coping with this. They often fail to see this as 'learning' in the educational sense, but it exists all the same. We shall look in more detail at the special features of the adult learning process, but here we must note two points: that each of the participants has developed such a style already; and that the styles that exist in our adult groups are varied.

Over the years, each of our adult student participants has developed their own strategies and patterns of learning, which they have found help them to learn most easily, most quickly and most effectively. Learning changes are not brought about without effort, and the process can be painful; it takes an investment of time and emotions, and, once done, no one wants to do it again. We all thus seek ways to ease the pain, shorten the time taken to master the necessary new material, and make the gains acquired more permanent. Experience has taught us what strategies we can adopt to achieve these ends.

Each of us learns in our own way, according to our particular aptitudes and experience. Some handle figures more easily than others. Some have fostered different methods for memorising facts (addresses, telephone numbers, etc.). Some need to see the written page in order to comprehend more fully rather than rely on the spoken word. Languages particularly throw up differences of approach in this respect. Some learners need a book and practise sounds from written words, finding it hard to react to spoken words, while others respond easily to oral tuition; both are valid methods of learning languages, and we should not try to force any learner into adopting a particular style because we prefer it to any other. We must thus remember that our student participants all have their own ways of dealing with learning needs, and opportunities to exercise these have to be created if new learning is to take place.

The pace of learning of each student participant also varies. In general, in those areas where the participants can call upon a good deal of experience — social relationships and roles, for instance — or where they may have direct experience of the subject-matter, they tend to learn fast, a good deal faster than young people, provided that the new material does not conflict with existing knowledge. But where they have less experience on which to fasten the new material — languages, for example, or computer studies — especially if it calls for extensive memorising, they tend to learn more slowly and have greater difficulty in mastering the material than their younger counterparts.

Such matters are central to our concerns as teachers. There is a wide range of learning styles within any group of adult learners, and we need to devise methods that give each of the participants full scope for exercising their own particular learning method, and as far as possible not impose our own upon them.

Implications for the teacher of adults

We can see, then, that teachers of adults, especially those who teach in groups, are faced with a difficult task from the start. Unless the group is narrowly conceived (as in some forms of industrial training), our student participants will consist of a wide variety of people all bringing their own advantages and disadvantages to the learning situation.

- Some are more adult than others; some are still searching in education for dependency, others for autonomy.

- All are growing and developing, but in different directions and at a different pace.

- Some bring a good deal of experience and knowledge, others bring less; and there are varying degrees of willingness to use this material to help the learning process.

- They have a wide range of intentions and needs, some specific, some more general and related to the subject-matter under discussion, and others unknown even to themselves.

- They are all at different points in the continuum between those who require to be taught everything and those who wish to find out everything for themselves; and they each have some consciousness of what they can and cannot do in the way of learning.

- They all have competing interests of greater importance than their learning.

- And they have all by now acquired their own ways of learning, which vary considerably the one from the other.

It is easy to view all of this in negative terms, to see most of what we have discussed as hindrances to learning. The pressure from competing interests, the worry and anxiety especially about their learning abilities, based as they often are on misconceptions as to what education involves, the problem of coping with unlearning and the attack on the personality that this can at times imply — all of these may seem to make the task of the teacher of adults particularly difficult. We must not be surprised if some of the student participants do not move as fast as we would wish them to; if they have difficulty in grasping some of the material that *we* find so easy and have so carefully constructed for them; if they show a lack of responsiveness to all our promptings to engage more wholeheartedly with the subject-matter of the class. We must not be put off if some of the learners require us to demonstrate or lecture when we would rather that they practise for themselves or discuss.

But there are many aspects of this discussion that give cause for hope. Within the group is a well of resources that we can use. Some of these can be quickly identified: the wealth of knowledge, skills and experience gathered together in one room; the fact that all the student participants, whether they know it or not, are already engaged in some form of learning; the awareness, however dim, of purpose and need; the greater use of reasoning powers, and the fact that adult students, when provoked, 'accept' the teacher's word less readily (those of us who prefer to demonstrate and to lecture, to perform rather than to watch, to listen to our own voice rather than to the voice of the learners, will not see this as a resource); the desire of many of the learners to apply what they learn one day to their lives the very next day and the fact that (unlike full-time students) they are in a position to do so. All these factors can be seen as combining to form a powerful aid to learning.

We need to try to identify both those factors that prevent us from being fully effective in the teaching-learning process and those resources that we can bring into play in order to overcome the obstacles. In adult education, our students are not there just to be taught; they are our greatest resource in the learning process.

Application

It should be important to you, as you look through this material, to relate it to your own experience. You may find it helpful to write down what assumptions you made about the potential student participants for the course you have chosen as your own, what characteristics they bring with them to your course. It may be possible for you, if you actually ran a course, to test this against the group that materialised so that you can assess how accurate your first thoughts were.

A second useful exercise at this stage is set out for yourself the range of helps and hindrances that you think your students will bring with them to the programme of study. Most of us do this without being fully conscious of it; to make it a deliberate process will help to bring into focus those whom we hope to help to learn.

Acknowledgements

1. From: Wood, John, *How Do You Feel? A Guide to Your Emotions*. Prentice-Hall, Inc.

2. Laing, R.D. *Knots*. Tavistock Publications Ltd.

Further reading

Allman P (1983) The nature and process of adult development, in M. Tight (ed) *Education for Adults*. Croom Helm, Beckenham.

Chickering A W (1977) *Experience and Learning: An Introduction to Experiential Learning*. Change Magazine Press, New Rochelle, NY.

Chickering A W and Havighurst R W (1981) The life cycle, in A. W. Chickering (ed) *The Modern American College: Responding to the New Realities of Diverse Students and a Changing Society*. Jossey Bass, San Francisco, CA.

Cross K P (1981) *Adults as Learners: Increasing Participation and Facilitating Learning*. Jossey Bass, San Francisco, CA.

Evans P (1975) *Motivation*. Methuen, London.

Giles K (1981) *Personal Change in Adults*. Open University Press, Milton Keynes.

Jarvis P (1987) *Adult Education in its Social Context*. Croom Helm, Beckenham.

Keeting M T (ed.) (1976) *Experiential Learning: Rationale Characteristics and Assessment*. Jossey Bass, San Francisco, CA.

Kidd J R (1973) *How Adults Learn*. Association Press, New York.

Knowles M S (1990) *The Adult Learner: a Neglected Species*. Gulf, Houston, TX.

Knox A (1977) *Adult Development and Learning*. Jossey Bass, San Francisco, CA.

Levinson D (1978) *The Seasons of a Man's Life*. Knopf, New York.

Levinson D (1986) *The Season of a Woman's Life*. Knopf, New York.

Miller H L (1964) *Teaching and Learning in Adult Education*. Macmillan, London.

Pressey S, Kuhlen R (1957) *Psychological Development through the Lifespan*. Harper, New York.

Rayner E (1971) *Human Development: an Introduction to the Psychodynamics of Growth Maturity and Ageing*. Allen and Unwin, London.

Rogers J (1989) *Adults Learning*. Open University Press, Milton Keynes.

Sheehy C T (1976) *Passages: Predictable Crises of Adult Life*. Dutton, New York.

2. Introduction: The Art and Science of Helping Adults Learn
Malcolm S. Knowles

This is a very personal book — a collection of descriptions by people who have personally applied the andragogical model. It seems fitting, therefore, that I present my current thinking about adult learning as a personal account of my wanderings through the morass of learning theory; for, like the wanderings of Odysseus, mine were circuitous, not a direct flight. I see this chapter as a way of introducing newcomers to the world of andragogy with a route map, but those who are already familiar with this world may want to scan the chapter to note certain changes in my current views of adult education.

My first experiences with adult learners

My experience with adult education began in 1935. I had prepared in college for a career in the U.S. Foreign Service, but when I graduated I was informed by the State Department that only the most urgent vacancies were being filled and that only those who had passed their exams in 1932 were being considered. So I had to get a "holding" job for at least three years to support a new wife and hoped-for family. The job I got was as director of related training for the National Youth Administration (NYA) in Massachusetts. The NYA was a work-study program for unemployed youth between the ages of eighteen and twenty-five, with the mission of increasing their employability; I was put in charge of the study half of the program.

I had no formal qualifications for this job outside of leading some boys' clubs in a settlement house. Nonetheless, I sensed that a vocational training program for unemployed youth would have to be different from the prescriptive academic courses that I had taken, although I didn't know in what ways. I tried to find a book that would tell me how to conduct a program of this sort, and I couldn't find one. So I sought out people who were directing adult education programs — including the director of the Boston Institute for Adult Education, a director of adult education in a public school, and a couple of deans of evening colleges — and formed an advisory council to give me guidance. At their suggestion I made an informal survey of a sample of employers to find out what jobs were open and what skills they required. Then I organized courses to provide these skills, employed instructors, found locations for the courses to meet, and published a descriptive brochure. The response to the program was enthusiastic, and many of the youths (especially those between twenty-one and twenty-five years of age) began getting jobs. I loved what I was doing, but I didn't know that it had a name. Then, around 1937, someone asked me what I did. When I told him, he said, "Oh, you are an adult educator." So now I had an identity. He also told me that there was a national organization, the American Association for Adult Education, that was holding

Reprinted with permission from *ANDRAGOGY IN ACTION: APPLYING MODERN PRINCIPLES OF ADULT LEARNING* by Malcolm S. Knowles. Copyright © 1984 Jossey-Bass Inc., Publishers, 350 Sansome Street, San Francisco, CA 94104. 001 (800) 956-7739.

its annual conference in New York in several weeks. I attended the conference and was impressed with the people I met there and with their ideas about the differences between adult learners and school children. At that point I joined the association and notified the State Department that I had changed my career goals to adult education and was no longer available for the Foreign Service.

During my five years with the NYA, I observed that some teachers were more effective than others in working with young adults; and I began developing some generalizations — for instance, that the more effective teachers were more interested in their students as persons, were more informal in their manner, involved students more in participatory activities, and gave them more helpful support. But my understanding of the emerging theory of adult education came from two individuals and their books. The single most influential person in guiding my thinking was Eduard C. Lindeman, whose book *The Meaning of Adult Education* (1926) enlightened me about the unique characteristics of adults as learners and the need for methods and techniques for helping them learn. Lindeman was at that time director of educational projects for the Works Projects Administration and thus was in a sense my supervisor. We spent many hours together, discussing what adult education was all about, and I regarded him as my mentor. Dorothy Hewitt, director of the Boston Center for Adult Education, which provided informal courses to the citizens of Boston, was a member of my advisory council and showed me step by step how she planned and managed her program. The book she co-authored with Kirtley Mather, *Adult Education: A Dynamic for Democracy* (1937), served as my how-to-do-it manual. I still reread these two books periodically for inspiration and reinforcement. I marvel that these two early pioneers — especially Lindeman — had insights about adult learning that only recently have been verified by research.

In 1940 I was invited to become director of adult education at the Huntington Avenue YMCA in Boston, and I found myself in possession of a built-in laboratory for applying ideas I was picking up from people and publications and for experimenting with new ideas. *The Journal of Adult Education*, published by the American Association for Adult Education, and the *Adult Education Bulletin*, published by the Department of Adult Education of the National Education Association, were rich sources of information. Both of them frequently ran articles by "successful" teachers of adults ("successful" being defined as the ability to attract and retain students) describing how differently they treated adults from the way children and youth are traditionally treated in school and college. It is interesting to me now, in retrospect, that although there was general agreement among adult educators that adults are different from youth as learners, there was no comprehensive theory about these differences. The literature was largely philosophical and anecdotal and at most provided miscellaneous principles or guidelines.

Getting an academic foundation

In 1944 I enlisted in the U.S. Navy and during the next two years had more time to read and think than I had ever had before in my life. I devoured all the books in print about adult education and started trying to work out a comprehensive theory about it. In 1946 I became director of adult education at the Central YMCA in Chicago and enrolled in the graduate program in adult education at the University of Chicago for my master's and doctor's degrees. I was greatly influenced by the intellectual rigor and teaching style of my major professor, Cyril O. Houle. He related to his students as colleagues and demonstrated that principles of adult education could be applied even in a traditional university. At this time also, I experienced the challenge of being a truly self-directed learner in a seminar with Arthur Shedlin, an associate of Carl Rogers.

For my master's thesis, I decided that I would attempt to bring together all the insights, principles, and practices regarding the education of adults that I had garnered from the literature, from other adult educators, and from my own experience, as at least a first step in constructing a comprehensive theory of adult education. When I was about half way through it, Cyril Houle informed me that he had been talking with the editor of Association Press about projects his students were working on and that the editor had expressed an interest in seeing the outline and first couple of chapters of my thesis. As a result, my first book was published in 1950 under the title *Informal Adult Education*. I had been trying to identify the essence of adult education, the thing that made it different from traditional education, and the best I could come up with was "informal." I still had not developed a comprehensive, coherent, integrated theory. But it was a step in that direction.

Into the larger world of adult education

In 1951 I became executive director of the newly formed Adult Education Association of the U.S.A., and my line of vision shifted from individual learners in particular programs to the broad scope of the adult education movement. But three forces kept me thinking about the adult learner. One was my doctoral studies at the University of Chicago, through which I became familiar with the formal theories of learning. My strongest impression was that these theories had all been based on research on animals (mostly rodents, at that) and children, and I had trouble seeing their relevance to what I had observed about learning by adults. In fact, it dawned on me that the educational psychologists had not been studying learning at all, but reactions to teaching. The second force was the research that Cyril Houle was engaged in at the time regarding how "continuing learners" — people who have engaged in systematic learning on their own — go about learning. The results of his study were published in a monograph under the title *The Inquiring Mind* in 1961, and had the effect of redirecting subsequent research by adult education researchers, especially Allen Tough, to focus on the internal dynamics of learning in adults. The third force was my participation in the human relations laboratories of the National Training Laboratories (NTL) Institute of Behavioral Sciences in Bethel, Maine. From this experience I derived a deep understanding and appreciation of the forces affecting learning that are at work in groups and in larger social systems.

In 1960 I was invited to Boston University to start a new graduate program in adult education. During the next fourteen years, I had a laboratory where I could apply principles of adult learning in a university setting; I had time and motivation for doing research; and I had doctoral students to extend and deepen the research. During this period a theoretical framework regarding adult learning evolved. But I didn't have a label for it that would enable me to talk about it in parallel to the traditional pedagogical model. (Incidentally, "pedagogy" is derived from the Greek words *paid*, meaning "child," and *agogos*, meaning "leader of." So pedagogy literally means "the art and science of teaching children.)

I found the solution in the summer of 1967, when a Yugoslavian adult educator, Dusan Savicevic, attended my summer session course on adult learning and at the end of it exclaimed, "Malcolm, you are preaching and practicing andragogy." I responded, "Whatagogy?" because I had never heard the term before. He explained that European adult educators had coined the term as a parallel to pedagogy, to provide a label for the growing body of knowledge and technology in regard to adult learning, and that it was being defined as "the art and science of helping adults learn." It made sense to me to have a differentiating label, and I started using the term in 1968, in articles describing my theoretical framework for thinking about adult learning.

In 1970 I put it all together in a book, *The Modern Practice of Adult Education: Andragogy Versus Pedagogy*. The "versus" was in the title because at that point I saw the two models, pedagogy and andragogy, as dichotomous — one for children, the other for adults. During the next ten years, however, a number of teachers in elementary, secondary, and higher education who had somehow been exposed to the andragogical model told me that they had experimented with applying (or adapting) the model in their practice and had found that young people learned better, too, when the andragogical model was applied. On the other hand, many teachers and trainers working with adults cited circumstances — especially in basic skills training — where the pedagogical model seemed to be required. So the revised edition of the book, published in 1980, had the subtitle *From Pedagogy to Andragogy*.

Toward a theory of adult learning

During the two decades between 1960 and 1980, we gained more knowledge about the unique characteristics of adults as learners and their learning processes than had been accumulated in all previous history. Houle's seminal study in 1961 had stimulated a rash of research by adult educators (Boud, 1981; Boyd, Apps, and Associates, 1980; Cross, 1981; Houle, 1980; Howe, 1977; Knox, 1977; Long, Hiemstra, and Associates, 1980; Smith, 1982; Tough, 1967, 1979, 1982). But knowledge was flowing from other social science disciplines as well. Clinical psychologists and psychiatrists were learning about how to help people change their behavior (Bandura, 1969; Maslow, 1962, 1970, 1971; Rogers, 1951, 1961, 1969, 1980); and, since education also is concerned with behavioral change, their findings were relevant to adult learning. Developmental psychologists were discovering that there are predictable developmental stages during the adult years as well as through adolescence and that the transitions from one stage to another are one of the chief triggers of readiness to learn (Baltes, 1978; Erikson, 1959; Goulet and Baltes, 1970; Havighurst, 1970; Knox, 1977; Levinson, 1978; Lidz, 1968; Neugarten, 1964, 1968; Pressey and Kuhlen, 1957; Sheehy, 1974; Stevens-Long, 1979). Social psychologists were discovering how the conditions of our environment — such as color, population density, stress, social norms, social class, race, and group processes — affect learning (Barker, 1978; Birren, 1969; Bronfenbrenner, 1979; David and Wright, 1975; Deutsch and others, 1968, Lewin, 1951; Moos, 1976, 1979; Moos and

Insel, 1974) and how change can be brought about in environments (Arends and Arends, 1977; Bennis, Benne, and Chin, 1968; Eiben and Milleren, 1976; Greiner, 1971; Hornstein and others, 1971; Lippitt, 1969, 1973; Martorana and Kuhns, 1975; Zurcher, 1977). Sociologists were adding to our knowledge about how institutional policies and procedures (concerning, for instance, admissions, registration, financial matters, and reward systems) affect learning (Barrett, 1970; Boocock, 1972; Corwin, 1974; Etzioni, 1961, 1969).

Clearly, by 1970 — and certainly by 1980 — there was a substantial enough body of knowledge about adult learners and their learning to warrant attempts to organize it into a systematic framework of assumptions, principles, and strategies. This is what andragogy sets out to do. I don't know whether it is a theory; this is a controversial issue, which Cross (1981, pp. 220–228) discusses lucidly and objectively. I feel more comfortable thinking of it as a system of concepts that, in fact, incorporates pedagogy rather than opposing it — a notion that I will develop more fully later. First, I must clarify my current thinking about the pedagogical and andragogical models.

Traditional learning — the pedagogical model

The pedagogical model is the one we have all had the most experience with. In fact, it is the only way of thinking about education that most of us know, for it has dominated all of education — even adult education until recently — since schools started being organized in the seventh century. Stated in their purest and most extreme form, these are the assumptions about learners inherent in the pedagogical model:

1. *Regarding the concept of the learner (and therefore, through conditioning in prior school experience, the learner's self-concept):* The learner is, by definition, a dependent personality, for the pedagogical model assigns to the teacher full responsibility for making all the decisions about what should be learned, how and when it should be learned, and whether it has been learned. The only role for the learner, therefore, is that of submissively carrying out the teacher's directions.

2. *Regarding the role of the learner's experience:* Learners enter into an educational activity with little experience that is of much value as a resource for learning. It is the experience of the teacher, the textbook writer, and the audiovisual aids producer that counts. Accordingly, the backbone of pedagogical methodology is transmission techniques — lectures, assigned readings, and audiovisual presentations.

3. *Regarding readiness to learn:* Students become ready to learn what they are told that they have to learn in order to advance to the next grade level; readiness is largely a function of age.

4. *Regarding orientation to learning:* Students enter into an educational activity with a subject-centered orientation to learning; they see learning as a process of acquiring prescribed subject matter content. Consequently, the curriculum is organized according to content units and is sequenced according to the logic of the subject matter.

5. *Regarding motivation to learn:* Students are motivated primarily by external pressures from parents and teachers, competition for grades, the consequences of failure, and the like.

This may sound like a caricature, but think back to all the teachers you have had. Didn't most of them operate on the basis of these assumptions? Of course, there have always been great teachers who experimented with other assumptions, but in my experience they were few and far between. In fact, teachers have been under pressure from their systems to be loyal to these assumptions, often in the name of "academic standards."

A new approach to learning — the andragogical model

In contrast — and in equally pure and extreme form — the assumptions inherent in the andragogical model are these:

1. *Regarding the concept of the learner:* The learner is self-directing. In fact, the psychological definition of adult is "One who has arrived at a self-concept of being responsible for one's own life, of being self-directing." When we have arrived at that point, we develop a deep psychological need to be perceived by others, and treated by others, as capable of taking responsibility for ourselves. And when we find ourselves in situations where we feel that others are imposing their wills on us without our participating in making decisions affecting us, we experience a feeling, often subconsciously, of resentment and resistance.

This fact about adult learners presents adult educators with a special problem. For even though adults may be totally self-directing in every other aspect of their lives — as workers, spouses, parents, citizens, leisure-time users — the minute they walk into a situation labeled "education," "training," or any of their synonyms, they hark back to their conditioning in school, assume a role of dependency, and demand to be taught. However, if they really are treated like children, this conditioned expectation conflicts with their much deeper psychological need to be self-directing, and their energy is diverted away from learning to dealing with this internal conflict. As they have become aware of this problem, adult educators have been devising strategies for helping adults make the transition from being dependent learners to being self-directed learners. It has become increasingly widespread practice to include an orientation to self-directed learning at the beginning of an educational activity or program (see Knowles, 1975; [and selections 6 and 8 in Chapter Two; selections 1, 2, 3, and 8 in Chapter Three; selections 1 and 3 in Chapter Four]).

2. *Regarding the role of the learner's experience:* The andragogical model assumes that adults enter into an educational activity with both a greater volume and a different quality of experience from youth. The greater volume is self-evident; the longer we live, the more experience we accumulate, at least in normal lives. The difference in quality of experience occurs because adults perform different roles from young people, such as the roles of full-time worker, spouse, parent, and voting citizen.

This difference in experience has several consequences for education. First of all, it means that, for many kinds of learning, adults are themselves the richest resources for one another; hence the greater emphasis in adult education on such techniques —

28

group discussion, simulation exercises, laboratory experiences, field experiences, problem-solving projects, and the like — that make use of the experiences of the learners. In addition, the differences in experience assure greater heterogeneity in groups of adults. The range of experience among a group of adults of various ages will be vastly greater than among a group of twelve-year-olds. Consequently, in adult education greater emphasis is placed on individualized learning plans, such as learning contracts (Knowles, 1975, 1980; [see also Chapter Two, selections 1, 6, and 8; Chapter Three, selections 1 and 5; Chapter Four, selection 3; Chapter Five, selections 1 and 3]). But there is a possible negative consequence as well. Because of their experience, adults often have developed habitual ways of thinking and acting, preconceptions about reality, prejudices, and defensiveness about their past ways of thinking and doing. To overcome this problem, adult educators are devising strategies for helping people become more open-minded (Benne, Bradford, and Lippitt, 1975; Davis and Scott, 1971; Ray, 1973).

There is a more subtle and perhaps even more potent consequence of adults' greater experience: it becomes increasingly the source of an adult's self-identity. Let me illustrate this point. If I had been asked when I was ten years old "Who are you?" I would have explained: "My name is Malcolm Knowles, the son of Dr. A. D. Knowles, a veterinarian; I belong to the Presbyterian Sunday School; I live at 415 Fourth Street, Missoula, Montana; and I attend school at the Roosevelt Grammar School on Sixth Street." My self-identity would be derived almost exclusively from external sources — the name I was given by my parents, my father's vocation, my religious affiliation, my residence, and my school. If I had been asked the same question at age forty, I would have given my name and then recounted the positions I had held with the NYA, the YMCA, the AEA, and so on. Like other adults, I would derive my self-identity from my experience. So if in an educational situation an adult's experience is ignored, not valued, not made use of, it is not just the experience that is being rejected; it is the person. Hence the great importance of using the experience of adult learners as a rich resource for learning. This principle is especially important in working with undereducated adults, who, after all, have little to sustain their dignity other than their experience.

3. *Regarding readiness to learn:* The andragogical model assumes that adults become ready to learn when they experience a need to know or do something in order to perform more effectively in some aspect of their lives. Chief sources of readiness are the developmental tasks associated with moving from one stage of development to another; but any change — birth of children, loss of job, divorce, death of a friend or relative, change of residence — is likely to trigger a readiness to learn. But we don't need to wait for readiness to develop naturally; there are things we can do to induce it, such as exposing learners to more effective role models, engaging them in career planning, and providing them with diagnostic experiences in which they can assess the gaps between where they are now and where they want and need to be (Knowles, 1980).

4. *Regarding orientation to learning:* Because adults are motivated to learn after they experience a need in their life situation, they enter an educational activity with a life-centered, task-centered, or problem-centered orientation to learning. For the most

part, adults do not learn for the sake of learning; they learn in order to be able to perform a task, solve a problem, or live in a more satisfying way. The chief implication of this assumption is the importance of organizing learning experiences (the curriculum) around life situations rather than according to subject matter units. For example, courses that might be titled "Composition I," "Composition II," and "Composition III" in a high school might better be titled "Writing Better Business Letters," "Writing for Pleasure and Profit," and "Improving Your Professional Communications" in an adult education program. I had a terrible time learning to use the computer on which I am writing this chapter because the instructional manual set out to teach me about computers rather than teaching me how to use the computer to compose a chapter.

Another implication is the importance of making clear at the outset of a learning experience what its relevance is to the learner's life tasks or problems. We have a dictum in adult education that one of the first tasks of a facilitator of learning is to develop "the need to know" what will be learned (see Freire, 1970; Knowles, 1980).

5. *Regarding motivation to learn:* Although it acknowledges that adults will respond to some external motivators — a better job, a salary increase, and the like — the andragogical model predicates that the more potent motivators are internal — self-esteem, recognition, better quality of life, greater self-confidence, self-actualization, and the like (Herzberg, 1966; Maslow, 1970). Program announcements are accordingly placing increasing emphasis on these kinds of outcomes.

Choosing which model to use

As I have said, I now regard the pedagogical and andragogical models as parallel, not antithetical. For centuries educators had only one model, the pedagogical model, to go on. Now we have two sets of assumptions about learners. In some situations, such as when learners of whatever age are entering a totally strange territory of content or are confronting a machine they have never seen before, they may be truly dependent on didactic instruction before they can take much initiative in their own learning; in such situations the pedagogical assumption of dependency is realistic, and pedagogical strategies would be appropriate. In many more instances, however, especially with adult learners, the andragogical assumptions would be realistic — particularly if the learners have had some orientation to self-directed learning — and andragogical strategies would be appropriate. There is growing evidence [see Chapter Seven, selections 1, 2, and 3] that the andragogical assumptions are realistic in many more situations than traditional schooling has recognized. For example, children are very self-directing in their learning *outside of school* and could also be more self-directed in school. Children and youth bring *some* experience with them into an educational activity, and this experience could be used as a resource for some kinds of learning. Children and youth also are more ready to learn when they experience a "need to know" than when they are told they have to learn, and we can expose them to life situations through which they will become aware of what they need to know. Finally, children and youth are naturally more motivated by intrinsic rewards than by external pressures; it is schools that have conditioned them to be otherwise [see Chapter Seven, selection 1].

Implications for program design

The pedagogical and andragogical models result in two very different approaches to the design and operation of educational programs. The basic format of the pedagogical model is a *content plan*, which requires the teacher to answer only four questions:

1. What content needs to be covered? The implication is that it is the teacher's responsibility to cover — in the classroom or through assigned reading — all the content that students need to learn. So the pedagogue constructs a long list of content items to be covered. (This requirement seems to me to place an unfair burden on the teacher to master all the content and to doom the students to be limited to the teacher's resources.)

2. How can this content be organized into manageable units, such as fifty-minute, three-hour, or one-week units? So the pedagogue clusters the content items into manageable units.

3. What would be the most logical sequence in which to present these units? It is the logic of the subject matter that determines the sequence, not the readiness of the learners or other psychological factors. So, in mathematical or scientific content programs, the sequence is typically from simple to complex; in history it is chronological.

4. What would be the most efficient means of transmitting this content? With highly informational content, the preferred means would probably be lecture or audiovisual presentations and assigned reading; if the content involves skill performance, it would probably be demonstration by the teacher and drill by the students.

In contrast, the basic format of the andragogical model is a *process design*. The andragogical model assigns a dual role to the facilitator of learning (a title preferred over "teacher"): first and primarily, the role of designer and manager of processes or procedures that will facilitate the acquisition of content by the learners; and only secondarily, the role of content resource. The andragogical model assumes that there are many resources other than the teacher, including peers, individuals with specialized knowledge and skill in the community, a wide variety of material and media resources, and field experiences. One of the principal responsibilities of the andragogue is to know about all these resources and to link learners with them.

An andragogical process design consists of seven elements:

1. *Climate setting*. What procedures would be most likely to produce a climate that is conducive to learning? In my estimation, a climate that is conducive to learning is a prerequisite to effective learning; and it seems tragic to me that so little attention is paid to climate in traditional education. I attach so much importance to climate setting that I devote about 10 per cent of the time available in an educational activity to this element, and most of the case descriptions [in this book] do, too. In planning procedures for climate setting, I give attention to two aspects of climate: physical environment and psychological atmosphere.

In regard to *physical environment*, the typical classroom setup, with chairs in rows and a lectern in front, is probably the least conducive to learning that the fertile human brain could invent. It announces to anyone entering the room that the name of the game here is one-way transmission, that the proper role of the student is to sit and listen to transmissions from the lectern. I make a point of getting to a meeting room before the participants arrive, and if it is set up like a classroom I move the lectern to a corner and put the chairs in one large circle or several small circles. My preference is to have the participants sitting around tables, five or six to a table. I also prefer meeting rooms that are bright and cheerful, with colorful decor.

Important as physical climate is, *psychological climate* is even more important. Here are the characteristics of a psychological climate that is conducive to learning as I see it:

- A *climate of mutual respect.* People are more open to learning when they feel respected. If they feel that they are being talked down to, ignored, or regarded as dumb, and that their experience is not valued, their energy is spent dealing with this feeling more than with learning.

- A *climate of collaborativeness.* Because of their conditioning in their earlier school experience, in which competition for grades and teachers' favor was the norm, adults tend to enter into any educational activity with a rivalrous attitude toward fellow participants. Since, for many kinds of learning in adult education, peers are the richest resources for learning, this competitiveness makes those resources inaccessible. For this reason the climate-setting exercise with which I open all my workshops and courses puts the participants into a sharing relationship from the outset.

- A *climate of mutual trust.* People learn from those they trust more than from those they mistrust. And here we who are put in the position of teacher or trainer of adults are at a disadvantage, for students in schools learn at an early age that on the whole teachers are not very trustworthy. For one thing, they have power over students; they are authorized to give grades, to determine who passes or fails, and otherwise to hand out punishments and rewards. For another thing, the institutions in which they work present them in their catalogues and program announcements as authority figures. And it is built into the bloodstreams of those who grew up in the Judeo-Christian democratic tradition that authority figures are to be mistrusted, at least until they are tested and their degree of trustworthiness determined. In my workshops I try to convey in various ways (for instance, by encouraging participants to make decisions and by lending them my books) that I trust participants and hope thereby to obtain their trust.

- A *climate of supportiveness.* People learn better when they feel supported rather than judged or threatened. I convey my desire to be supportive by accepting learners with an unqualified positive regard, matching any diagnosis of a weakness with a valuing of a strength, empathizing with their problems or worries, and defining my role as that of a helper. But I also organize them into peer-support groups and coach them on how to support one another.

- *A climate of openness and authenticity.* When people feel free to be open and natural, to say what they really think and feel, they are more likely to be willing to examine new ideas and risk new behaviors than when they feel the need to be defensive. In school we often have to pretend to know things that we don't or to think things that we don't or to feel things that we don't, and this interferes with learning. If the teacher or trainer demonstrates openness and authenticity in his or her own behavior, this will be the model that participants will adopt.

- *A climate of pleasure.* Learning should be one of the most pleasant and gratifying experiences in life; for, after all, it is the way people can become what they are capable of being — achieving their full potential. It should be an adventure, spiced with the excitement of discovery. It should be fun. I think it is tragic that so much of our previous educational experience has been a dull chore.

- *A climate of humanness.* Perhaps what I have been saying about climate can be summed up with the adjective "human." Learning is a very human activity. The more people feel that they are being treated as human beings, the more they are likely to learn. Among other things, this means providing for human comfort — good lighting and ventilation, comfortable chairs, availability of refreshments, designation of nonsmoking areas, frequent breaks, and the like. It also means providing a caring, accepting, respecting, helping social atmosphere.

  [A climate-setting exercise designed to bring these characteristics into being is described in Chapter Four, selection 6, and other climate-setting strategies are described in Chapter Two, selection 8; Chapter Three, selections 7 and 8; and Chapter Eight, selection 2.]

2. *Involving learners in mutual planning.* What procedures can be used to get the participants to share in the planning? I sometimes have subgroups choose a representative to serve on a planning committee to meet with me to discuss where we should go next. Frequently I will present several optional possibilities for activities and ask the groups to discuss them and report their preferences. There is a basic law of human nature at work here: people tend to feel committed to any decision in proportion to the extent to which they have participated in making it; the reverse is even more true — people tend to feel uncommitted to any decision to the extent that they feel others are making it for them and imposing it on them.

3. *Involving participants in diagnosing their own needs for learning.* What procedures can be used for helping learners responsibly and realistically identify what they need to learn? One of the pervasive problems in this process is meshing the needs the learners are aware of (felt needs) with the needs their organizations or society has for them (ascribed needs). A variety of strategies are available, ranging from simple interest-finding checklists to elaborate performance assessment systems, with a balance between felt needs and ascribed needs being negotiated between the facilitator and the learners. I frequently use a model of competencies, which reflects both personal and organizational needs, so that the learners can identify the gaps between where they are now and where the model specifies they need to be (see Knowles, 1980, pp. 229–232, 256–261, 369, 371).

4. *Involving learners in formulating their learning objectives.* What procedures can be used to help learners translate their diagnosed needs into learning objectives? See the following section on learning contracts.

5. *Involving learners in designing learning plans.* What procedures can be used to help the learners identify resources and devise strategies for using these resources to accomplish their objectives? See the following section on learning contracts.

6. *Helping learners carry out their learning plans.* See the following section on learning contracts.

7. *Involving learners in evaluating their learning.* Evaluation of the accomplishment of objectives by individual learners is treated in the following section. But evaluation is also concerned with judging the quality and worth of the total program. Assessing individuals' learning outcomes is a part of this larger evaluation, but more than this is involved in this process. This book is not the place to go into detail about the complex process of program evaluation, but I would be remiss if I neglected to call my readers' attention to the fact that a major turn in our very way of thinking about evaluation has been in progress in the last few years. This turn, away from almost exclusive emphasis on quantitative evaluation toward increasing emphasis on qualitative evaluation, is described in Cronbach and others, 1980; Guba and Lincoln, 1981; Kirkpatrick, 1975; and Patton, 1978, 1980, 1981, 1982.

Using learning contracts to provide structure

Learning contracts are an effective way to help learners structure their learning. Some people have difficulty with the term "contract" because of its legalistic flavor and substitute "learning plan" or "learning agreement" for it. But "learning contract" is the term most often found in the literature.

The procedure I use in helping learners design and execute learning contracts is as follows: (1) Each learner translates a diagnosed learning need into a learning objective that describes the terminal behavior to be achieved (which is appropriate for most basic skills learning) or the direction of improvement in ability (which is appropriate for more complex learnings). (2) The learner next identifies, with the facilitator's help, the most effective resources and strategies for accomplishing each objective. (3) The learner then specifies what evidence will be collected for indicating the extent to which each objective was accomplished. (4) Finally, the learner specifies how this evidence will be judged or validated. After the learners have completed a first draft of their contracts, they review the drafts with small groups of peers and get their reactions and suggestions. Then I review the contracts to make sure that the required objectives of the program are included, to suggest other resources, and to determine whether I can agree with the learners' proposals for collecting and validating evidence of accomplishment. Once I approve a contract, the learner proceeds to carry it out, with me always available as a consultant and resource. The resources specified in the contracts include group activities; information inputs by me or other specialists, peers, or individuals in the community; and independent study. When the contracts are fulfilled, the learners present me with their "portfolios of evidence," which often include papers, tapes, rating scales by judges or observers, and oral presentations. I indicate whether I accept the portfolio as fulfilling the contract or, if not, what additional evidence is required for my acceptance.

I use learning contracts in almost all of my practice. Students contract with me to meet the requirements of the university courses I teach. (Incidentally, even though there may be a number of unnegotiable requirements, the means by which students accomplish required objectives can be highly individualized.) Students going out on field experiences, such as practicums or internships, contract with me and the field supervisor — a three-way contract. I also use contracts in short-term workshops, but in these the learners leave the workshop with a contract specifying how they are going to continue to learn on their own. Finally, I use learning contracts in the in-service education programs I am involved in; many physicians, nurses, social workers, managers and supervisors, and educators are using learning contracts for their continuing personal and professional development.

More detailed descriptions of contract learning can be found in Knowles, 1975, pp. 25–28; 1978, pp. 127–128, 198–203; 1980, pp. 243–244, 381–389; [and in Chapter Two, selections 1, 6, and 8; Chapter Three, selections 1 and 5; and Chapter Five, selections 1 and 3, in this book].

Ways of using andragogy for education and training

The andragogical model has been widely adopted or adapted in a variety of programs — from individual courses at every level of education to total programs of in-service education, undergraduate education, graduate education, continuing education, human resources development, continuing professional education, technical training, remedial education, and religious education. It appears in almost every kind of institution, including elementary and secondary schools, community colleges, colleges and universities, business and industry, government agencies, health agencies, professional societies, churches, and voluntary organizations — in North America and around the world. "Andragogy" was so recently introduced into our literature (a decade and a half ago), though, that it does not yet appear in a dictionary. But it will before long.

As Cross (1981, pp. 227–228) states, "Whether andragogy can serve as the foundation for a unifying theory of adult education remains to be seen. At the very least, it identifies some characteristics of adult learners that deserve attention. It has been far more successful than most theory in getting the attention of practitioners, and it has been moderately successful in sparking debate; it has not been especially successful, however, in stimulating research to test the assumptions. Most important, perhaps, the visibility of andragogy has heightened awareness of the need for answers to three major questions: (1) Is it useful to distinguish the learning needs of adults from those of children? If so, are we talking about dichotomous differences or continuous differences? Or both? (2) What are we really seeking: Theories of learning? Theories of teaching? Both? (3) Do we have, or can we develop, an initial framework on which successive generations of scholars can build? Does andragogy lead to researchable questions that will advance knowledge in adult education?" Actually, a growing amount of research is being done, which I shall summarize in [the last chapter]. But I agree that andragogy's greatest impact has been in action.

References

Arends R I, Arends J H (1977) *Systems Change Strategies in Educational Settings*. Human Sciences Press, New York.

Baltes P D (ed) (1978) *Life-Span Development and Behavior*. Vol 1, Academic Press, New York.

Bandura A (1969) *Principles of Behavior Modification*. Holt, Rinehart and Winston, New York.

Barker R G *et al.* (1978) *Habitats, Environments, and Human Behavior: Studies in Ecological Psychology and Eco-Behavioral Science*. Jossey-Bass, San Francisco.

Barrett J H (1970) *Individual Goals and Organizational Behavior*. Institute for Social Research, University of Michigan, Ann Arbor.

Benne K, Bradford L P, Lippitt R (1975) *The Laboratory Method of Changing and Learning*. Science and Behavior Books, Palo Alto, Calif.

Bennis W, Benne K, Chin R (1968) *The Planning of Change*. Holt, Rinehart and Winston, New York.

Birren F (1969) *Light, Color, and Environment*. Van Nostrand Reinhold, New York.

Boocock S S (1972) *An Introduction to the Sociology of Learning*. Houghton Mifflin, Boston.

Boud D (1981) *Developing Student Autonomy in Learning*. Nichols, New York.

Boyd R D, Apps J W *et al.* (1980) *Redefining the Discipline of Adult Education*. Jossey-Bass, San Francisco.

Bronfenbrenner U (1979) *The Ecology of Human Development*. Harvard University Press, Cambridge, Mass.

Corwin R G (1974) *Education in Crisis: A Sociological Analysis of Schools and Universities in Transition*. Wiley, New York.

Cronbach L J *et al.* (1980) *Toward Reform of Program Evaluation: Aims, Methods, and Institutional Arrangements*. Jossey-Bass, San Francisco.

Cross K P (1981) *Adults as Learners: Increasing Participation and Facilitating Learning*. Jossey-Bass, San Francisco.

David T G, Wright B D (eds) (1975) *Learning Environments*. University of Chicago Press, Chicago.

Davis G A, Scott J A (1971) *Training Creative Thinking*, Holt, Rinehart and Winston, New York.

Deutsch M *et al.* (1968) *Social Class, Race, and Psychological Development*. Holt, Rinehart and Winston, New York.

Eiben R, Milliren A (eds) (1976) *Educational Change: A Humanistic Approach*, University Associates, La Jolla, Calif.

Erikson E (1959) *Identity and the Life Cycle*. Psychological Issues Monograph 1, International Universities Press, New York.

Etzioni A (1961) *A Sociological Reader on Complex Organizations*. Free Press, New York.

Freire P (1970) *Pedagogy of the Oppressed*. Seabury Press, New York.

Goulet L R, Baltes P B (1970) *Life-Span Developmental Psychology*. Academic Press, New York.

Greiner L E (ed) (1971) *Organizational Change and Development*. Irwin, Homewood, Ill.

Guba E G, Lincoln Y S (1981) *Effective Evaluation: Improving the Usefulness of Evaluation Results Through Responsive and Naturalistic Approaches*. Jossey-Bass, San Francisco.

Havighurst R (1970) *Developmental Tasks and Education* (2nd ed), McKay, New York.

Herzberg F (1966) *Work and the Nature of Men*. World Publishing, Cleveland.

Hewitt D, Mather K F (1937) *Adult Education: A Dynamic for Democracy*. Appleton-Century-Crofts, New York.

Hornstein J A *et al.* (1961) *Social Intervention*, Free Press, New York.

Houle C O (1961) *The Inquiring Mind*. University of Wisconsin Press, Madison.

Houle C O (1980) *Continuing Learning in the Professions*. Jossey-Bass, San Francisco.

Howe M J A (ed) (1977) *Adult Learning: Psychological Research and Applications*. Wiley, New York.

Kirkpatrick D L (1975) *Evaluating Training Programs*. American Society for Training and Development, Washington, D.C.

Knowles M S (1975) *Self-Directed Learning: A Guide for Learners and Teachers*. Follett, Chicago.

Knowles M S (1970) *The Modern Practice of Adult Education: From Pedagogy to Andragogy* (2nd edn), Follett, Chicago. (Originally published 1970.)

Knox A B (1977) *Adult Development and Learning: A Handbook on Individual Growth and Competence in the Adult Years*. Jossey-Bass, San Francisco.

Levinson D J (1978) *The Seasons of a Man's Life*. Knopf, New York.

Lewin K (1951) *Field Theory in Social Science*. Harper & Row, New York.

Lidz T (1968) *The Person: His Development Throughout the Life Cycle*. Basic Books, New York.

Lindeman E C (1926) *The Meaning of Adult Education*. New Republic Press, New York.

Lippitt G (1969) *Organizational Renewal*. Appleton-Century-Crofts, New York.

Lippitt G (1973) *Visualizing Change*. NTL National Learning Resources, Fairfax, Va.

Long H B, Hiemstra R *et al.* (1980) *Changing Approaches to Studying Adult Education*. Jossey-Bass, San Francisco.

Martorana S V, Kuhns E (1975) *Managing Academic Change: Interactive Forces and Leadership in Higher Education*. Jossey-Bass, San Francisco.

Maslow A (1962) *Toward a Psychology of Being*. Van Nostrand, New York.

Maslow A (1970) *Motivation and Personality*. Harper & Row, New York.

Maslow A (1971) *The Farther Reaches of Human Nature*. Viking Press, New York.

Moos R H (1976) *The Human Context: Environmental Determinants of Behavior*. Wiley-Interscience, New York.

Moos R H (1979) *Evaluating Educational Environments: Procedures, Measures, Findings and Policy Implications*. Jossey-Bass, San Francisco.

Moos R H, Insel P M (1974) *Issues in Social Ecology*. National Press Books, Palo Alto, Calif.

Neugarten B L (1964) *Personality in Middle and Later Life*. Lieber-Atherton, New York.

Neugarten B L (ed) (1968) *Middle Age and Aging*. University of Chicago Press, Chicago.

Patton M Q (1978) *Utilization-Focused Evaluation*. Sage, Beverly Hills, Calif.

Patton M Q (1980) *Utilization Evaluation*. Sage, Beverly Hills, Calif.

Patton M Q (1981) *Creative Evaluation*. Sage, Beverly Hills, Calif.

Patton M Q (1982) *Practical Evaluation*. Sage, Beverly Hills, Calif.

Pressy S L, Kuhlen R G (1957) *Psychological Development Through the Life Span*. Harper & Row, New York.

Ray W S (1973) *Simple Experiments in Psychology*. Behavioral Publications, New York.

Rogers C A (1951) *Client-Centered Therapy*. Houghton Mifflin, Boston.

Rogers C A (1961) *On Becoming a Person*. Houghton Mifflin, Boston.

Rogers C A (1969) *Freedom to Learn*. Merrill, Columbus, Ohio.

Rogers C A (1980) *A Way of Being*. Houghton Mifflin, Boston.

Sheehy G (1974) *Passages: Predictable Crises of Adult Life*. Dutton, New York.

Smith R M (1982 *Learning How to Learn*. Cambridge, New York.

Stevens-Long J (1979) *Adult Life: Developmental Processes*. Mayfield, Palo Alto, Calif.

Tough A M (1967) *Learning Without a Teacher*. Ontario Institute for Studies in Education, Toronto.

Tough A M (1979) *The Adult's Learning Projects*. (2nd edn) Ontario Institute for Studies in Education, Toronto. (Originally published 1971.)

Tough A M (1982) *Intentional Changes: A Fresh Approach to Helping People Change*. Follett, Chicago.

Zurcher L A (1977) *The Mutable Self: A Concept for Social Change*. Sage, Beverly Hills, Calif.

3.   In Defence of Andragogy
Part 2: An Educational Process
Consistent with Modern Nursing's Aims
Frank Milligan

In 1987 the English National Board (1987) made it clear that it supported a move towards an andragogical approach to nurse education. Recently such moves have been questioned as has the validity of andragogy (Darbyshire, 1993). In response to such challenges this paper extends some of the arguments made in the article 'In defence of andragogy' (Milligan, 1995). It is argued that andragogy provides a framework within which care and other crucial aspects of the nurse–patient/client relationship can be mirrored and thereby facilitated in future practitioners.

In the socialization processes inherent in nurse education, care is surely difficult to teach or facilitate unless the philosophy and methods are consistent with such ends. Furthermore, it is frequently argued that as educationalists we need to be consistent in our approach to students with that which we hope to see in their future practice (Bevis & Murray 1990). Andragogy offers a medium through which this can be facilitated. It is essentially a humanistic educational process that values the individual. The power relationship between the educator and student is much more horizontal than is found in the historically common hierarchical educational relationship.

An educational process based upon andragogy therefore mirrors important parts of the nurse–patient/client relationship. It offers a theory of education consistent with the aims of modern day nursing practice. We should seek to improve our understanding of andragogy and no longer conceptualize it as one end of a false dichotomy with pedagogy.

Introduction

There are some important questions that ought to be considered in relation to the concept of andragogy. Why is it so unpopular? (see Darbyshire, 1993). Why does it not yet appear in the Oxford English Dictionary? And will nursing, and the contribution it makes to health and health care, benefit from the ongoing debate on the relevance and use of andragogy?

I will argue that andragogy, as a discrete field of adult education, exists in the sense of a useful educational process that is of increasing importance to nurse education. It offers an educational process consistent with modern nurse education's aims and should be valued for this. It will also be made clear that andragogy per se is not my main concern in terms of promoting a particular educational theory, but the emphasis on educational process that andragogy brings at this moment (as opposed to the

Frank Milligan: 'In Defence of Andragogy. Part 2: An Educational Process Consistent with Modern Nursing's Aims' in *NURSE EDUCATION TODAY* (1997), 17(6), pp. 487–493. Reprinted by permission of the publisher Churchill Livingstone.

historical institutionalized obsession with educational outcome) that is seen to be of fundamental value to nursing education.

I will start by outlining the concept of andragogy, followed by what I feel are some common misconceptions in relation to it. The importance of educational processes that are consistent with modern nursing's aims will then be highlighted, as will the notion that andragogy offers the most effective method available to ensure that nurse education facilitates effective practice in what is invariably an unpredictable future for nursing and the health service. The work of John Dewey is referred to in relation to this final point.

A brief outline of the theory of andragogy

My own conception of andragogy has evolved primarily from the work of Malcolm Knowles (1985, 1990), the Nottingham Andragogy Group (1983) and other works cited here, and can be summarized thus: the facilitation of adult learning that can best be achieved through a student-centred approach that, in a developmental manner, enhances students' self-concept and promotes autonomy, self-direction and critical thinking.

Although Knowles, an educationalist from the USA, is commonly seen as the main developer of andragogy (Jarvis, 1984), it is in fact historically a European concept that has been studied and developed widely (Richardson & Lane, 1993). It is clear that Knowles' work is only one interpretation of andragogy and European (Savicevic, 1991), US (De La Haye *et al.* 1994), and UK developments (Nottingham Andragogy Group, 1983), amongst others, can be found. I will, however, briefly outline the five key assumptions upon which Knowles (1985) bases andragogy, and use them to develop some important arguments with regard to a clearer understanding of the concept and some of the common misconceptions made in relation to it. The assumptions are as follows:

1. *The concept of the learner.* That the adult learner is self-directed, although Knowles noted that people's experiences of education frequently lead to a more dependent stance being taken by them.

2. *The role of the learner's experience.* Adult learners are seen to have a greater volume, and different quality of experience than younger learners. This difference in quality is based upon their roles as workers, family members, being a parent, etc.

3. *Readiness to learn.* That adults '. . . become ready to learn when they experience a need to know or do something in order to perform more effectively in some aspect of their lives' (Knowles, 1985, p. 11). Adult students become ready to learn when they see a need in relation to being able to do particular things (Chandler, 1992).

4. *Orientation to learning.* This tends to be task or problem centred, therefore learning should be organized around life, or what might be termed real situations. Knowles asserts that adults do not, for the most part, learn for the sake of learning.

5. *Motivation to learn.* Although the last two assumptions seem to imply a quite conservative, in other words work-based approach to motivation (Jarvis, 1985), Knowles makes a point of identifying humanistic needs as being important motivators: '. . . that the more potent motivators are internal, self-esteem, recognition, better quality of life, greater self-confidence, self-actualisation, and the like' (Knowles, 1985, p. 12).

The examination of andragogy is now enhanced through analysis of some common misconceptions in relation to it.

Common misconceptions!

There has been recent debate on the value, or otherwise, of andragogy and more specifically Knowles' conception of it (Darbyshire, 1993; Milligan, 1995). I will now extend this debate by highlighting what I feel are some common misconceptions made in relation to andragogy.

The first, and philosophically the most important misconception is that andragogy is the dichotomous opposite of pedagogy (De La Haye *et al.* 1994). This presentation is quite common (McPherson & Lorenz, 1985; Darbyshire, 1993; Richardson & Lane, 1993). Such a dichotomy can be found in the earlier writings of Knowles, but his conceptualization changed as he accepted that pedagogy and andragogy should be seen as parallel and not dichotomous opposites (Knowles, 1985). It is perhaps more appropriate to conceptualize andragogy as a discrete field of adult education within the broad remit of pedagogy (the art and science of teaching (Oxford English Dictionary, 2nd edn, 1989), (Savicevic, 1991; Milligan, 1995).

The second common misconception is that it is frequently assumed that student centredness, and the goal of achieving self-directedness in students, means leaving students to it! Indeed, I am aware of courses philosophically based upon andragogy that did just that. Students from the very start of the course were left to get on with it with very little, if any guidance; they were, it might be said, left to 'sink or swim'. Andragogy is frequently seen, under such circumstances, to be an excuse for lecturers to reduce their effort and workload. The volume and quality of work available on facilitating student centredness strongly mitigates against such a simplistic view being taken. Good examples include the works of Grow (1991), Slevin & Lavery (1991), and Higgs (1993). Grow identifies four learner states (dependent learner, interested learner, involved learner, self-directed learner) and compares these with different teaching styles. The grid that is developed (Grow, 1991) shows that different learning states require different teaching styles and that self-directedness is something that needs to be fostered and worked towards by both student and lecturer. In fact, Grow asserts that the learners state is more important in choosing the appropriate teaching methods than the subject matter! Higgs (1993) also makes it clear that learners need to learn how to learn independently, and this requires guidance from an educator skilled in such matters (Slevin & Lavery, 1991).

Another important issue to consider when reservations about the viability of student centredness are raised is that of the educationalists' own educational (sic) experiences, and those of the students (Higgs, 1993). Much of what both groups have experienced will simply not have involved student centredness, as Knowles (1985), Heron (1989) and Higgs (1993) all note. Heron (1993), in a provocative chapter on educational assessment and the power relationship it frequently operates within, highlights the oppressive nature of much so-called educational activity. Control, all too often and frequently inappropriately, lies solely with the educator rather than shared with the student.

The third major misconception is that andragogy is not possible within the constraints of modern nurse education. Even those nurse educationalists I have met who have been positive and active in their use of andragogy have felt that it has its limits in pre-registration education due to the constraints of the need to meet the occupational criteria of the course. In a sense this illustrates the point just made, that because the process of pre-registration courses frequently operates within an unequal power relationship in favour of the educator, handing over a significant degree of responsibility to the student seems inappropriate.

The fourth major misconception is that andragogy is *The* art and science of teaching adults; that it encompasses the whole field of adult learning and the many various and diverse so-called educational activities that take place within this. Although such interpretations can be found (Savicevic, 1991), albeit rarely, there are strong grounds upon which this can be challenged, namely that andragogy is an educational theory; it is primarily concerned with education and not training or vocationalization. The philosophical differences here are reasonably clear and explained within the works of Moore (1986) and Peters (1974), and as Quicke (1989) asserts, vocationalization is not education!

Moore (1986) claims that the educated person has intellectual abilities that have been developed so that they are sensitive to matters of moral and aesthetic concern. In examining the historical bonds between education and preparation for employment, Watts (1985) defines education as being concerned with: the development of the individual's full range of abilities and aptitudes; the cultivation of spiritual and moral values; the nurturing of imagination and sensibility, and the transmission and interpretation of culture. Within Watts' work this is then balanced against the need to prepare people for work-based roles, a vocational purpose that Watts notes sits uneasily with some educationalists.

The status of some subjects tends to be measured by how academic they are, and clear vocational links frequently carry little status for this reason (Watts, 1985). Vocational, in this sense, refers to common work roles. It is the difference between more practical training for such work roles, for example National Vocational Qualifications (NVQs) (Burke, 1989), and the education that is commonly associated with, for example, professions such as medicine and law, that perhaps best illustrates the point being made here. The former may fail to meet these definitions of education (Moore, 1986; Watts, 1985) if they do not reflect pertinent controversies and arguments inherent in the subject, and relate these to the students own cultural meaning (Quicke, 1989). Such a process is similar to that described by Mezirow (1983) as perspective transformation, in which individuals achieve new insights into their own position through actively questioning this position in relation to their understanding of the material being studied. I do not infer that law and medicine necessarily achieve this, but they are commonly considered to be 'an education'.

Within vocational work there is more concern with the practical achievement of tasks than questioning of the validity, cultural and historical place of those tasks. Therefore the narrower aims of training and vocationalization generally fail to meet the criteria given here to qualify them as education, and will consequently not be andragogical, as andragogy values the individual and that individual's personal growth and does meet the criteria given here.

Although, as Knowles makes clear, andragogy is very much concerned with work and the practicalities of preparation and development for work roles, implicit to this goal is enhancement of the individual's self-concept and understanding of the world. Such understanding involves an acknowledgement that the educational is political (Freire, 1985), a notion not evident within vocational education today which reflects a 'new Right' move towards removing such sociopolitical challenges from a range of curricula (Dale, 1985; Quicke, 1989; Milligan, 1995; Crawford, 1995). Indeed, Crawford (1995) notes, in reviewing conflicts around the history content of the National Curriculum, that arguments put forward by the Right have an ideological emphasis that far outweighs their educational substance. Furthermore, he asserts that critiques of the Right and education have been sacrificed for a conception of cultural cohesion that is based upon false assumptions. It seems that the 'the educational is political', and political enough to draw significant political attention!

To over-simplify what is a complex argument, vocationalization and training endeavour to fit people to particular tasks and jobs. Education is a means through which an *improved* person is assisted in their preparation for life and the roles it entails (admittedly work-related on many occasions). Therefore, it can be argued that andragogy does not logically encompass all activities that go under the banner of adult education, simply because some of these are not education! They are training and vocationalization. Andragogy is a particular educational approach to facilitating adult learning. I leave it to the reader to consider the implications of a growing trained, vocational workforce within nursing that does not have the sociopolitical awareness fostered through more critical educational methods, such as those inherent in Project 2000 (UKCC, 1987) curricula.

Educational process and the problem of our own educational histories

The importance of an educational process that is consistent with the aims of nurse education will be made clear through the example of our own educational histories. Process, for the purposes of this paper, is defined as the activities that take place within a curriculum in terms of the manner in which the content is defined, delivered and worked on and through by the students and teaching staff. It refers to the broad range of methods through which a particular course is operationalized. What educational histories are also requires some explanation. By this I mean the previous experiences that people have gone through (including the socioeducational milieu within which they operate), under the heading of education, that affect their current performance and perceptions of what might happen in educational settings.

Quite a lot of my work as a nurse educator has involved introducing people to teaching/facilitating learning for what is often the first time. It is common for these individuals to state that what stresses them is 'standing up in front of students'; 'having to be up the front'. Similarly they are worried about being asked questions; 'what if I don't know the answer'. It is also interesting that when people enter a lecture theatre for a lecturer or paper, many will invariably sit at the back.

All these, I suggest, are symptomatic of traditional, didactic educational experiences; someone stood up at the front and talked at you. You expected them to know the answers because they were knowledgeable about their field and you sat far enough back to ensure it was unlikely you would be asked a question. That distance, so evident when you speak in a lecture theatre, is symbolic of the distance that existed between the teacher and the student. There was no need for proximity, in either a physical or more educational sense; involvement was not important. Dennison & Kirk (1990) challenge that such methods must have held some attraction for those that subsequently moved into education, otherwise why did they make the move? In terms of process, very little interaction is involved and it is inherently passive for the student. In terms of power, it most obviously lies with the lecturer (Heron, 1993).

Andragogy and the process of nurse education

Substantial arguments have been made elsewhere to support the use of andragogy in nurse education (for example, ENB 1987; Richardson, 1988; Burnard, 1991). Here I will concentrate on some issues related to the assumptions, mentioned earlier, that Knowles (1985) based his conception of andragogy on, and reflect further upon what has been noted with regard to educational histories.

The process of achieving a self-directed learner seems entirely consistent with what is required of current nurse practitioners. They are now expected to record and monitor their own occupational development (UKCC, 1995). Furthermore, due to the quickly changing nature of health practice, its organization, management and the treatment and methods used within it, constant revision of what is relevant knowledge is necessary. The pace of these changes will inevitably continue to increase due to the information technology explosion. Also, self-directedness in learners clearly mirrors independence on the part of the patient in the nurse/patient relationship. In particular situations patients/clients will become most dependent, but the goal of independence, of establishing a flattened power relationship through which the patient establishes some control over their destiny remains.

Knowles' second assumption with regard to the quantity and quality of life experience appears consistent with a great deal of modern nurse education. There has been an increasing emphasis on the value of experiential work in the education of nurses (Richardson, 1988; Burnard, 1991) culminating in the move towards reflective practice (Bound et al. 1988; Johns, 1995). Furthermore, the personal element of knowledge, which is very much derived from an individual's previous and ongoing experience, is highlighted by Barbara Carper (1978). Her work is used with some success with all levels of student nurse, pre and post registration, in my own department.

The third assumption, readiness to learn, indicates that motivation is initiated through a need to know about something. Students usually come into nursing in a highly motivated state. They are keen and frequently want to 'get on with it'. However, I wonder if there is sometimes a failure to indicate clearly to students what is required of nurses in practice. With the move towards more student time being spent on theory in the early part of Project 2000 courses, as opposed to practice, there is a risk that motivation can be adversely affected. More subtly, do we know what nursing is? Are we confident about this so that we can, through theory, explain nursing?

Again, reflective practice offers a medium through which practice can be emphasized, and the use of narrative (Darbyshire, 1994) offers a means through which the everyday, yet special work of nursing can be illustrated and valued. Such approaches should enhance students' readiness to learn and are again an integral part of the work with students in the department.

There are few problems with accepting Knowles' fourth assumption, that learning ought to be [a] problem, and what I will term practice related. Again, reflective practice (Schön, 1988) including diary and/or journal writing, the use of case studies and critical incident analysis all offer methods which will try to integrate theory and practice; seek to elucidate learning from experience.

In the fifth assumption, by taking such a humanistic stance Knowles offers a challenge; trust students to study what they see as relevant. If, as in assumption 3, the roles of the nurse are made clear and, as in assumption 4, the problems inherent in nursing practice are evident, then the motivation to achieve a satisfying level of practice should be generated within the individual undertaking study.

In terms of trying to relate andragogy to the concept of care, this seems possible at two levels. Firstly, in terms of mirroring the qualities or values inherent within care, and more simply, in an effort to be consistent with what is commonly required of nursing practice. Elsewhere I have shown similarities between the work of the Nottingham Andragogy Group (1983) and Boykin & Schoenhofer's (1990) work on caring in nursing (Milligan, 1995). Mayerhoff (cited in Dunlop, 1986) saw trust as an important issue in care, and it has been shown here to be an element within the process of andragogy. More broadly, it is evident that the relationship between the student and the educator should be based upon sharing responsibility, and this includes the negotiation of aims and methods of achieving those aims. Again, these mirror important aspects of nursing practice.

John Dewey and the task that faces nurse education

Having claimed that nurse educationalists need to be able to clarify for students the purposes and future of nursing, and having hinted that some may not be best placed to do this, I will now explain, using the work of John Dewey, why this is perhaps a difficult task.

John Dewey was a US philosopher and educationalist in the early part of this century, who was very much interested in the democratic conception of education and also wrote of the central value of reflection in education. I would like briefly to transpose some of his ideas onto nurse education.

Education, when undertaken as Dewey saw fit, was consistent with democracy, a concept at least superficially compatible with good nursing practice. For a society to be considered a democracy it must support effective education. However, there was a tension for the democracy in the educational processes used in that Dewey felt that these methods could not simply pass on directly the values/knowledge, etc. that were common and thought to be of worth to that democratic society. This was due both to the transient nature of knowledge, a problem more recently highlighted by the likes of Knowles (1985), Rogers (1983), and Schön (1988), and the problem of simply repeating what is, or has been, common and found within the society. Just because it is common does not mean that in the longer term it will remain the best or most effective knowledge or value(s). Dewey saw such an attitude as being important in that education risked becoming indoctrination.

Change was seen as an important element of democratic societies. To quote Dewey: 'Particularly it is true that a society which not only changes but which has the ideal of such change as will improve it, will have different standards and methods of education from one which aims simply at the perpetuation of its own customs' (Dewey, cited in Sidorsky, 1977). It was seen as essential, therefore, that education prepared people for change.

Dewey also broadly argued that the democratic spirit, which in essence would be an important element of the educational process, be exhibited in the classroom: 'Any education given by a group tends to socialise its members, but the quality and value of the socialisation depends upon the habits and aims of the group' (Dewey, cited in Sidorsky, 1977, p. 220), supporting the arguments made here that nurse education processes need to be consistent with practice.

It is important to ponder the potential depth of the educational problem clarified by Dewey. It is implied that the educational process needs to contain qualities that will enable the student to operate within a system that may be very different to that known by the educationalist. Educationalists in Dewey's view cannot simply repeat what has been common and of relevance to them. With this argument in mind the importance of any substantial emphasis on educational outcome fades. Outcomes for Dewey seem to be acknowledged as anything but fixed. Process, and the flexibility and honesty of this process, seem to surface clearly. To overstate the point, Dewey simply seemed to be saying that a democracy is frequently not clear about where it is going, but the honesty of such an admission was more important than the admission itself.

Taking this in the light of the comments made with regard to Dewey's perceived need for education to facilitate change, not perpetuate what has been common, a challenge of some substance for nurse education becomes clear, namely that educationalists are required to facilitate the preparation of practitioners who will be (to be realistic already frequently are) radically different to themselves. I suggest that Dewey's work, as described here, has a resonance [for] nurse education today; that Project 2000 (UKCC, 1987) marks a significant move away from the 'perpetuation of customs' that has historically been common in nursing education. That Project 2000 is symptomatic of a more questioning, more critical stance in nurse education and nursing practice and that nursing is undergoing a significant period of change (as is health care generally), perhaps even a paradigm shift in change in which an adherence to the value of educational process, as opposed to outcomes, is desirable if not essential.

Furthermore, the arguments made earlier in relation to the influence of the 'new Right' in education are inconsistent with Dewey's emphasis on the significance of change and democratic spirit within education. This leads to the question of whether nursing can continue to support the dichotomy created between the vocational NVQ system and education for practitioners who will register?

There are quite clear outcomes required of nurse education, the most important of which are those defined by statute (Nurse, Midwives and Health Visitors approval order 1989). In addition, it is apparent from curricular documents for Project 2000 courses that outcomes can clearly be defined for pre-registration nurse education. However, it is also evident from such documents, especially when looked at historically, that what is required of both students and nurse educators very quickly changes, and there is no reason to suppose that the pace of the change will slow, in fact it will almost certainly increase. Using andragogical methods will facilitate self-directedness and the confidence that goes with this in students, allowing them to adapt more effectively to changes that will occur in nursing and health care practice. The importance of outcomes is therefore acknowledged, but it is the methods through which they are achieved that is seen to be of real importance.

Conclusion

One of the tasks of this paper has been to substantiate the continuing and perhaps even the growing use of the theory of andragogy. I have clarified here what I feel are clear misconceptions behind some of the arguments used to diminish the value of the theory of andragogy. Some of the underlying assumptions of andragogy have been outlined and clearly linked to some important aspects of nurse education and nursing practice. Furthermore, the influence of our own educational experiences has been briefly explored, and the common association that is found, one of distance and a power relationship in favour of the educator, was shown to be inconsistent with that which is required of modern nursing.

Reluctance on the part of some educators to move towards a considered student-centred approach (by this I mean a stance supported by relevant educational literature and research) is in part due to their own educational histories and their reluctance to see power in the educational relationship move towards the student. They also perhaps, through the students, reflect the subservience historically found in the doctor/nurse relationship. Slevin & Lavery (1991, p. 376) concluded that, 'Teachers will have to be more willing to take risks in allowing students greater responsibility for their own learning', when arguing for a more student-centred approach to nurse education. I suggest that such risks are proportional to the understanding, or lack of understanding that is conveyed to students in making clear to them what is relevant to nursing and nursing practice.

Andragogy is consistent with nursing care and nursing work, the relationship and actions commonly undertaken between nurses and patient/clients, because: it places more power in the hands of students; it asks students to take responsibility for a good deal of their learning; it involves them; and, perhaps most importantly, it encourages educators to trust them. To be brief, it treats them like adults.

Perhaps the real value of the theory of andragogy is that it simply offers another perspective on education. It offers one more lens through which to view pedagogy; *the art and science of teaching*. It values the process of educational activity above that of outcome although the latter remains a practical necessity. Some of the resistance to andragogy in pre-registration nurse education has been on the grounds of the need to dictate an outcome — the registered nurse. It has been argued here, substantiated by the work of Dewey, that we, nursing and nurse education, have a very difficult task in trying to predict accurately what will be required of tomorrow's nurse. Therefore, an emphasis on educational process is not only desirable and adaptive, it is necessary and the most potent means of achieving effective nursing in the future. It is through an adaptive educational process that we will be able to effectively meet the outcomes of tomorrow.

References

Bevis E O, Murray J P (1990) The essence of the curriculum revolution: emancipatory teaching. *Journal of Nurse Education* 29 (7): 326–331.

Boud D, Keogh R, Walker D (eds) (1988) *Reflection: turning experiences into learning*. Kogan Page, London.

Boykin A, Schoenhofer S (1990) Caring in nursing: analysis of extant theory. *Nursing Science Quarterly* 3 (4): 149–155.

Burke J (ed) (1989) *Competency based education and training*. Falmer Press, London.

Burnard P (1991) *Learning human skills*, 2nd edn. Butterworth Heinemann, Guildford.

Carper B (1978) Fundamental patterns of knowing in nursing. *Advances in Nursing Science* 1(1): 13–23.

Chandler T (1992) Planning for teaching. In: S M Hinchliff (ed) *The practitioner as teacher*. Scutari Press, Oxford.

Crawford K (1995) A history of the Right: the battle for control of National Curriculum history 1989–1994. *British Journal of Educational Studies* 43(4): 433–456.

Dale R (1985) The background and inception of the technical and vocational education initiative. In: R Dale (ed) *Education, training and employment; towards a new vocationalism*. Open University/Pergamon Press, Oxford.

Darbyshire P (1993) In defence of pedagogy: a critique of the notion of andragogy. *Nurse Education Today* 13: 328–335.

Darbyshire P (1994) Reality bites. *Nursing Times* 90(40): 31–33.

De La Haye B L, Limerick D C, Hearn G (1994) The relationship between andragogical and pedagogical orientations and the implications for adult learning. *Adult Education Quarterly* 44 (4): 187–200.

Dennison B, Kirk R (1990) *Do, review, learn, apply: a simple guide to experiential learning*. Blackwell Education. Wiltshire.

Dunlop M J (1986) Is a science of caring possible? *Journal of Advanced Nursing* 11(6): 661–670.

ENB (1987) *Managing change in nurse education*. ENB, Milton Keynes.

Grow G O (1991) Teaching learners to be self-directed. *Adult Education Quarterly* 41(3): 125–149.

Freire P (1985) *Pedagogy of the oppressed*. Pelican, Suffolk.

Heron J (1989) *The facilitators' handbook*. Kogan Page, Guildford.

Heron J (1993) Assessment revisited. In: D Boud (ed) *Developing student autonomy in learning*, 2nd edn. Kogan Page, Chippenham.

Higgs J (1993) Planning learning experiences to promote autonomous learning. In: D Boud (ed) *Developing student autonomy in learning*, 2nd edn. Kogan Page, Chippenham.

Jarvis P (1984) Andragogy — a sign of the times. *Studies in the Education of Adults* 4: 32–39.

Jarvis P (1985) *The sociology of adult and continuing education*. Croom Helm, London.

Johns C (1995) Framing learning through reflection within Carper's fundamental ways of knowing in nursing. *Journal of Advanced Nursing* 22: 226–234.

Knowles M (1985) *Andragogy in action*. Jossey-Bass, USA.

Knowles M (1990) *The adult learner; a neglected species*, 4th edn. Gulf, USA.

McPherson R B, Lorenz J A (1985) The pedagogical and andragogical principle — the consummate teacher. *NASSP Bulletin*: 55–60.

Mezirow J (1983) A critical theory of adult learning and education. In: M Tight (ed) *Education for adults; adult learning and education*. Croom Helm, London.

Milligan F J (1995) In defence of andragogy. *Nurse Education Today* 15: 22–27.

Moore T W (1986) *Philosophy of education: an introduction*. Routledge and Kegan Paul, London.

Nottingham Andragogy Group (1983) *Towards a developmental theory of andragogy*. Department of Adult Education, University of Nottingham.

Nurses, Midwives and Health Visitors Approval Order Statutory Instruments (1989) The nurses midwives and health visitors (registered fever nurses amendment rules and training amendment rules) approval order 1989. Statutory Instruments No 1456, HMSO, London.

Peters R S (1974) *Ethics and education*. Unwin, London.

Quicke J (1989) The 'new Right' and education. In: B Moon, P Murphy, J Raynor (eds) *Policies for the curriculum*. Hodder and Stoughton, Suffolk.

Richardson M (1988) Innovating andragogy in a basic nursing course: an evaluation of the self-directed independent study contract with basic nursing students. *Nurse Education Today* 8: 315–324.

Richardson M, Lane K (1993) Andragogical concepts for teachers of adults. *Catalyst for Change* 22: 16–18.

Rogers C (1983) *Freedom to learn for the 80s*. Charles Merrill, USA.

Savicevic D M (1991) Modern conceptions of andragogy: a European framework. *Studies in the Education of Adults* 23 (2): 179–201.

Schön D A (1988) *Educating the reflective practitioner*. Jossey Bass, San Francisco.

Sidorsky D (1977) *John Dewey: the essential writings*. Harper and Row, New York.

Slevin O D'A, Lavery M C (1991) Self-directed learning and student supervision. *Nurse Education Today* 11: 368–377.

United Kingdom Central Council for Nursing, Midwifery and Health Visiting (1987) Project 2000: the final proposals: project paper 9. UKCC, London.

United Kingdom Central Council for Nursing, Midwifery and Health Visiting (1995) PREP and you: maintaining your registration. Standards for education following registration. UKCC, London.

Watts A G (1985) Education and employment: the traditional bonds. In: R Dale (ed) *Education, training and employment; towards a new vocationalism*. Open University/Pergamon Press, Oxford.

4. Experiential Learning and Andragogy — Negotiated Learning in Nurse Education: A Critical Appraisal

Philip Burnard

Andragogy and experiential learning have frequently been cited as recommended approaches to aspects of nurse education. This paper offers a critical appraisal of the two approaches and offers suggestions as to how a negotiated nursing curriculum may be developed.

Introduction

Andragogy and experiential learning are two fairly contemporary approaches to aspects of nurse education. Both have their advantages and disadvantages but both, combined, can offer a powerful means of equipping learner nurses with a range of practical, intellectual, social and interpersonal skills. This article considers critically the two approaches and then offers an outline for their combined use.

Experiential learning

Experiential learning has received considerable coverage in the recent literature on nurse education (Raichura, 1987; Tomlinson, 1985; Kagan, Evans & Kay, 1986; Miles, 1987). The theoretical literature seems to use the term in two different ways. One approach involves the concept of life as a learning process and thus experiential learning is learning through the process of living, working and generally relating to the world. This approach to the concept of experiential learning is best exemplified by Keeton and his associates (1976).

The other approach is via humanistic psychology and emphasises subjective experience, personal interpretation and the education of the emotions. This approach is best exemplified in the writings of Kilty (1983), Shaffer (1978) and Heron (1973, 1982, 1977).

One of the problems with Heron's work is that it is insufficiently referenced and thus it is difficult to place his work in context. He seems to draw from a wide variety of sources, including encounter, gestalt and humanistic psychology. He has recently made his interest in mysticism and transpersonal psychology more overt (1987). Through the Human Potential Research Project at the University of Surrey, he has had much to do with influencing the ways in which nurse tutors have adopted the experiential learning approach to nurse education.

Apart from these two main themes in the experiential learning literature, there are also some 'hybrids'. Kolb (1984), for example, combines some of the 'learning through the process of living' approach with ideas from Carl Rogers and Carl Jung and applies,

Philip Burnard: 'Experiential Learning and Andragogy — Negotiated Learning in Nurse Education: A Critical Appraisal' in *NURSE EDUCATION TODAY* (1989), 9, pp. 300–306. Reprinted by permission of the publisher Churchill Livingstone.

almost paradoxically, a fairly rigorous quantitative approach to researching his theoretical constructs. Boydel's (1976) theoretical approach also seems to stand outside the mainstream humanistic approach and yet does not fit completely into the first approach either.

Experiential knowledge

The present writer has proposed the idea of experiential learning being defined through a theory of knowledge (1987). Three types of knowledge have been proposed: propositional, practical and experiential knowledge. Propositional knowledge is 'textbook' knowledge of facts, theories and models. Practical knowledge is knowledge revealed through practice — for example the demonstration of successfully giving an injection or the demonstration of effective counselling skills. Experiential knowledge is *personal* knowledge, gained through direct encounter with a person, place or thing. It is that knowledge that we 'know' for ourselves and that cannot easily be transmitted to other people. Experiential learning, then, is *any learning which increases the facilitation of experiential knowledge*. In this way, it is differentiated from traditional learning methods which, arguably, have mostly been concerned with the development of propositional or practical knowledge.

Tutors' views of experiential learning

This, then, is a brief overview of the literature. Nurse tutors, it would seem are less certain about how to define experiential learning. In the present writer's ongoing research into the field, it is emerging that nurse educators interpret the concept of experiential learning in widely differing ways (Burnard, 1989). Some, for instance, see it only as a means of teaching certain topics, notably interpersonal skills. Others see it as applicable to all nursing topics including law and anatomy and physiology. Some see the approach as being concerned with learning from practical experience (including clinical placements) whilst others see it as more concerned with 'personal' learning and self awareness. Yet others view experiential learning as being concerned mainly with role play and compare and contrast it to more 'traditional' methods such as the lecture. Some are fairly zealous in their adoption of experiential learning and base their entire curriculum on it, whilst others see it as one teaching method amongst a range of teaching methods.

Both the literature and the tutors that the present writer has talked to are in agreement on two issues: that experiential learning is concerned with personal experience and with 'practice' rather than theory. Sometimes those issues are overlaid with fairly complicated theories about the person — often humanistic or transpersonal. In other cases, the approach is essentially pragmatic: the progress of learning by doing is a practical aid to developing certain skills.

In passing, it is interesting to reflect on why the humanistic and transpersonal themes have emerged in nurse education at this time, given that they developed and perhaps reached a peak in the 1960s. Much of the 'classic' humanistic theory was worked out in the 60s (Rogers, 1967; Rodzak, 1969). Humanistic psychology has had little impact on traditional academic psychology, as the late Carl Rogers noted recently (1985), and the encounter movement is certainly less pervasive than it used to be.

At least two, very speculative, reasons for the current interest in the humanistic approach to experiential learning in nurse education can be mooted. One concerns the age of nurse tutors. Because of the career path leading to the post of nurse tutor, many tutors will be of an age where they can recall the 60s and may have 'brought with them' the attitudes and values of that period. The second, is the publication of the 1982 syllabus of training for psychiatric nursing students (ENB, 1982). This syllabus was formulated, to some degree, by people who had a considerable interest in humanistic psychology. Many aspects of the syllabus reflect the humanistic approach and the syllabus has been influential in aspects of nurse education beyond psychiatric nursing. The syllabus is also unusual in that it recommends that experiential learning methods be used.

Andragogy

Andragogy, a term associated with Malcolm Knowles (Knowles, 1978, 1980, 1984), though used before his time, is one used to differentiate the theory and practice of adult education from pedagogy — the theory and practice of the education of children. Knowles claimed that adults differed in some fundamental ways from children and, therefore, required a different educational system. Such a system included the ideas that:

– adult education should be grounded in the participants wealth of prior experience,

– adults need to be able to apply what they learn,

– adult education should be an active rather than a passive process.

Out of these ideas, Knowles drew up a method of conducting adult education sessions.

One objection that may be raised about Knowles' theory is that the ideas identified above may be applicable, also, to children. If this is the case, it is difficult to see how he can argue for a discreet theory of adult education based on these principles. Knowles acknowledges this problem and, in later writing, tends to describe andragogy as an attitude towards education rather than as being a discreet theory of adult education. This argument and others relating to andragogy have been well described by Jarvis (1983, 1984) and Brookfield (1987).

Andragogy has much in common with the student-centred learning approach of the late Carl Rogers (1984). This is not surprising as both Knowles and Rogers were influenced, through their respective professors of education, by John Dewey, the pragmatist and philosopher of education (Dewey, 1966, 1971; Kirschenbaum, 1979). It also has much in common with many of the approaches to experiential learning, emphasising, as they do, the centrality of personal experience and subjective interpretation.

Another observation that may be made about both andragogy and experiential learning is that they are both very American in their approach. The American educational system, influenced as it has been by Dewey's work, has always tended towards a more student-centred, individualistic approach to education. It was something of a surprise, therefore, for the present writer to find little or no evidence of experiential learning methods being regularly used in the parts of California, Florida and New England, visited early in 1987 (Burnard, 1987). The accent, there, was very much on learning to pre-set, prescribed objectives. In California, particularly, 'experiential learning' was something associated with the encounter movement of the 1960s. On the east coast, and particularly around New York, humanistic psychology was often not recognised as a separate school of psychology at all. Whether or not all this means that we are behind or ahead of the Americans in terms of modern approaches to nurse education, is a moot point. Some would argue that we have arrived at student-centred learning rather late in the day. Others would no doubt argue that we are putting into practice what American educators have been preaching for years.

Application

How, then, may aspects of experiential learning and andragogy usefully be combined in nurse education? Such a combination needs to take into account certain basic principles such as negotiation, the importance of personal experience and the use of self and peer assessment. What must also be borne in mind, however, is that learner nurses and nurse tutors have to work to a prescribed syllabus of training laid down by the English and Welsh National Boards. This fact makes nurse education somewhat different to many of the experiential learning training workshops at which all of the content may arise out of participants needs and wants. Many nurse tutors may encounter problems in translating workshop experience into practice because of this fact. Also, there is a large difference between using experiential learning methods in a 2-day to 1-week training workshop and using them on a regular basis throughout a 3-year-programme.

Figure 1 offers a tentative cycle which acknowledges both the principles of andragogy and the principles of experiential learning, as outlined by Kolb (1984), Heron (1973) and others (Burnard 1985, 1987, 1989; Burnard & Chapman, 1988).

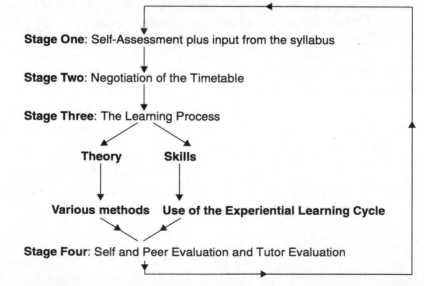

Stage One: Self-Assessment plus input from the syllabus

Stage Two: Negotiation of the Timetable

Stage Three: The Learning Process

Theory   **Skills**

Various methods   **Use of the Experiential Learning Cycle**

Stage Four: Self and Peer Evaluation and Tutor Evaluation

Figure 1   **A cycle for combining andragogy and experiential learning in nurse education**

In stage one, two things happen. First, the students identify their own learning needs through direction from the tutor and in line with the 'learning contract' approach described by Knowles (1975). Second, the tutor identifies certain learning needs out of the prescribed syllabus. The students can draw from their previous ward experience, here, and may find a 'brainstorming' session a useful means of generating topics.

Thus, in stage two, a timetable is negotiated. It will consist of the two elements described above and may be divided into a 'theory' element and a 'skills' element. The skills element may include both practical nursing skills and interpersonal skills, as appropriate. Again, it will be remembered that the content of this theory and skills mix will arise jointly out of the expressed needs of the students and the suggested ideas of the nurse tutor.

The theory element may then be learned using a whole range of educational approaches, including the traditional ones of lecture and seminar, as required. However, for the skills element, it is recommended that the experiential learning cycle be followed. Such a cycle is illustrated in Figure 2. Its use has been described, in detail, elsewhere (Burnard, 1987).

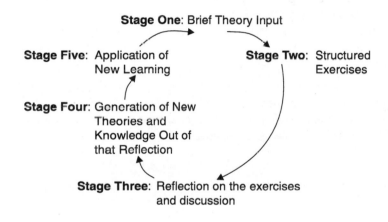

Figure 2   An experiential learning cycle

Self and peer evaluation

Following the learning of both theory and practice, learners are called upon to self and peer evaluate their new learning. Again, this has been described elsewhere (Burnard, 1987; Kilty, 1978). Essentially, the aim is to encourage learner autonomy by developing in those learners the ability to check the learning development of themselves and their colleagues. At this stage, too, it is usually necessary (if not mandatory) to include the more 'objective' evaluation processes that are instigated by tutors: examination, tests, questionnaires, check lists and so forth.

Out of this evaluation phase can emerge and evolve a new assessment phase and thus the cycle continues.

Student-centred learning

The cycle, briefly outlined here incorporates the student-centred, negotiating approach of andragogy with the accent on personal experience and self and peer evaluation of experiential learning. It also acknowledges that learner nurses need to work to a syllabus and that nurse tutors can contribute much to effectively planning a course of study around such a syllabus. In this cycle, 'negotiation' means just that — the programme emerges out of the experience and knowledge of both students and tutors. In recent years it has been almost as if tutors were required to remain quietly in the background and ensure that they never inflicted their views on their learners! Whilst it would be difficult to sensibly advocate a return to the days of a totally prescribed course of training, it seems reasonable to acknowledge the educational skill of tutors in helping students to build an effective programme of nursing education.

Perhaps, then, it is a question of developing a balance between what Heron (1986) calls 'following' and 'leading'. Following involves taking the lead from the students, using their experience and ideas. Leading, on the other hand, means making suggestions and using structure to help the students. Together, these methods can ensure balance and symmetry in the nurse education programme. If the programme involves too much 'following' or is too student-directed in its methods, it will be unbalanced. On the other hand, if it involves too much 'leading or is too teacher-directed in its methods, it will also be unbalanced.

Having said this, the attitude towards nurse education should always remain student centred. The issue is not whether or not the tutor or the student should serve as the focal point of the educational process but the means by which the students educational needs are identified and satisfied. In this sense, then, the focus remains the student. Figure 3 identifies this dialectical relationship.

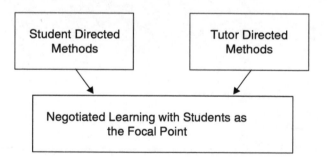

Figure 3   Combining student-directed and teacher-directed methods

Objections

There may, of course, be some practical objections to this combined approach. First, the approach takes time, it is far easier and less time consuming if the tutor prepares the timetable and the lessons. However, the negotiated approach is likely to yield a more appropriate timetable, geared to this group of students, at this time.

Second, it is likely that many students have been socialised into a more teacher-directed and teacher-centred approach. In the present writer's experience it takes time for such students to adapt to the approach suggested here but when they do, they seem to prefer it to the more traditional approach. Some, of course, do not prefer it and it seems reasonable to take into account the needs and wants of the other-directed student. Not everyone, after all, is necessarily self-directed (Reisman, 1950).

Third, there is the question of 'getting through the syllabus'. This seems a sensible issue to consider as, like it or not, students have to sit examinations during and at the end of their training. Whilst the literature on the question of content in the curriculum offers various views of what should, could or may be included in a nurse training course (Cork, 1987; Greaves, 1987; Beattie, 1987), in the end, all schools of nursing are constrained, at least to some degree, by syllabuses prescribed by the National Boards (this may, of course, change with the introduction of the recommendations of Project 2000). If the negotiated approach, as indicated here, is used and the syllabus is repeatedly referred back to as a sourcebook for guidance, then such problems should not arise. The accent, here, is on negotiation: the tutor should be free to recommend that certain aspects of the syllabus be introduced at certain stages of training. As we noted above, the student-centred approach to education should never mean that the tutor is redundant in the educational process and she should feel free to exercise judgement in such aspects of curriculum planning. In the end, however, no course of training, traditional or negotiated, ever covers every aspect of the syllabus.

As we move into the late 1980s it is important that our teaching and learning methods remain up-to-date. It is hoped that the combined approach described here can serve as a practice guide to negotiating some aspects of nurse education programmes.

References

Beattie A (1987) Making a curriculum work. In P Allan and M Jolley (eds) *The Curriculum in Nursing Education*. Croom Helm, London.

Boydel T (1976) *Experiential learning*. Manchester Monograph No 5, Department of Adult and Continuing Education, University of Manchester.

Brookfield S D (1987) *Developing critical thinkers: challenging adults to explore alternative ways of thinking and acting*. Open University, Milton Keynes.

Burnard P (1985) *Learning human skills. A Guide for Nurses*, Heinemann, London.

Burnard P (1987) Self and peer assessment. *Senior Nurse* 6: 5, 16–17.

Burnard P (1987) A study of the ways in which experiential learning methods are used to develop interpersonal skills in nurses in Canada and the USA. Florence Nightingale Memorial Committee, London.

Burnard P (1987) Towards an epistemological basis for experiential learning in nurse education. *Journal of Advanced Nursing* 12, 189–193.

Burnard P (1989) Exploring nurse educators' views of experiential learning: a pilot study. *Nurse Education Today* 9: 1, 39–45.

Burnard P (1989) *Counselling skills for health professionals*. Chapman and Hall, London.

Burnard P, Chapman C M (1988) *Professional and ethical issues in nursing: the code of professional conduct.* Wiley, Chichester.

Cork M (1987) Approaches to curriculum planning. In B. Davis (ed) *Nursing Education, Research and Developments.* Croom Helm, London.

Dewey J (1916; 1966) *Democracy and education.* Free Press, New York.

Dewey J (1938; 1971) *Experience and education.* Collier Macmillan, New York.

English and Welsh National Boards for Nursing, Midwifery and Health Visiting (1982) Syllabus of training: part 3 (Registered Mental Nurse).

Greaves F (1987) *The nursing curriculum: theory and practice.* Croom Helm, London.

Heron J (1973) Experiential training techniques. Human Potential Research Project, University of Surrey, Guildford.

Heron J (1982) Education of the affect. Human Potential Research Project, University of Surrey, Guildford.

Heron J (1977) Behaviour analysis in education and training. Human Potential Research Project, University of Surrey, Guildford.

Heron J (1987) *Confessions of a Janus brain.* Endymion Press, London.

Heron J (1986) Six category intervention analysis. Human Potential Research Project, University of Surrey, Guildford.

Jarvis P (1983) *The theory and practice of adult and continuing education.* Croom Helm, London.

Jarvis P (1984) *The sociology of adult and continuing education.* Croom Helm, London.

Kagan C, Evans J, Kay B (1986) *A manual of interpersonal skills for nurses: an experiential approach.* Harper and Row, London.

Keeton M *et al* (1976) *Experiental learning.* Jossey Bass, San Francisco, California.

Kilty J (1978) Self and peer assessment. Human Potential Research Project, University of Surrey, Guildford.

Kilty J (1983) Experiential learning. Human Potential Research Project, University of Surrey, Guildford.

Kirschenbaum H (1979) *On becoming Carl Rogers.* Dell, New York.

Kolb D (1984) *Experiential learning.* Prentice Hall, New Jersey.

Knowles M S (1975) *Self directed learning.* Cambridge, New York.

Knowles M S (1978) *The adult learner: a neglected species.* Gulf, Houston, Texas.

Knowles M S (1980) *The modern practice of adult education.* 2nd edn, Follett, Chicago.

Knowles M S (1984) *Andragogy in action: applying modern principles of adult education.* Jossey Bass, San Francisco, California.

Miles R (1987) Experiential learning in the curriculum. In: P Allan and M Jolley (eds), *The Curriculum in Nurse Education.* Croom Helm, London.

Raichura L (1987) Learning by doing. *Nursing Times* 83: 13, 59–61.

Riesman D (1950) *The lonely crowd.* Yale University Press. New Haven, Connecticut.

Rogers C R (1967) *On becoming a person.* Constable, London.

Rogers C R (1984) *Freedom to learn for the eighties.* Merrill, Columbus, Ohio.

Rogers C R (1985) Towards a more human science of the person. *Journal of Humanistic Psychology* 25: 4, 7–24.

Roszak T (1969) *The making of a counter culture: reflections on the technocratic society and its youthful opposition.* Doubleday, New York.

Shaffer J B P (1978) *Humanistic psychology.* Prentice Hall, New Jersey.

Tomlinson A (1985) The use of experiential methods in teaching interpersonal skills to nurses. In: C. Kagen (ed) *Interpersonal Skills in Nursing: Research and Applications.* Kogan Page, London.

5. Teaching and Learning: A Climate of Change

Susan Major

We cannot teach another person directly, we can only facilitate his or her learning.

This paper stems from the author's experience on a Community Practitioner Teacher (CPT) course. It was in November 1988 that the course members were first exposed to various teaching and learning methods that had been developed around the experiential and student centred approaches. Experiential learning (EL) in particular may be argued as very different from most teaching and learning methods we are used to. This implies that traditional teaching and perhaps traditional nursing cannot be compatible with student centred and patient centred approaches. This ostensible incompatibility calls for a climate of change which will eventually shift the teaching and the practice from 'doing for' to 'doing with'.

It is evident that more educationalists have questioned the credibility of traditional methods of learning. The 'traditional' or expository teaching and learning has been described by Ausubel (1) as the 'presentation of the entire content of what is to be learned to the learner in its final form'. The learner plays a passive role, digesting the knowledge given to him by the teacher. Learning outcome is determined by what is accurate as defined and desired by the teacher.

On the other hand McEvoy (2) proposed that new models of learning should be adopted to make the learning process interesting, imaginative, and capable of critical reflection. This approach requires the student to be actively involved in the teaching and learning act, to determine for himself/herself the value of his/her experience and to share knowledge with colleagues.

This approach can also be argued to be central to experiential learning (EL).

It is difficult to attribute the EL model to any one pioneer, as in recent years numerous models of EL have been developed. Needles to say, definitions have been varied and wide. For instance, Rogers (3) defines EL as a learning experience with qualities of personal involvement. It takes into account both feeling and cognitive aspects of the person. Burnard (4) checked student nurses' perception of EL and found such definitives as:

• Learning through practice

• Learning without text book

• Learning without chalk and talk

• Warning through role play

Susan Major: 'Teaching and Learning: A Climate of Change' in *NURSING STANDARD* (1989), Vol. 4, No. 3, pp. 36–38.

The advent of EL

EL origins can be traced back to the 1940s. Perhaps Lewin's (5) work on action research and T groups (training groups) provided the foundation.

The 'T group' was discovered when Lewin, along with his colleagues, set up a training programme on group interactions. The programme centred around experiential activities such as discussion and role play. Staff and participants were treated equally, while their activities were observed by researchers. Normally, evening sessions gave Lewin and his staff an opportunity for feedback. However, by chance, three participants were allowed to join in on one such evening session. These participants concluded that they had learnt from the experience of sitting in. The staff also agreed that there was more insight and usefulness in such experiential reflections. This was the inception of the EL model, although further contributions to the EL model followed. The well known work of Kolb and Fry (6) is based on Lewin's ideas.

Kolb and Fry suggest that the basic perception of EL is misleadingly simple, that is change, growth and learning occur through a sequence of four logical stages of progression which can be summarised thus:

1. Concrete experience

2. Collating data and making observations about the experience

3. Analysing the data to formulate conclusions and feedback

4. Change in behaviour, to facilitate choice of new experience.

See Figure 1 for the EL cycle.

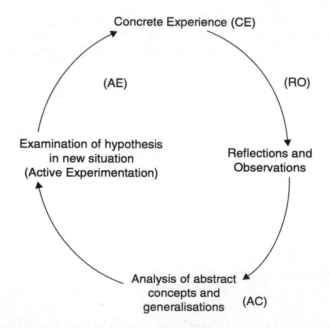

Figure 1   The EL Cycle: adapted from Kolb and Fry

According to Kolb and Fry, the development of EL starts with the concrete experience (CE) of here and now. This forms the foundations for stage two, reflecting and observing (RO). This subsequently leads to the abstract conceptualisation (AC) (stage three) from which a new naive experimentation (AE) may result (stage four).

Kolb and Fry out of their description of Lewin's work suggested that learning was helped in an environment where there is dialectic tensions and conflict between immediate concrete experience and analytic detachment. That is, by addressing the issues of the experience (CE) in open forum, where one can be challenged and aroused (RO), a cognitive awareness may result (AC). The creation of this cognitive awareness may be experimented with later (AE). Kolb and Fry further suggest that the acquisition of knowledge and skills are achieved through confrontation within the four angles of EL. To elaborate they identity four 'abilities' required by the student for effective learning. Concrete experience abilities, reflective observation abilities, abstract conceptual abilities and active experimentation abilities. However, the student will not learn unless he/she is able to judge the experience or mediate over it for meaning and form aims with reference to aspirations and calculations. Kolb and Fry see the students role as moving in fluctuating degrees from actor to observer, that is from specific involvement to the general analytic detachment. The role of the teacher becomes that of facilitator. The overall experience is the outcome of continually changing cognitive processes.

The EL process can be applied to any learning situation provided it is well understood, particularly by the teacher [or] facilitator.

The author has used counselling as an area of study to highlight the use of EL during a student's (mental health) field work placement. Student participation is increased by working through the themes of the nursing process. Emphasis is placed on the students' ability to learn. They are given the opportunity to reflect, process, interpret and apply meaning to their experience (RO–AE).

The EL stages can be seen as such:

Concrete Experience (CE): It is assumed that the student has been introduced to counselling during a theoretical block in college. In particular, they should be familiar with a model of counselling and be able to draw on the theoretical material implicit in the model. Selected reading, for instance Egan (7), Rogers (8) and Nelson-Jones (9), would be necessary. This experience provides the basis for reflection and observation.

Source of motivation

Reflection and observation: This stage may be seen as an introduction to EL activities. The student, in an attempt to get to know the team may engage in a group discussion where exchange of experiences and expression of attitudes and opinions can be voiced. Boydell (10) indicates that learning is achieved through the interaction and association with people who eventually become a source of motivation. Furthermore, he points out that the advancement and possession of knowledge, and its interpretation, depends on the strength of interpersonal relationships maintained with other well motivated people.

Abstract conceptualisation (AC): Out of the students' ability or inability to reflect and observe their past experiences (inductive reasoning), should come the desire to develop a knowledge/theoretical base (deductive reasoning) to provide a foundation for future practice. Learning will take place through further reading, student led case presentations with key areas of counselling skills being identified for discussion, role play, video tape recordings, psycho drama and so on. For instance, the CPT (facilitator) may invite the student (actor) to role play a situation that may illustrate communication techniques for example, reflecting:

Client (student): Do you think I should leave my job?

Counsellor (CPT): Do you think you should leave your job?

Active Experimentation (AE): The student will be invited to 'take on' a client for counselling sessions under the direct supervision of his/her CPT. For the purpose of this paper, the client contact will enable the student to follow the sequence of the learning cycle, nursing process and the counselling cycle (Figure 2).

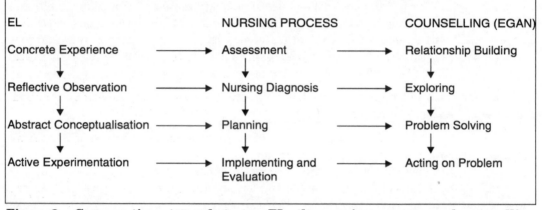

Figure 2   Comparative stages between EL, the nursing process and counselling
Source: SF Major (1989) unpublished.

Elaborating, the concrete experience (CE) will be viewed in two parts. Firstly as experience before the placement and secondly as the initial contact with the client (assessment), where trust, warmth and respect (relationship building) may develop.

The reflecting and observing (RO) will take place between the client and counsellor (student). They may identify (nursing diagnosis) and explore the problems that arise out of the assessment and plan further interventions.

The ability to draw conclusions (AC) can be seen as problem solving with the client formulating ideas that may resolve conflicts.

The active experimentation (AE) assumes that the client is now able to act upon the problems and examine the change that has occurred, hence evaluation.

It is not uncommon for nurses who undertake post basic courses based on experimental philosophies to feel apprehensive at the prospect of being responsible for their own learning. After all, so many have been previously taught using traditional expository teaching methods. But how does EL differ from the traditional approaches?

Traditional models assume that:

- the teacher is the expert, with a reservoir of knowledge that is tapped by the student.

- the possession of expertise can make claims to primacy, that is the teacher not only has a hierarchial authority, but is seen as a total resource, deemed necessary for the learning process to be achieved.

- students may interpret learning as memorising, that is they merely retain knowledge until it is required for external evaluation.

By contrast, EL assumes that:

- the teacher is a facilitator of learning, with attitudinal resources that help initiate a relationship between himself and the learner.

- learning is self-initiated, students are expected to take on responsibility for their own learning.

- learning is a meaningful experience. It allows students to develop their own level of inquiry, sanction and be critical of their own experience.

- the learner is seen as a 'whole' person, with both the psychological and intellectual components being identified for learning to take place.

These assumptions are not exhaustive, but serve to highlight some of the fundamental differences between traditional and experiential learning.

It can be argued that the advent of the 1982 Mental Nursing Syllabus, the shift from training to education, the proposals of Project 2000 aimed at producing a knowledgeable doer and the profession's desire to advocate continuous assessment in clinical practice, can only be truly realised under a climate of change. Central to this climate of change is questioning the hidden values and assumptions about teaching and learning. More importantly, clinical facilitators (supervisors) should realise they cannot teach another person direct but can only encourage and motivate his/her learning. It is, therefore, the facilitators task to create a climate conducive to experiential learning and other problem-solving approaches.

Conclusion

The purpose of this paper has been to emphasise the shift from traditional learning/ teaching methods to experiential means. The EL self directed approach has been questioned by nurses who see it as too radical a shift from the expository teaching methods. Maybe the traditional teacher and the traditional nurse feels more comfortable controlling his/her student and patient. In either case, a real shift to experiential learning and patient centred care can only be realised when the anxiety if not compulsion 'to do for' is replaced by the desire 'to do with'. EL requires 'doing with' and doing with enhances meaningful learning, problem-solving potential, and intrinsic motivation for professional development.

References

1. Ausubel D P (1968) *Educational Psychology: a cognitive view*. Holt, Rinehart, Winston.

2. McEvoy P (1989) 'A new model for learning'. *Senior Nurse*, Vol 9, No 2.

3. Rogers C R (1969) *Freedom to learn*. Merrill, Colombus, Ohio.

4. Burnard P (1989) 'Psychatric nursing students perception of EL'. *Nursing Times*, Jan 14.

5. Lewin K (1948) *Resolving social conflicts: selected papers on group dynamics*. New York: Harper PA 22:4891.

6. Kolb D A, Fry R (1975) 'Towards an applied theory of experiential learning'. In: G L Cooper (ed), *Theories of group processes*. John Wiley and Son, London.

7. Egan G (1986) *The skilled helper*. Brooks/Cole Publishing Co, California.

8. Rogers C R (1951) *Client centered therapy*. Constable and Co Ltd, London.

9. Nelson-Jones R (1982) *The theory and practice of counselling psychology*. Cassell, London.

10. Boydell T (1976) 'Experiental learning'. Manchester Monograph 5, Dept. Adult Education, University of Manchester.

How Adults Learn

Theories of learning are the province of educational psychologists who have long sought the definitive answer as to how and why learning takes place. In a nursing and midwifery education context there is no single theory which provides all the answers to questions relating to learning. We have tried to acknowledge in this section the breadth and diversity of theories which may impact on nurses and midwives learning but, as in other sections, the extracts and articles chosen are merely the tip of a very large iceberg and further reading will be required if you wish to broaden and deepen your knowledge base.

Honey and Mumford (1992) contend that learning is such a fundamental process that many people take it for granted and pay little or no attention to how it actually occurs and the factors which affect it. Facilitators of learning ignore the theoretical basis of the learning process at their peril. They are in danger of assuming that learning occurs automatically and fail to recognise the key role they have to play in influencing the effectiveness of any potential learning experience. There has been an attempt in identifying extracts for this section to choose those which best relate theory to practice so that you can make best use of learning opportunities as they arise within your own practice environment.

McMillan and Dwyer (1990) suggest that facilitators of learning need to ask themselves the basic question: *"Is what I am doing helping the student to learn?"* All too often facilitators, in the words of Honey and Mumford (1990), *"assume that learners are empty buckets to be filled up by the teaching method the facilitator favours"*. The fact that the buckets are different sizes, and/or leak or are upside down is conveniently overlooked. It is essential that facilitators are aware of individual learning styles and the possible impact on the learning process for both the student and themselves. Quinn (1995) stresses that there is little to be gained by a facilitator considering theories of learning in isolation from the individual learner and the context in which he/she is operating.

It is appropriate to review various approaches to learning so that the most suitable is adopted for a given situation. Behavioural, cognitive and humanist perspectives are explored in a number of extracts which highlight their relevance for facilitating in clinical practice. Learning is an innate part of human development but the facilitator has a contribution to play in enabling learners to learn effectively and efficiently through experience.

References

Honey P, Mumford A (1992) *The manual of learning styles*. Peter Honey, Maidenhead.

Quinn F M (1996) *The principles and practice of nurse education*. Chapman and Hall, London.

McMillan M A, Dwyer J (1990) Facilitating a match between teaching and learning styles. *Nurse Education Today*. June. 10(3): 186–192.

6.   Setting the Scene for Learning Styles
Peter Honey and Alan Mumford

Learning is such a fundamental process that many people take it for granted, conveniently assuming that by the time they are adults they have learned how to learn and need no further assistance with the process. Thus lecturers concentrate on lecturing and assume students are skilled at such learning activities as listening, note taking, researching, essay writing and revising. Trainers too often assume that learners are empty buckets waiting to be filled up by the training method the trainer favours. The fact that the buckets are different sizes, and/or leak and/or are upside down is conveniently overlooked.

Yet it is patently clear that people vary not just in their learning skills but also in their learning styles. Why otherwise might two people, matched for age, intelligence and need, exposed to the same learning opportunity react so differently? One person emerges enthusiastic, able to articulate and implement what has been learned. The other claims it was a waste of time and that nothing has been learned. The question we all face is why, with other factors apparently constant, one person learns and the other does not? This Manual aims to show that the reason for the divergence stems from unspoken preferences about how to learn. Perhaps the learning opportunity involved 'having a go' by being pitched in at 'the deep end' with minimal guidance. It so happened that this suited one person's style but not the other who preferred to learn by being given some information and ideas on how to act before 'having a go'.

The term learning styles is used as a description of the attitudes and behaviours which determine an individual's preferred way of learning. Most people are unaware of their learning style preferences. They just know vaguely that they feel more comfortable with, and learn more from, some activities than others. Trainers often realise people learn differently, but may not be sure how and why. In this Manual we show how learning styles can be identified and how this can help both trainer and learner.

The case for helping people to be more effective learners ought to be self evident, yet many trainers still give insufficient recognition to it. It is perhaps **the** most important of **all** the life skills since the way in which people learn affects everything else. We live in the post industrial 'information' age where data have a shorter shelf-life and where transformational changes are less predictable and occur more rapidly than ever before. Clearly learning is the key, not just to surviving but to thriving on all these changes. So this Manual gives help on the crucial issue of learning to learn, thus enabling people to continue to learn long after an event which a trainer has designed.

Peter Honey and Alan Mumford: 'Setting the Scene for Learning Styles' from *THE MANUAL OF LEARNING STYLES* (1989), pp. 1–8. Published by Peter Honey, Ardingly House, 10 Linden Avenue, Maidenhead, Berks SL6 6HB. © 1989 Peter Honey and Alan Mumford.

What is learning?

Learning has happened when people can demonstrate that they know something they didn't know before (insights and realisations as well as facts) and/or when they can do something they couldn't do before (skills). We learn in two substantially different ways. Sometimes we are 'taught' through formal structured activities such as lectures, case studies and books. We also learn from our experiences, often in an unconscious, ill defined way. Learning dedicated to the acquisition of knowledge is both more familiar and more straightforward than experiential learning. It is more familiar not because we necessarily do it more often, but because most people associate the word 'learning' with the acquisition of facts rather more than with the messier process of learning from day to day experiences. As we shall see, learning style preferences have implications for **all** types of learning.

The range of influences on learning

The history of the development of ways to help people learn how to be more effective is relatively short; perhaps fifty years in the UK and a little longer in the USA. One of the constant features in that history has been the discovery of a succession of what were claimed to be uniquely appropriate 'methods'. Lectures were abandoned and replaced by case studies. Books about human relations techniques were replaced by T Groups. Structured training need analyses gave way to individual commitment to self development. The problem of ineffective learning remains, because all these 'solutions' dealt too exclusively with teaching methods and not with differences in individual approaches to learning.

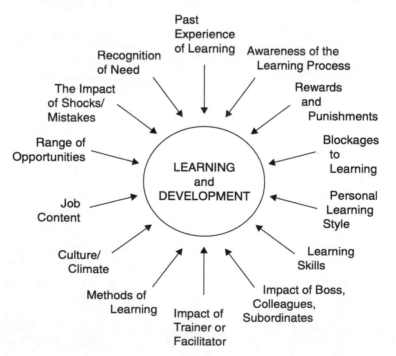

This Manual is about the contribution which can be made to effective learning by an understanding and use of individual styles of learning. We are, however, clear that we are describing one of several major aspects which must be 'right' before effective learning occurs. We are not adding another innovation and claiming that without it nothing useful will be done; we are saying that with attention to individual learning styles, much more effective learning can take place.

In order to emphasise the importance of placing learning styles in the total learning context, it is worth remembering the large number of factors which influence the extent of learning. The following diagram shows just some of the many influences on what is learned or not learned.

This helps to put this Manual into its proper perspective since it can be seen that it focuses on just one of the range of influences; personal learning style. However, the learning cycle and learning styles are particularly important for the trainer because they fall within an area that the trainer can directly influence.

Learning as a continuous process

Learning is a life-long process. It never makes sense to say we have learned all there is to learn or that our learning is complete.

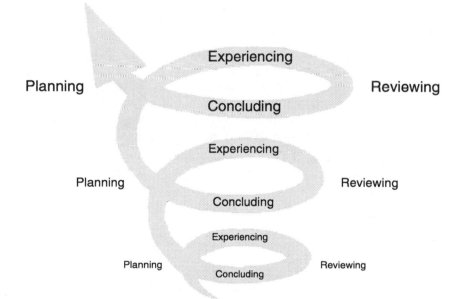

The continuous process is rather like the coils in a spring or, as Professor John Morris has described it, a never-ending spiral. Each coil of the spring or loop in the spiral has four distinct stages on each cycle.

Our description of the stages in the learning cycle originated from the work of David Kolb. Kolb uses different words to describe the stages of the cycle and four learning styles. The similarities between his model and ours are greater than the differences.

However, since we first published the Learning Styles Questionnaire in 1982 many users have found it enjoys a greater face validity with learners mainly because, unlike Kolb, we refrain from asking direct questions about how people learn. We based it instead on what managers and professional people do.

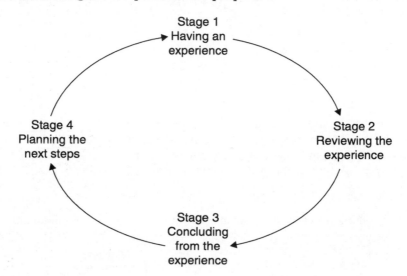

A learner can start anywhere on the cycle because each stage feeds into the next. A person could for example, start at stage 2 by acquiring some information and pondering it before reaching some conclusions, stage 3, and deciding how to apply it, stage 4. On the other hand someone could start at stage 4 with a technique that they plan to incorporate into their *modus operandi*. Using the technique would then be at stage 1 in the cycle before reviewing how it worked out, stage 2, reaching conclusions stage 3, and modifying the technique in the light of the experience, stage 4.

This continuous, iterative process is so fundamental that it underpins many other approaches. The scientific method is one example. Many problem solving/decision making processes also map onto the stages in the learning cycle as do the methods of continuous improvement in Total Quality Management.

Ways of distorting the learning cycle

The four stages, experiencing, reviewing, concluding and planning are mutually supportive. None is fully effective as a learning procedure on its own. Each stage plays an equally important part in the total process (though the time spent on each may vary considerably).

Most people, however, develop preferences which give them a liking for certain stages over others. The preferences lead to a distortion of the learning process so that greater emphasis is placed on some stages to the detriment of others. Here are some typical examples:

- Preferences for experiencing such that people develop an addiction for activities to the extent that they cannot sit still but have to be rushing around constantly on the go. This results in plenty of experiences and the assumption that having experiences is synonymous with learning from them.

- Preferences for reviewing such that people shy away from first hand experiences and postpone reaching conclusions for as long as possible whilst more data are gathered. This results in an 'analysis to paralysis' tendency with plenty of pondering but little action.

- Preferences for concluding such that people have a compulsion to reach an answer quickly. This results in a tendency to jump to conclusions by circumventing the review stage, where uncertainty and ambiguity are higher. Conclusions, even if they are the wrong ones, are comforting things to have.

- Preferences for seizing on an expedient course of action and implementing it with inadequate analysis. This results in a tendency to go for 'quick fixes' by overemphasising the planning and experiencing stages to the detriment of reviewing and concluding.

Learning styles

Learning styles are the key to understanding these different preferences. Learning styles, in common with any other style, have in themselves been learned as people repeated strategies and tactics that were found to be successful and discontinued those that were not. In this way preferences for certain behaviour patterns develop and become habitual. These styles tend to be strengthened as people gravitate towards careers that are compatible with their preferred *modus operandi*.

Here are paragraphs describing four learning styles.

Activists

Activists involve themselves fully and without bias in new experiences. They enjoy the here and now and are happy to be dominated by immediate experiences. They are open-minded, not sceptical, and this tends to make them enthusiastic about anything new. Their philosophy is: *"I'll try anything once"*. They tend to act first and consider the consequences afterwards. Their days are filled with activity. They tackle problems by brainstorming. As soon as the excitement from one activity has died down they are busy looking for the next. They tend to thrive on the challenge of new experiences but are bored with implementation and longer term consolidation. They are gregarious people constantly involving themselves with others but, in doing so, they seek to centre all activities around themselves.

Reflectors

Reflectors like to stand back to ponder experiences and observe them from many different perspectives. They collect data, both first hand and from others, and prefer to think about it thoroughly before coming to any conclusion. The thorough collection and analysis of data about experiences and events is what counts so they tend to postpone reaching definitive conclusions for as long as possible. Their philosophy is to be cautious. They are thoughtful people who like to consider all possible angles and implications before making a move. They prefer to take a back seat in meetings and discussions. They enjoy observing other people in action. They listen to others and get the drift of the discussion before making their own points. They tend to adopt a low profile and have a slightly distant, tolerant, unruffled air about them. When they act it is part of a wide picture which includes the past as well as the present and others' observations as well as their own.

Theorists

Theorists adapt and integrate observations into complex but logically sound theories. They think problems through in a vertical, step by step, logical way. They assimilate disparate facts into coherent theories. They tend to be perfectionists who won't rest easy until things are tidy and fit into a rational scheme. They like to analyse and synthesise. They are keen on basic assumptions, principles, theories, models and systems thinking. Their philosophy prizes rationality and logic. *"If it's logical it's good"*. Questions they frequently ask are: *"Does it make sense?" "How does this fit with that?" "What are the basic assumptions?"* They tend to be detached, analytical and dedicated to rational objectivity rather than anything subjective or ambiguous. Their approach to problems is consistently logical. This is their 'mental set' and they rigidly reject anything that doesn't fit with it. They prefer to maximise certainty and feel uncomfortable with subjective judgements, lateral thinking and anything flippant.

Pragmatists

Pragmatists are keen on trying out ideas, theories and techniques to see if they work in practice. They positively search out new ideas and take the first opportunity to experiment with applications. They are the sort of people who return from management courses brimming with new ideas that they want to try out in practice. They like to get on with things and act quickly and confidently on ideas that attract them. They tend to be impatient with ruminating and open-ended discussions. They are essentially practical, down to earth people who like making practical decisions and solving problems. They respond to problems and opportunities 'as a challenge'. Their philosophy is: *"There is always a better way"* and *"If it works it's good"*.

Each style 'connects' with a stage on the continuous learning cycle. People with Activist preferences, with their 'I'll try anything once' approach, are well equipped for Experiencing. People with Reflector preferences, with their predilection for mulling over data, are well equipped for Reviewing. People with Theorist preferences, with their need to tidy up and have 'answers', are well equipped for Concluding. Finally, people with Pragmatist preferences, with their liking for things practical, are well equipped for Planning. The diagram below shows the learning styles positioned around the learning cycle.

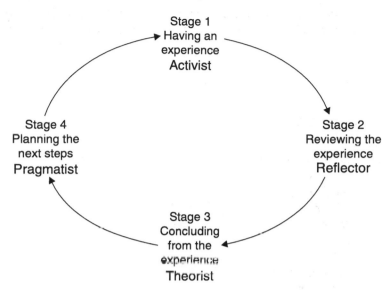

This Manual

This Manual, the third edition, is again practical rather than theoretical. After ten years' experience by ourselves and others, it shows that learning activities can be designed to encompass the full cycle. We can also confirm that people are helped to be more effective learners if they are aware of their learning style preferences. The questionnaire results provide a starting point, not a finishing point because knowledge of learning styles is only useful if it is applied rather than merely recorded. [In the chapters that follow] we describe how this can be done. The most significant uses explored in this Manual are:

*   Increased awareness of learning activities which are congruent or incongruent with a person's dominant style(s).

*   A better choice by trainers and learners of those activities, leading to more effective and more economical learning provision. Avoidance of inappropriate learning experience is both good in itself and less likely to lead to the Shakespeare effect, where inappropriate early experiences put young people off for life.

*   An identification of ways in which a person's less effective learning processes and skills can be improved.

*   Advice on how the different learning styles of trainers, learners, bosses and subordinates influence the way they help others to learn.

This edition of the Manual improves on earlier editions in a variety of ways amongst them being:

*   Fuller descriptions of how to introduce, administer, score and interpret the Learning Styles Questionnaire.

- Expanded examples of how to use learning styles to design programmes and learning to learn sessions.

- More 'norms' for additional occupational groups and updated norms calculated from a data base which has expanded over a ten year period.

- A more comprehensive bibliography of books, articles and papers on learning styles.

Reference

Kolb D (1984) *Experiential Learning: Experience as a Source of Learning and Development.* Prentice Hall, New Jersey.

7. Facilitating a Match between Teaching and Learning Styles

Margaret A. McMillan and Jeanette Dwyer

As a result of educator/student interactions within a particular course, both parties anticipate that some learning will occur, some change in behaviour will have taken place and some personal growth will be evident. In order to facilitate such change every educator ought to reflect on personal practice and ask 'Is what I am doing helping the student to learn?' The answer to this question firstly should come from the student and secondly should further prompt the educator to ask 'Do I need to change my style of teaching to match the learning needs of these students?'

In searching for an answer to these questions it is suggested that the teacher would need to reflect on just what constitutes teaching and learning styles. Then one might need to investigate the possibility of matching teaching style with the students' learning styles.

This paper looks at the perceived need to identify different approaches to learning and the potential for matching teaching and learning styles. It is suggested that a facilitative approach to teaching, such as that used at Macarthur Institute of Higher Education in Australia, will accommodate students' learning needs.

Introduction

Particular approaches to teaching and learning are frequently advocated in curriculum documents. For example problem based learning (PBL) methodology is applied to the nursing curriculum used at Macarthur Institute of Higher Education (MIHE), which is located in the south west of Sydney in New South Wales (NSW) Australia. There is an assumption by proponents of particular teaching/learning strategies that exposure to course content, delivered to students in a particular way, will cause the student to learn. Whether or not this is so is dependent on a number of factors. One needs to consider the validity of the course aims and objectives, the individual characteristics of the students, the context of learning and the personality and needs of the educators themselves. The possibility of matching teaching and learning styles is complex in reality and begs the question, 'Is there any value in attempting a match between styles of teaching and learning?' The answer is possibly not; the issue is really one of recognising the need to challenge the students to identify and find answers to their own learning difficulties. Then the educator needs to capitalise on the student's greater personal responsibility for learning by continually monitoring student progress and guiding the student through the process of learning. Brookfield (1989) suggests that 'anchors' can then be put down when the expanse of the unknown warrants deeper investigation. The teaching style should be facilitative, encompassing a variety

Margaret A. McMillan and Jeanette Dwyer: 'Facilitating a Match between Teaching and Learning Styles' in *NURSE EDUCATION TODAY* (1990), 10, pp. 186–192. Reprinted by permission of the publisher Churchill Livingstone.

of strategies through which the facilitator can be sufficiently flexible in response to perceived student needs.

The teaching/learning environment

To look at the learning environment one should begin with the key players, that is the teacher and the student, and then look at the educational climate and the style or approach of the players to the task at hand, that is, learning. Partridge (1983) discusses teaching and learning styles and suggests that the advantage of matching the two is obvious given that the interaction between teacher and learner will be more comfortable and that learning will probably occur more 'efficiently and effectively'. He suggests however that in order to match teaching and learning styles, four factors should be considered, the:

1. developmental level of the learner

2. subject matter to be learned

3. surrounding context and

4. goals of education.

Focusing more on the mature age learner, Lindeman (1926; in Knowles, 1984) discussed learning styles in terms of key assumptions concerning the adult. These assumptions relate to the motivation arising from relevant and interesting experiences that meet perceived personal needs, a life centred orientation to learning and a need for self direction. Also warranting consideration is the notion that individual differences increase with age and provision must therefore be made for differences in style, time, place, and pace of learning.

It becomes readily apparent that achieving a match between teaching and learning styles is complex. However the summary of learning style research provided by Dunn *et al* (1981) suggests that learning styles within an individual are not permanently fixed and can therefore be affected by a teaching style. Given the many potential differences in learning, it can be seen that matching or mismatching styles in teaching can have definite effects on the learner. This point of view is supported by Witkin (1978) who writes:

> 'It is easy to see that a teachers' cognitive style can influence his way of teaching, that a students' cognitive style may influence his way of learning and that a match or mismatching of cognitive style between teacher and student may determine how well they get along, with important consequences for the learning process.'

The chicken or the egg

It is difficult to determine whether teachers adapt to students' learning needs or students' respond to teacher implied strategies for learning through the use of specific instructional techniques. Teaching styles can greatly advantage or disadvantage the extent of learning given the power of either the more didactic styles or those where students themselves identify and pursue personal learning goals. A report on surveys related to student learning difficulties (File, 1984) considers teacher-student interaction and notes:

> '. . . the link that is made between learning difficulties and teaching practice is evident in both the way in which students conceptualize difficulties and perhaps more importantly in the remedies that they suggest.'

It is in relation to students' ideas on personal learning difficulties that Brookfield (1989) sounds a cautionary note. When discussing research on student learning he notes that much of the research on adult student learning is based on the *teachers'* perception of learning rather than reports of the *students'* experiences. This leaves a wealth of evidence regarding potential match/mismatch untapped and has important implications for the teacher-students relationship.

Baird (1973) considers student perceptions of teacher behaviour to have a distinct effect on the student. This view is supported by Ramsden (1979; cited in Entwistle, 1981) who found that:

> '. . . students adapt their learning strategies to the perceived demands of lecturers and departments.'

Hence students who perceive that their learning difficulties arise from poor teaching techniques suggest remedial strategies for the teacher rather than acknowledging inadequacies within themselves in coping with the tertiary environment. It is therefore possible that the necessity for teachers and learners to recognise that learning difficulties rather than learning styles ought to be the focus of attention when considering learning outcomes. This argument appears to be supported by Anderson and Bruce (1979) who comment that:

> '. . . improvement in education results as educators consciously examine the needs of students and determine appropriate instructional treatment with specific objectives.'

The potential for matchmaking

Factors to be considered in any attempt to match teaching and learning styles are economic, feasibility, resource availability and class size. Obviously, the larger the class, the more difficult it would be to match styles of teaching with the potential variety in the learning styles. Dixon (1985) suggests that:

> '. . . what would seem on the surface to be a simple one to one correspondence between a learner's style and an appropriate instructional methodology is in reality very complex.'

Dixon notes that an individual may actually have more than one preferred learning style which may even vary from subject to subject. Should it be possible to reduce class size, the other factors come into play. Is it economically feasible to have a larger number of classes with fewer students in each so that the teaching/learning style can more readily be matched? The answer is more likely to be yes if:

1. the budget allows this to occur

2. sufficient teachers are available

3. classroom space is available

4. literary resources are simple

5. timetabling of teachers, students, rooms and equipment does not overlap.

Brookfield (1989) further highlights the complexity of achieving a match between the two. He notes that one needs to consider the nature of the task at hand, the political ethos, prior experience of both student and education, the personality of the teacher and the needs of all individuals in a group. These factors coincide with those cited by Partridge (1988), that is goals, subject matter, content and the developmental levels of the learners.

The identification of student learning styles

If it is held that matching teaching and learning styles will, given the complexity of the task, result in a positive learning outcome, one needs to consider whether specific learning styles of students can be identified and how the information will subsequently be used. Dixon (1985) suggests the use of learning style instruments that have already been developed. She then proposed that:

> '. . . the learner be responsible for using the learning styles information
> and that the instructor assume responsibility for creating an environment
> in which the resulting diversity can be accommodated.'

In this way, students become aware of the diversity in learning styles among individuals and more aware of their own style(s) of learning. Dixon (1985) does point out however that such activities can have negative effects on the student. If numerical ratings are used, it is possible for students to devalue their learning ability or be categorised by staff peers or even themselves into one specific learning style, again limiting the cognitive development associated with learning.

Brookfield (1989) is sceptical about the oversimplification which can occur when one attempts to recognise appropriate learning styles. He suggests that learners do not always know best. Teachers therefore should concentrate on providing students with a benchmark against which learning can be measured. It would seem then that staff/teachers should retain the responsibility for adapting their teaching style to students' learning style. However student awareness of the diversity in approaches to teaching and learning can only enhance the interaction between the student and teacher.

The Macarthur Nursing Program

Macarthur offers several nursing programs each of which uses PBL methodology in curriculum implementation. One of these courses is the pre-service Diploma of Applied Science (Nursing) (DAS(N)). This course attracts a student population of which 50% are categorised as of mature age and 50% are of non Anglo-Saxon origin. The majority of students are drawn from an area in the south west of Sydney which is considered to be socially and educationally disadvantaged, particularly in relation to availability of health and education resources.

These people may have a minimal exposure to formal education, may be intimidated by entry to tertiary education and may be coming to terms with English as a second language. Some may have experienced what they personally describe as a sense of failure in facets of their daily lives, including education achievement. The situation for many students is that there is a need for change; a need for personal growth. Their entry to tertiary education however may initially cause them to feel even more uneasy about their recent decision to pursue higher education. The philosophy of this School of Nursing suggests that the problem based learning (PBL) strategy used in the implementation of the program would appear to be well suited to accommodate the needs of adult learners from such diverse backgrounds. Ryan (1987) sees problem based learning as a:

> '. . . distinctly student-centred mode of learning . . . while on the one hand considerable freedom is given to the students to pursue self-directed learning, on the other hand considerable contact with faculty is maintained . . . guiding and challenging their linking by way of carefully worded questioning.'

It appears that age and developmental level are crucial factors when discussing the adult learning environment such as that at Macarthur (Lindeman, 1926; Dunn *et al.* 1989; Knowles, 1984; Brookfield, 1989). If motivation relates to satisfying learning needs and interest then the extent of motivation to learn will depend on the ability of the adult to identify their personal learning needs. Experience is seen as the 'richest' resource of learning, but the availability of life situations appropriate to subject matter to be learned may vary greatly with the adult age continuum. Whilst recognising that adults have a deep need to have a capacity for self-directedness, learning cannot be assumed in either the younger or the older adult. Consideration of the factors needed for adult learning strategies are pertinent when one considers the population from which Macarthur nursing students are drawn. By capitalising on the perceived need to learn and the richness of personal experiences shared within a group, one can turn previously considered negative experiences into positive ones. The difference in ages can also be accommodated by the use of small groups of individuals working together. MIHE Nursing Course Assessment document (1988) states that the self directed approach to study used in PBL not only increases the students' confidence in their own academic ability but also their capacity to learn in 'novel' situations. There is an acceptance by advocates of PBL for the need to self-evaluate and engage in the process of lifelong learning.

The same emphasis in PBL on development of self-directedness, the capacity to learn in novel situations, the need to continually self evaluate and to have a commitment to ongoing learning is important in preparing a professional nurse for practice in a dynamic work environment.

Facilitation versus teaching

Fischer and Fischer (1979, quoted in Conti 1985) define teaching style as:

> '. . . distinctive qualities of behaviours that are consistent through time and carry out from situation to situation . . . style thus refers to a

persuasive quality of teaching behaviour that persists even though the content that is being taught may change.'

The distinctive style advocated by the Macarthur Nursing Program is that of facilitator. An MIHE document (1989) describes facilitation as:

'. . . a balance between confrontation and support in which students assume a major responsibility for their own learning and the tutor's role is to debate, challenge, question, probe, encourage, guide, negotiate and mediate in an environment of mutual trust and cooperation.'

It goes on to report that:

'. . . the facilitative process is effective in both the classroom and clinical nursing setting and is used in both simulated and actual situations.'

The success in matching teaching styles with individual adult learning styles will depend on the teacher's ability to perform as *facilitator* of learning and the student's readiness to engage in an enquiry oriented interaction with the teachers and accept challenges to already well developed patterns of thinking, the result of a lifetime of experience. Should these aspects of the learning situation exist the availability of resource options, including the teacher, can only be seen as advantageous to the learner. By allowing for maximum learning opportunities at a pace suitable to the learner, one can as Brookfield (1986) suggests:

'. . . help them to realize that the bodies of knowledge accepted truths, commonly held values and customary behaviours comprising their world are contextual and culturally constructed.'

Disadvantages arise when the teacher lacks abilities or skills in facilitation and/or the student is not ready to participate in a self-directed learning mode. One cannot assume that students will automatically become self-directed in their learning. If staff are to encourage and guide students in a particular direction there is an obvious need for staff to take the initiative in student guidance. This means there is an implicit inequality in student/staff relationships, an inequality which is a reflection of the real world. The facilitator however should work on creating a learning environment in which collaboration or collegiality is encouraged. Most importantly the facilitator has to be seen as authentic, having a sound knowledge base and an interest in meeting the student's needs.

It is suggested that the facilitator's role, one of resource person, enhances the likelihood of a match between expectations of the students and the facilitator as there is an acceptance of co-learning in areas of knowledge deficit.

We would argue that students can be introduced to a style of learning that is compatible in broad terms with the teaching style. If the style of teaching is such that it allows for a range of individual learning styles, the student may have sufficient latitude in selecting a learning style suitable to his or her individual preferences.

Feasibility of PBL

Mennin and Martinez-Burrola (in Kaufman, 1985) look at the evaluation at programs using PBL. This study compares the cost of operating a problem-based program with those associated with the more traditional. It was found that:

> '. . . faculty time devoted to PBL was no greater than that devoted to conventional education.'

This finding together with the Macarthur experience in program implementation would seem to address some of the arguments and complexities of applying appropriate instructional methodology to the task of meeting students' needs. Macarthur proposes that it is possible to reduce class sizes for those new students who need more guidance and structure whilst at the same time cater for the greater capacity for self direction of the more senior students. Careful timetabling can also ensure that no overlap occurs in relation to the demands placed on facilitators, students and resources such as classroom space. The demands on resources are not markedly different from those of a traditional program. The same budgetary constraints apply no matter what the methodology.

Staff employed within the School of Nursing at Macarthur come from a variety of backgrounds. Some have limited knowledge of the facilitative skills that are advocated with the problem based teaching/learning strategy. As discussed previously the student body has a large number of mature age students but ranges from the young adult, straight from high school and probably accustomed to a very teacher-centred or high structured learning situation, to those older adults who may or may not have a limited formal education.

Therefore, the extent of student self-directed learning skills will vary. Perceived student deficiencies in learning skills are dealt with in first year when basic enquiry and processing skills are developed. Staff needs for the required teaching methodology are met through staff development sessions.

Although such strategies do not entirely eliminate the potential for mismatch in teaching and learning styles the likelihood of staff/students' needs is enhanced.

Conclusion

There is much support for matching teaching and learning styles where optimum efficiency and effectiveness in learning are issues. While there are undoubted advantages, such a pursuit would not only be resource intensive but would also impose budgetary constraints and still may not achieve learning goals. A compromise may exist in a teaching style that allows some degree of freedom in adaptation to individual needs. The responsibility for learning lies with the students. The teacher, being responsible for setting a benchmark for growth, monitoring progress and intervening at the appropriate time.

Matching of teaching and learning styles may have some undesirable effects in that it might leave the learner poorly equipped to adapt with different teaching styles that could be encountered in the future. There is also the potential to mask learning difficulties. The successful matching of styles requires that adequate methods to determine specific learning preferences in students are available and that teachers have the ability to adapt their approach in response to individual student needs. Educators must be prepared to be flexible and to continually review their own practice.

The adoption of a facilitative style of teaching and encouraging student self-directedness in learning, appears to allow for individual differences in learning for a varying age group. The student can develop skills of conceptualisation allowing for a transfer of knowledge to novel situations and gain a sense of academic achievement. Consideration must be given to any weakness in approach to learning within the individual student, by working with the student to identify personal problems and potential solutions.

The nature of the Macarthur nursing program using PBL would appear to address the development of enquiry (problem solving) skills which not only apply to problem-solving in the nursing context but also in relation to their everyday experiences which in turn encompasses approaches to study commitments.

References

Andersen W R, Bruce S W. A plan for matching learning and teaching, student learning styles: diagnosing and prescribing programs. V A National Association of Secondary School Principles, Reston.

Baird L L (1973) Teaching styles: an exploratory study of dimensions and effects. *Journal of Education Psychology* 64, 1: 15–21.

Brookfield S D (1986) *Understanding and facilitating adult learning.* Jossey Bass, London.

Brookfield S D and Brundage D (1989) Current thinking on adult learning: implications for higher and continuing education. Tertiary Education Research Centre Seminar, University of New South Wales, Sydney, Australia.

Conti G J (1985) The relationship between teaching style and adult student learning. *Adult Education Quarterly* 35, 4: 220–228.

Dixon N M (1985) The implementation of learning style information. *Lifelong Learning*, Vol I, March, 16–27.

Dunn R. *et al* (1981) Learning style researchers define differences differently. *Education Leadership* 38. 5: 372–375.

Dunn R S, Dunn K J (1979) Learning styles/teaching styles: should they . . . can they . . . be matched? *Educational Leadership* 36, 4: 238–244.

Entwistle N (1981) *Styles of learning and teaching.* John Wiley and Sons, New York.

File J (1984) Student learning difficulties and teaching methods. *Studies in Higher Education* 9.2: 191–194.

Kaufman A (1985) (ed) *Implementing PBL: lessons from successful innovations.* Springer, New York.

Knowles M (1984) *The adult learner: a neglected species.* Gulf Publishing Co, London.

Macarthur Institute of Higher Education (1988) School of Nursing and Health Studies, Bachelor of Applied Science (Nursing) Course Assessment Documentation to the New South Wales Higher Education Board. Sydney, Australia.

Partridge R (1983) Learning styles: review of selected models. *Journal of Nursing Education* 22, 6: 243–248.

Ryan C (1987) Individual differences and problem solving ability. Unpublished Masters thesis, Faculty of Education, University of Sydney, New South Wales, Australia.

Schipper L. Innovative teaching. *Improving College and University Teaching* 32: 1 54–57.

Stone D R, Neilsen E C (1982) *Educational Psychology: the development of teaching skills*. Harper and Row, New York.

Macarthur Institute of Higher Education (1989) Diploma of Applied Science (Nursing) Review. Sydney, Australia.

Witkin H A (1978) *Cognitive style in academic performance and in teacher-student relations in individual learning*. Jossey Bass, San Francisco.

8. An Investigation into whether Nurse Teachers take into Account the Individual Learning Styles of their Students when Formulating Teaching Strategies

Caroline M. Dux

Many factors have an effect on ways students learn, but differences in learning styles may not be reflected in the way they are taught. A small study of the learning styles of 119 students and 13 nurse teachers was carried out as part of a Certificate of Education Course. In addition a short questionnaire was used to determine teachers preferred teaching styles.

The data collected demonstrated that the groups sampled did not express a very strong preference for any one learning style, but for a combination of styles as did the teachers sampled.

The author concludes that nurse teachers should examine more closely the reasons why they favour one strategy over another. This in turn should make learning more challenging and rewarding for the students and teachers.

Introduction

From both the theoretical and practical experiences of education and teaching encountered during a Certificate of Education Course I became increasingly interested in the different factors which are related to how and when student nurses learn. I felt it would be useful to examine the individual learning style of students and teachers in one College of Nurse Education, and to discover if these are similar, and whether there is a relationship between learning styles of students and teaching methods used.

The concept of learning styles in education is significant, because of its relevance to factors which determine individuals' preferred ways of coping with problem solving situations, and hence learning. As Child states:

> 'The style of the learner is only part of the story — Another important part is the style of the teacher and the impact this has upon the learners' performance.' (Child, 1986)

In the following 'students' are student nurses and 'teachers' are nurse teachers.

Caroline M. Dux: 'An Investigation into whether Nurse Teachers take into Account the Individual Learning Styles of their Students when Formulating Teaching Strategies' in *NURSE EDUCATION TODAY* (1989), 9, pp. 186–191. Reprinted by permission of the publisher Churchill Livingstone.

Learning styles

There are a number of factors which contribute to how an individual benefits from a particular learning experience. These include teaching styles, teaching methods, motivation, attention, previous education, and sociological factors, as well as individual learning styles. In a learning situation, involving two students who have equal educational and sociological backgrounds, one student may seem to learn from the situation, and the other not. Research by Joyce and Hudson (1968) involving medical students showed that the best examination results were achieved when teachers and students had similar learning styles. Lovell (1986) suggests that when students encounter a learning situation that suits their learning style, they are more likely to learn from it, than if these are ignored.

By the time students enter nursing, they each have different interests, skills, abilities, knowledge, experiences, attitudes and motivation; each will learn different things, at different paces, in different settings, and with a different sense of involvement. These factors will affect learning styles, as will their personality and intelligence. It is important therefore for nurse teachers to be aware of and respond to the individual needs of the students, including their preferred learning styles. The emphasis is, increasingly on a problem solving approach to learning, to complement the nursing process approach used in the clinical environment. As not all students have learning styles which would benefit from this approach, there is a need to examine individual learning styles.

Honey and Mumford (1982) said that

> 'with attention to individual learning styles, much more effective learning can take place.'

The research by Hudson (1968) and Parlett (1969) is particularly relevant to contemporary nurse education. They describe a trend towards student-centred progressive learning, as opposed to a more traditional teacher-centre approach in which the teacher is seen as a facilitator. Although the individual learning styles of the students need to be identified, this approach could reduce the conflict which tends to occur between what is taught in the 'School' and the reality of what happens on the ward. Unfortunately, in most Schools of Nursing, due to shortages of teaching staff, traditional attitudes and the constraints placed by the curriculum and time table, teachers are either unable or unwilling to adapt their teaching.

However nurse education is gradually moving away from a more traditional to a more progressive philosophy, in which theoretical input is correlated more closely with a practical application, both in the classroom and the clinical situation. Hopefully, this approach will displace the traditional teaching style where the imparting of knowledge didactically is seen as teaching, whether or not the students can apply the material in the written or clinical situation. It might also help reduce the wastage rates of students during training — in 1987, 500 students left training each month in England (Rogers, 1987). In America, a survey in 1987 showed that in one New York hospital alone, decreasing applicants to nursing and increasing numbers leaving had led to a 13.6% vacancy rate, compared to 6.3% the previous year (Moccia, 1987).

To help meet the needs of the students and to enable them to benefit from this changing philosophy, their needs and those of their teachers should be identified. In this way teachers learn to meet the new demands made on them through adapting traditional formal teaching strategies to more progressive ones. Nurse teachers learning styles could then be related to those of their students to achieve improved learning.

The study

The Learning Styles Questionnaire (LSQ) used in this study was developed by Honey and Mumford (Honey & Mumford, 1982). They based their LSQ on the Learning Style Inventory developed by Kolb (Kolb, 1979).

The study was a small one involving 119 students and 13 teachers in one College of Nursing Education (the main limitation to the study being one of time).

The study was designed to discover whether teachers use methods which typically benefited those students with certain learning styles only, and whether these teaching methods reflect the teacher's own personal learning styles and/or those of the students. It was also hoped to see whether learning styles of students change during their training.

To discover the preferred learning styles, the Honey and Mumford Learning Styles Questionnaire (LSQ) was used (Honey & Mumford, 1982). To determine the preferred teaching methods of the teachers, a simple short additional questionnaire was devised and attached to each LSQ given to teachers. The supplementary questionnaire being re-designed following a pilot study, and was kept short to help increase response rates.

The 80 items on the LSQ are mostly couched in behavioural terms and describe an action that the individual might or might not take. The LSQ gives general trends to learning styles and attributes four items to the learning styles demonstrated by the answers to the LSQ:

Activist: Enjoy the here and now, dominated by immediate experiences, tend to revel in the short term crisis.

Reflectors: Like to stand back and ponder on experience and observe them from different perspectives. They collect data and analyse it before coming to any conclusion.

Theorists: Are keen on basic assumptions, principles, theories, models and systems thinking. They prize rationality and logic.

Pragmatists: Positively search out new ideas and take the first opportunity to experiment.

During the actual study, each group of students entering the College of Nurse Education over a 2-month period was personally approached. The aim of the study was explained and their co-operation requested; confidentiality being assured. This personal approach appears to have had a beneficial effect on the response rates.

119 LSQs were given to students, 110 returned = 92% Response Rate.

13 LSQs were given to teachers, 11 returned = 85% Response Rate.

A cross section of all available students was sampled, and at least one set from each year was represented in the study, including one post basic group.

Results

The data collected was compared for analysis to the general norms of the Manual of Learning Styles (Honey & Mumford, 1982). Analysis of the data showed that one style did not always predominate, but that those sampled exhibited a combination of styles, one of which may have been more prominent than others. Those profiles showing moderate or strong preferences for all four styles indicated that the person was said to be an all rounder, adaptable to new and different learning situations, and would as such benefit from new learning experiences (Honey & Mumford, 1982). Those profiles which showed low preferences in all four styles, indicated that the person was either too selective in answering the LSQ or had a low interest in learning.

The more junior students appeared not to have formed definite preferred learning styles and exhibited a preference for many single or combinations of styles. This could indicate that they would be more responsive to different methods of teaching and learning experiences than the student that indicates a very definite preference for one style.

This apparent feature, if proved significant using a much larger sample, could be used to help plan learning strategies for junior students and for sessions on learning skills.

Figures 1 and 2 show the percentage of those demonstrating very strong/strong preferences for each style. Of the 10 groups 70 have a preference for the activist style of learning, either on its own or in conjunction with one or more styles (Figure 1). The group showing the lowest preference for the activist style are the post basic learners and the ENB Intensive Care Course 100, who, through the nature of their work, need to be able to respond appropriately in any given situation. This group did however demonstrate a very strong/strong preference for the reflector mode of learning (Figure 1). This, when the nature of their work is considered, is a surprising finding, and one which should be tested in a larger study. It could perhaps have been predicted that the group would have been predominently theorists. Figure 2 showed that the pragmatist style was the one least preferred, which correlates well with the use of experiential methods, which seem to be less popular with students.

The data collected appears to show a general preference by students for activist and reflector styles of learning, which may be appropriate to the learning/work involved in nursing.

Figures 1 and 2 show that the sample groups did not exhibit any definite trends in increased/decreased preferences for any one learning style during their training. The learning styles of the teachers are more evenly balanced between the four styles than is seen amongst the students. In general, the learning styles of the teachers are similar to those of the students.

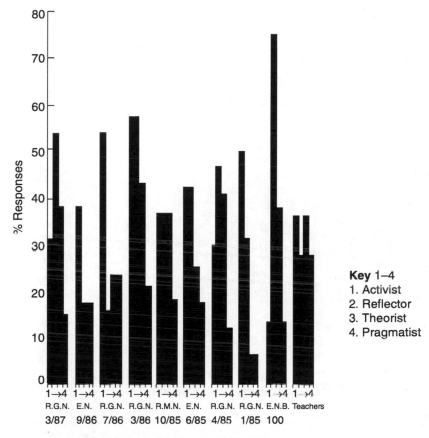

Figure 1   Preferences for different learning styles

An attempt was made to review preferred teaching methods in the light of the students' learning styles. During informal discussions with teachers, many admitted to planning sessions using an 'Ideal' method, usually involving more inductive techniques. In practice they had to use more traditional and less progressive methods. Resistance to change by the students was given as an explanation as well as the constraints of the timetable. During these discussions the teachers interviewed rarely gave any indication that they considered the needs of their students with regard to their preferred learning styles, when planning teaching strategies.

The supplementary questionnaire was designed to attempt to discover if these informal impressions could be supported by statistical evidence.

Table 1 shows the preferred teaching methods for the RGN and EN groups according to the order of preference as indicated by the teachers. One surprising finding was the comparability between the items listed in the top part of each list, which had not been anticipated.

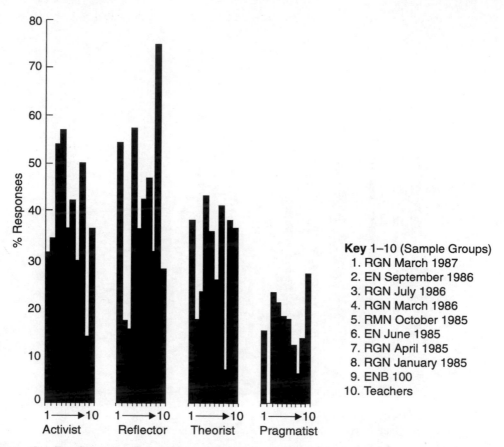

Figure 2   Preferences for different learning styles, by groups

The results showed that, despite an impression obtained during the informal discussions that only a few methods were used, a wide range of teaching strategies were being used.

The author stated before that nurse education is moving away from the traditional model to a more progressive one. These findings however, suggest the need for teachers, to be committed to this not only in theory but also in practice.

The learning styles of the groups sampled demonstrated a wide range and combination of preferred learning styles, but with no overall very prominent learning style. The apparent preference by the teachers for using self directed teaching methods, verbal exposition with question and answer sessions and group work, appears to relate well, not only to the learning styles of the teachers, but also the students. The latter relates well to the activist and reflector styles of learning.

Perhaps one surprising finding from Table 1 was the popularity of the lecture method. It had been anticipated from the LSQ responses and from the general trend towards progressive methods using less didactic teaching methods that lectures would be less frequently used.

Table 1 **Preferred teaching methods for the RGN and EN groups, according to the order of preference given by the teacher**

RGNs		ENs	
1	Self Directed learning, including worksheets	1	Self Directed
2	Verbal Exposition (± Questions)	2	Group Work
3	Controlled Discussion	3	Verbal Exposition (± Questions)
4	Question and Answer	4	Question and Answer
5	Group Work	5	Role Play
6	Role Play	6	Controlled Discussions
7	Buzz Groups	7	Buzz Groups
8	Lectures	8	Lectures
9	Simulation	9	Free Discussion
10	Free Discussion	10	Simulation
11	Games	11	Games
12	Audio Visual Aids	12	Problem Solving
13	Workshops	13	Audio Visual Aids
14	Demonstrating		
15	Case Discussion		
16	Problem Solving		
17	Experiential		
18	Hands On		

Conclusion

In conclusion, the data showed that the groups sampled did not show a very strong preference for one learning style, but rather for a combination of styles, as did those teachers sampled. The findings from the supplementary questionnaire indicated the need to examine further and in more depth, the reasons why teachers really choose one method rather than another, and when and if they adapt these.

One way to help reduce the wastage rates in nursing would be for teaching and education to meet the individual needs of each student, as well as the objectives of the course. Students and teachers might find the learning process more challenging and rewarding if this approach were adopted, and teaching to occur using an appropriate method, and not one that is used just because it has always been used for that purpose.

If it is accepted that teaching methodology should reflect a groups' learning styles, then if one group were shown to have strong preferences for activist and reflector styles, then teachers should perhaps adapt their strategies appropriately.

References

Child D (1986) *Psychology and the teacher*, 4th edn. Holt, Rinehart & Winston, London.

Honey P, Mumford A (1982) *The manual of learning styles*. Honey, Maidenhead.

Hudson L (1968) *Frames of mind*, 1st edn. Methuen, London.

Hudson L (1970) *The ecology of human intelligence*. Penguin, Harmondsworth.

Joyce C R B, Hudson L (1968) Student style and teaching styles — an experimental study. *British Journal of Medical Education* 2: 28–32.

Kolb D A *et al (1979) Organisational psychology — an experiential approach*, 3rd edn. Prentice Hall, London.

Lovell R B (1986) *Adult learning*, 4th edn. Croom Helm, Beckenham.

Moccia P (1987) The nature of the nursing shortage — will crisis become structure? *Nursing and Health Care* 8, 6: 321–322.

Parlett M R (1969) The syllabus-bound student. In: L Hudson *The Ecology of Human Intelligence*. Penguin, Harmondsworth.

Rogers R (1987) Nurses flee the profession. *Health Service Journal* 97, 16: 441.

Rosenfeld P (1987) Nursing education in crisis — a look at recruitment and retention. *Nursing and Health Care* 8, 5: 283–286.

9. Learning Theories Made Easy: Behaviourism

Gilean McKenna

The last few years have witnessed many developments in nurse education, particularly as links with higher education are strengthened. The clinical environment, however, remains a key area for learning, and practitioners continue to make a huge contribution to the education of both pre- and post-registration students. In order to maximise opportunities, a knowledge of learning theories is useful. This is the first of three articles explaining the different theories of learning. This week the behaviourist theories are described. The following weeks will discuss cognitive and humanist perspectives. The series of three articles uses a creative approach to explain the theories, and to highlight their relevance for teaching in clinical practice.

The Director of Nurse Education (DNE) at the St Elsewhere Academy of Nursing is trying a create the ultimate programme of nursing education. In order to ensure that the very highest standards of teaching and learning are achieved, she has decided to employ a theorist of learning.

The job has been advertised and three very different candidates, representing the schools of behaviourism, cognitivism and humanism, have been shortlisted for interview.

The first person to present a case was from the school of behaviourism. This man believed learning to be a change in observable behaviour, which occurred when a link or connection was made between two events — that is, a stimulus and a response. By manipulation of this link the behaviour could be altered. To support his argument for the behaviourist theory of learning, the candidate produced evidence from many early, noted psychologists.

Watson (1878–1958) observed the behaviour of animals and children, and concluded that the more frequently a stimulus–response (S–R) link occurred, the more likely it was to be established as learned behaviour.

To add to this concept, Guthrie's theory of contiguity was discussed. This theory stated that if a stimulus occurred at the same time as a response, the response would be repeated when the stimulus subsequently occurred again — that is, following repeated pairings, the stimulus and response would be linked together. For example, it may be desirable to pair handwashing and aseptic procedures together.

The next piece of work to be presented was by the Russian physiologist, Pavlov (1849–1936), who broke new ground with his theory of classical conditioning.

Gilean McKenna: 'Learning Theories Made Easy: Behaviourism' in *NURSING STANDARD* (1995), 9(29), pp. 29–31.

While experimenting with salivation in dogs, he linked one stimulus — meat powder, to a second stimulus — a bell sound, to produce a response of salivation. After conditioning, the dogs would salivate to the sound of a bell (conditioned stimulus), even in the absence of the meat powder (unconditioned stimulus). On this occasion the salivation is called a conditioned response. Pavlov found that once a response had been conditioned, it could then be produced by other stimuli, similar to the conditioned response. He called it generalisation.

The DNE looked puzzled. 'That may well be true, but what have salivating dogs got to do with the education of student nurses?'

The candidate smiled and proceeded to explain that, as parts of nursing and nurse education may be of a highly emotional nature, there is a place for classical conditioning in nurse education.

He referred to Woolfolk and Nicolich (1) who suggested that emotional responses to particular situations were learned, in part through classical conditioning. He continued by quoting Bernard Lovell: 'It is the kind of learning that underlies the acquisition of the emotional component of our attitudes' (2).

He added that an emotional response to an experience can be either positive or negative. A bad experience may well produce a physiological response of fear or anxiety.

For example, if a student is forced to participate in a role-play for a particular teacher, and is then humiliated for the performance, an anxiety response (sweaty palms, palpitations, dry mouth) may be evoked when role-play is next suggested in that class. Generalisation of this conditioned response may be exhibited if the student becomes anxious at the suggestion of role-play in another class.

Extinguishing fear/anxiety

Another use of classical conditioning in education is to extinguish already established fear/anxiety responses. If, for example, a student has had a bad experience giving an injection and now trembles at the thought of having to give one, the teacher must help him/her overcome the fear.

The performance may be broken down into small steps, perhaps starting with watching a video of injection techniques, or touching and handling syringes. As each step is achieved without the expected negative outcome, the student will gradually lose the fear anxiety/response associated with injections.

'All right,' said the DNE. 'I accept that classical conditioning has a place in nurse education, but it is rather limited. What else have you got to offer?' The man then rummaged in his briefcase and produced a rather large folder. His eyes lit up as he began to recite the findings of Thorndike and of Skinner.

Thorndike (1874–1949), through his theories of trial and error learning, suggested that learning occurred when a specific response became linked to a specific stimulus, by a process of trial and error, until the successful link was found. Unlike Watson, who was mainly concerned with the simultaneous presence of a stimulus and response,

Thorndike emphasised the importance of the end effect of the response, suggesting that a positive outcome to a response would result in that response being repeated.

This belief was reflected in Thorndike's law of effect, which stated that satisfying results serve to strengthen or reinforce S–R links. Dissatisfying outcomes did not necessarily extinguish the response, but did cause alternative responses to be found by 'trial and error'. Watson's work was supported, however, by Thorndike's law of exercise which stated that S–R links were strengthened by repeatedly occurring together, provided that positive reinforcement normally occurred.

The DNE summarised by saying: 'So in nursing education, although repetition and practice are very useful, it is knowledge of results that is crucial.' The man smiled in agreement and continued.

Like Thorndike, Skinner believed that it was the end result of behaviour that governed its repetition but rather than being a random response to a stimulus, he viewed behaviour as a deliberate action that was influenced by a positive or negative outcome, or reinforcement. From this principle Skinner formulated 'operant conditioning', which stated that behaviour was directed by its consequences, in order to bring about certain desirable objectives.

'I see, a little like Freud's belief that we go through life seeking pleasure and avoiding pain,' added the DNE.

Encouraged by this, the candidate continued to explain the effect of antecedents and consequences on behaviour.

Depending on the consequences, the repetition of behaviour can be increased or decreased. Positive or negative reinforcements are used to encourage the repetition of behaviour, and punishment can be used to eliminate or decrease a behaviour. Hence, behaviour can be controlled by its consequences.

Some behaviours may have to be achieved gradually, each step being shaped by its consequence, until the desired behaviour is elicited. To maintain the behaviour the reinforcements must continue.

The DNE butted in: 'So you are saying that, as soon as the reinforcement stops, so will the behaviour? That's no good. The teachers can't spend all their time reinforcing the students' every move.'

After a quick rustle of papers, the candidate produced a schedule of reinforcement, illustrating that frequent reinforcement is important when a new behaviour is being learnt, but that intermittent reinforcement is much more effective in maintaining that behaviour.

For example, when a student nurse is learning an aseptic dressing technique, the teacher may give praise for each step — preparing the patient, handwashing and so on — thus shaping behaviour until the complete procedure is able to be performed.

Then the praise should be given only for the complete, correct performance and become increasingly intermittent, in order to maintain the behaviour.

Cueing

The other way that teachers can influence behaviour is by giving information or cues prior to the behaviour being performed. Cueing is an example of how antecedents can be influenced positively, and serve to remind the learner of the appropriate or expected behaviour (for example, when the teacher mentions handwashing to a learner before he/she starts an aseptic procedure, or gives precise guidelines or criteria for a case-study).

Evidence of operant conditioning is also found in various forms of self-directed learning. Linear programmes and computerised study packs involve students with a sequence of questions. If students answer correctly, they are informed, that is, reinforced, and are able to move on to the next question. If they answer wrongly, they are also informed, given an explanation, and offered the chance to answer again until the correct answer is selected.

Bernard Lovell (2) suggested that Skinner's operant conditioning was the most significant single contribution to the theory of learning.

The DNE was clearly still not convinced. 'I can see that operant conditioning does have its uses,' she said. 'But isn't it very reliant on the student emitting some sort of behaviour first, before all these reinforcements can be used, and isn't all this a rather slow process?'

The candidate then reached for his final offering — the work of neobehaviourist Albert Bandura (3) and his theory of social learning or vicarious conditioning. This theory involves the observed behaviour of others and the consequences of those behaviours. If the consequences are perceived to be desirable, the behaviour may be copied or modelled. If the consequences are seen to be undesirable, the behaviour may be avoided. Hence, learning can occur vicariously, through the experience of others.

This theory differs from those previously discussed because learning may occur instantly. It also acknowledges the thinking process in that behaviour is influenced by the meaning attached to it and the perceived consequences.

The DNE appeared to be impressed. 'Yes, I can see that this is highly significant to nursing education, particularly as the behaviour, attitudes, and values of teachers or other role-models may be copied by the learners.'

The man nodded in agreement. He concluded by explaining that this is particularly significant in the clinical area, where any behaviour that is seen to be rewarded, for example, by patient satisfaction or peer admiration, is likely to be copied. When the copied behaviour is of a high standard, the role-modelling is highly effective and positive.

There may be dangers, however, when questionable practices are copied as there is limited discrimination between 'good' and 'bad' behaviour, and only perceived desirable or undesirable outcomes which result from the behaviour.

The DNE pondered for a few seconds: 'Thank you, I can see that there are some uses for classical, operant, and vicarious conditioning in nursing education. However, I'm not sure I like the idea of the students being motivated mostly by reinforcement, rather than learning by self-motivation. I want my nurses to think, and not just respond.'

'I'll be in touch when I have interviewed the other candidates for the post.'

References

1.   Woolfolk A E, Nicolich L M (1980) *Educational Psychology for Teachers*. Prentice-Hall, Englewood Cliffs, NJ.

2.   Bernard Lovell R (1987) *Adult Learning*. Croom Helm, London.

3.   Bandura A L (1977) *Social Learning Theory*. Prentice-Hall, Englewood Cliffs, NJ.

10.   Learning Theories Made Easy: Cognitivism

Gilean McKenna

This is the second of three articles explaining theories of learning with particular relevance to clinical areas. In the story so far, the Director of Nurse Education at the St Elsewhere Academy of Nursing is trying to create the ultimate programme of nursing education. In order to ensure that the very highest standards of teaching and learning are achieved, the DNE has decided to employ a theorist of learning. Last week she interviewed the candidate representing the school of behaviourism. This week, the candidate from the school of cognitivism makes his presentation.

The DNE welcomed the candidate into her office and began the interview. 'In your application you claim to have the ideal theory for the 21st century. You say that your theory will produce a truly educated nurse, who is knowledgeable, questioning, research-minded and able to problem-solve. Please tell me more.'

The young man leaned forward in his chair and began to explain enthusiastically that his theory was not like the behaviourist view, in which learning involves little thinking and is observed to be a change in behaviour. In contrast, the cognitive psychologists believe that learning is an internal purposive process concerned with thinking, perception, organisation and insight.

He referred to Woolfolk and Nicolich (1), who suggested that this type of learning could not be observed directly as it involved a change in the capability of the individual to respond. The learner was actively involved with problem-solving, seeking out new information, and drawing on past experience in order to gain understanding.

He began to state his case by explaining the significance of Gestalt psychology to the origins of cognitive learning theories.

Referring to Child (2), he described Gestalt, a German word that means pattern or form, and the work of the early Gestalt psychologists — Wertheimer (1880–1943), Kohler (1887–1967), and Koffka (1886–1941).

These men were initially concerned with the study of perception and their work emphasised the ability of the individual to organise and integrate what is perceived into an overall pattern or Gestalt.

Wertheimer believed that breaking down behaviour into constituent parts obscured the full meaning of the total behaviour. From this stemmed the Gestalt phrase: 'The whole is greater than the sum of its parts.'

Wertheimer believed that perceptions were organised by the individual, using the principle of 'pragnanz', into as simple a structure or form as possible, in order that

Gilean McKenna: 'Learning Theories Made Easy: Cognitivism' in *NURSING STANDARD* (1995), 9(30), pp. 25–28.

meaning could be imposed. Pragnanz was made up of four laws of perception — similarity, proximity, closure and continuity. Referring to Quinn (3), the candidate continued to explain how Koffka believed that these laws of perception could also be used as laws of learning, and from this grew the Gestalt theory of learning by insight.

Insightful learning occurs when a problem is suddenly solved by the restructuring of the component parts into new relationships, so they are perceived as a whole. Kohler demonstrated insightful learning in 1925, using a chimpanzee in a cage with some bananas suspended out of reach. The chimpanzee also had some boxes which, if stacked, could be used to reach the bananas. After various futile attempts, the chimpanzee suddenly perceived the relationship between stacking the boxes and reaching the bananas. This insight to the solution of the problem could be transferred and repeated in similar future situations. Thus learning had occurred.

Previous knowledge

The DNE grinned and said excitedly: 'Yes, I see. So this could apply to the situation where students cannot initially make any sense of the squiggles that make up an ECG rhythm strip. Then, when the students understand cardiac conduction, and relate the activity of the heart during the cardiac cycle to the ECG readings, they are able to understand the significance of the P wave and the QRS complex . . . But, hang on a minute, doesn't all this require previous knowledge?'

Pleased with this response, the candidate reached for his copy of Child (2) to explain that, rather than using mechanical repetition of stimulus-response bonds, insightful learning depends on the adaptation of past experience or existing knowledge to form new insights.

'Yes that is true, but how can nurse teachers use this in education?'

The candidate explained that a nurse teacher may use the principles of pragnanz to structure sessions so they are seen as a whole rather than as isolated facts.

For example, if a session on the structure and function of the respiratory tract is linked to a disorder such as bronchitis and to the activities of daily living, the students will then perceive the anatomy and physiology, the disordered condition, and the effect on the patient as a whole, rather than three unrelated units.

The use of problem-solving techniques may allow learners to undergo an insightful process. For example, rather than telling students about the nursing care of a patient with bronchitis, the teacher can explain the disordered physiology. The students can then work out what problems the patient may experience and identify the appropriate nursing care, relating all this to the physiology and to the patients they have nursed with this condition.

Bruner's theory of learning through discovery was introduced next. Bruner (4) suggested that the ultimate aim of teaching was to instill a general understanding of the structure of a subject.

He believed learning to be an active process, stimulated by curiosity. The knowledge is constructed by relating the incoming information to a previously acquired frame of reference. The frame of reference is a system of representation that gives meaning and organisation to knowledge and experience. There are three modes in Bruner's 'system of representation' — *enactive, iconic* and *symbolic*:

- The *enactive* mode of representation consists a habitual set of actions, known without the use of imagery or words, that are appropriate for achieving a certain result. This often applies to motor skills.

- The *iconic* mode is based on imagery, and used for knowledge, represented by images that 'stand' for a concept, but do not fully define it.

- The *symbolic* mode is the transformation of the iconic imagery into a symbolic system — usually language.

Although these three stages develop during childhood in the order presented, they extend more or less intact throughout adult life.

The DNE was becoming a little impatient. 'Will you please get to the point. What is the use of these icons and things to nursing education?'

The candidate quickly responded with an example of blood pressure recording. When a student initially learns the motor skill of measuring blood pressure, but has no concept at all of the significance of that recording, it will be an enactive representation. Later, as the student begins to grasp the concept of 'blood pressure', it may be in the image of a pump (the heart), connected to a series of narrowing and widening tubes (the blood vessels), with blood circulating around the body. This will be iconic representation. Eventually the student will reach the symbolic mode, being able to define blood pressure and describe the significance of cardiac output and peripheral resistance.

The DNE nodded approvingly. 'I see, so if a learner is having trouble grasping a concept, the teacher could help by using imagery or making analogies to everyday things that are understood — like comparing the effects of vasoconstriction to someone standing on the garden hose.'

The candidate nodded and proceeded to explain that as well as describing a hierarchical structure of learning — that is action, image, and symbol — Bruner also suggests there is a coding system that makes up the pattern of enactive, iconic and symbolic representations.

This coding system allows the thousands of perceived facts to be grouped and related to each other. This allows learners to go beyond the information given and formulate new ideas by deducing additional information from previously learned principles stored in the system.

For example, if given the specific information that hypovolaemic shock is caused by a reduced circulating volume, a learner with a sound understanding of the concept of blood pressure and its control will be able to deduce that this will lead to a reduced cardiac output and result in a decreased blood pressure and increased heart rate.

Learning by discovery

Sequence is important and sessions should be structured to make use of relevant existing knowledge. Bruner (4) advocates the use of a spiral curriculum, in which all important concepts and subjects are introduced in a simple form at a very early stage of the programme, and then built upon with more complex ideas.

The candidate then referred to the work of Bigge (5) to discuss the advantages of Bruner's theory of learning by discovery.

• Once a situation is mastered, the individual alters the way in which new situations are approached in the search for information, so the student learns how to learn.

• The student is encouraged to discover the value of intuitive guesses, and try out his/her own hypotheses.

• The student's ability and confidence in problem-solving will increase as he/she acquires understanding of basic concepts and the ability to transfer knowledge.

• There is increased self-motivation and accountability for learning.

• Curiosity is aroused and the student is encouraged to adopt a questioning, research-minded approach.

The DNE smiled smugly. 'That might well be so, but according to my friend Mr Myles (6), this approach to learning may be difficult to structure in large groups of mixed ability learners, and it can be very time consuming, as well as expensive getting lots of fancy equipment; not to mention that a few 'bright sparks' might be doing all the discovering, leaving the rest feeling bewildered. What else have you got to offer me?'

The candidate described the work of Ausubel (7), which suggests that students learn more efficiently when they are presented with material in an organised, sequenced form that can be assimilated to their previous knowledge. This is the basis of the theory of reception or assimilation.

Ausubel (7) believes that learning is a deductive process that should move from an initial understanding of general concepts, to an understanding of specifics. This is unlike Bruner (4) who suggests that learning occurs inductively, using specifics to discover general concepts.

He advocates a method of expository teaching in order to enhance 'meaningful learning'. This method of teaching is very closely linked to the students' previous knowledge, and involves high levels of interaction between the teacher and the students. Meaningful learning is suggested to be more efficient than rote learning, which is unlikely to be retained because it is not connected with existing knowledge.

Ausubel (7) describes a sequence of learning that considers the students' existing knowledge and the processes by which they are most likely to assimilate new material into their existing conceptual structures. This is achieved by the use of an advance organiser, followed by the subordinate content. Quinn (3) describes an 'advance organiser' as a concept that is introduced in advance of the new material in order to provide an anchoring structure for it. This conceptual statement may be in the form of prose or a diagrammatic flow-chart.

For example, when teaching about pressure sores, a broad statement can introduce the session, such as: 'Pressure sores are known as decubitus ulcers. They are skin ulcers which occur over bony prominences, due mainly to restricted mobility. They can be prevented by the principle of relieving pressure.' This can then be followed by the subordinate content such as the pathophysiology, aetiology and nursing care.

To emphasise this point, the candidate then quoted Bernard-Lovell, stating: 'The principle function of the advance organiser is to provide a scaffolding of ideas to bridge the gap between what the student already knows and what he/she needs to know before he/she can learn the new material in a meaningful fashion' (8).

The candidate continued by outlining the advantages of Ausubel's approach to teaching. First, it activates the relevant knowledge the student already has, and second, it enhances the assimilation of new knowledge into the established conceptual structure, which increases retention and makes rote learning unnecessary.

'Yes,' said the DNE, rubbing her chin thoughtfully. 'I suppose these advance organisers do help create the right learning set, and assist the student to focus on the relevant aspects of a session. In fact, I think they could even be a little more stimulating than the usual objectives that we churn out before a session. You don't seem very fond of rote learning, but I do believe that it has a place — how else do students recall the cranial nerves? Have you got any proof of the efficiency of this reception learning in nursing education?'

The candidate shook his head, but quickly pointed out the work of Woolfolk and Nicolich (1), which suggests that Ausubel's approach is particularly suitable when teaching the relationship between concepts, or for introducing novel or difficult material. It is also very appropriate for adult learners, who have a lot of previous knowledge and are able to manipulate ideas.

Information processing

Moving on, the candidate next introduced the work of Robert Gagné (9), concerning the information-processing model of learning based on the study of memory. An analogy is often made between a computer and the human mind, as both go through a similar process of gathering information from incoming stimuli, organising the information, that is, encoding it, retaining it, and, when needed, retrieving it.

The candidate explained that, although the other cognitive theorists acknowledge the importance of existing knowledge, the information process theorists emphasise the process of retaining and retrieving this knowledge.

Gagné (9) devised a model of learning and memory. He describes a process whereby stimuli from the environment affect the receptors and then enter the nervous system via a sensory register which codes the information into a patterned representation. The information remains in this form for fractions of a second, after which it is either lost through decay, or entered into short-term memory. Once in short-term memory it is coded into a conceptual form, where it remains for only a few seconds.

The short-term memory has a limited capacity to store about seven items. Rehearsal of the information may retain it for longer, or even allow it to be encoded into long-term memory.

From short-term memory the information is either lost through decay and interference, or it is once again transformed and organised, ready to enter the long-term memory, where it is stored for later recall.

Once in long-term memory, information is categorised, and the general meaning, rather than exact details, is stored.

The DNE now looked thoroughly confused, so the candidate produced a diagram to help clarify this model.

Retrieval of information depends on how it is stored in long-term memory, that is, the representation and organisation. As discussed previously, information that is linked or coded into the appropriate conceptual or cognitive structure is more likely to be recalled efficienctly.

Although information is thought to be stored permanently once it is entered into long-term memory, retrieval can be obscured by interference. Retroactive is the term used when new information interferes with old, and proactive describes old information interfering with new.

'How can nurse teachers use this?' asked the DNE enthusiastically.

The candidate said there were many ways teachers could maximise learning and retention.

First, the teacher can help students to focus attention selectively by changing the stimulus regularly and making use of colours, movement, voice and varying teaching methods. Novelty and humour can be very useful, but may also distract attention if not used carefully. The students can be given cues as to which points are particularly important. The teacher must also be aware of fatigue, limited attention spans, and the amount of new information being introduced, to prevent information overload.

Second, the teacher can help make new information meaningful by linking it to that already known — this may involve helping learners to retrieve the relevant previous knowledge.

Third, repetition of information can aid the encoding process. The spacing of the repetition or practice can be important.

'Thank you,' said the DNE. 'I have another appointment now, so we must end. I must admit that I am not too keen on learning outcomes. They seem a little too precise and related to objectives. But I am interested in some of your learning theories. I particularly like the sound of Bruner's ideas. I think that Ausubel's advance organisers are excellent and, of course, an understanding of perception, insight and memory is imperative.

'I have one final candidate to interview, so I'll be in touch with you after that.'

References

1. Woolfolk A E, Nicolich L M (1980) *Educational Psychology for Teachers*. Prentice-Hall, Englewood Cliffs, NJ.

2. Child D (1986) *Psychology and the Teacher*, 4th edn. Cassell, London.

3. Quinn F M (1980) *The Principles and Practice of Nurse Education*. Croom Helm, London.

4. Bruner J S (1966) *Towards a Theory of Instruction*. Belknap, Cambridge, Mass.

5. Bigge M L (1982) *Learning Theories for Teachers*, 4th edn. Harper and Row, New York.

6. Myles A (1987) Psychology and the curriculum. In P Allan, M Jolley (eds) *The Curriculum in Nursing Education*. Croom Helm, London.

7. Ausubel D P (1968) *Educational Psychology: A Cognitive View*. Holt, Rinehart and Winston, New York.

8. Bernard-Lovell R (1987) *Adult Learning*. Croom Helm, London.

9. Gagné R M (1975) *Essentials of Learning for Instruction*. Dryden Press, Hinsdale, Ill.

11. Learning Theories Made Easy: Humanism

Gilean McKenna

This is the last of three articles explaining theories of learning with particular relevance to clinical areas. In the story so far, the Director of Nursing Education at the St Elsewhere Academy of Nursing is trying to create the ultimate programme of nursing education. In order to ensure that the very highest standards of teaching and learning are achieved, the DNE has decided to employ a theorist of learning. She first interviewed the candidate representing the school of behaviourism and last week the cognitivist candidate made his presentation. The series now concludes with the humanist candidate — and the final decision.

The candidate representing the humanist theorists appeared relaxed and self-assured as he walked into the office. He shook the DNE's hand firmly, introducing himself as Bob, and asked her first name. The DNE appeared a little surprised by his lack of formality, but the man seemed pleasant and very knowledgeable as he explained his ideas for nursing education.

The humanist theory of learning is concerned with feelings and experiences, leading to personal growth and individual fulfilment. Maslow (1) made a significant contribution to the humanist approach with his theory of motivation and hierarchy of needs. In order to ascend to self-actualisation, lower level needs (that is, comfort and security), must first be partially satisfied.

The goal of education is therefore to assist the achievement of self-actualisation, and fulfil the maximum potential for personal growth. This is closely linked to the work of Carl Rogers and Malcolm Knowles.

Rogers (2), who advocated a student-centred approach to learning, identifies a continuum of meaning. At one end of the continuum is material which has no personal meaning. This learning involves only the mind and not feelings, that is, it has no relevance for the whole person and therefore becomes futile. At the opposite end of the continuum is significant, meaningful, experiential learning, which involves both thoughts and feelings.

Rogers (2) believes that significant, experiential learning has five qualities:

- It involves the whole person — both feelings and cognitive processes

- It is self-initiated, with a sense of discovery coming from within

- It is pervasive and makes a difference in the behaviour, attitudes and maybe the personality of the learner

Gilean McKenna: 'Learning Theories Made Easy: Humanism' in *NURSING STANDARD* (1995), 9(31), pp. 29–31.

- It is evaluated by the learner, who knows if his or her needs have been met or not

- The essence of it has meaning.

The teacher is primarily concerned with permitting the students to learn by feeding their own curiosity. The students are given responsibility and freedom to learn what they wish to learn, as they wish.

'Hold on for just one minute,' said the DNE. This idea sounds all very well for school children, but I have a set curriculum that must be met in order to conform to UKCC and ENB guidelines. How can I possibly allow the students to study whatever takes their fancy?'

Pleased that this issue had been raised, Bob explained that, in order to decrease student anxiety and frustration at not being spoon-fed, there is a need for a perceived structure in the form of limits and minimal requirements. This gives enough direction for work to commence, thus ensuring that the content requirements of the curriculum are fulfilled, but the process remains free.

'Do the students like this method?' asked the DNE. 'Isn't it easier for them to simply take notes from a lecture?'

Bob smiled. He agreed that, initially, the struggle for personal growth may be painful. It may even evoke student hostility and resentment, but in the long-term, true learning will take place above and beyond the set curriculum. This learning will be remembered, utilised and valued for years to come.

'Yes, I can see that you're possibly right, but doesn't it require a rather special type of teacher to do this?' questioned the DNE. 'Some of my tutors have been giving lectures for years, and would not be best pleased to give them up!'

Bob reassured her that it did indeed require a rather special teacher, one who had been through a process of self-discovery for him/herself and was prepared to become a 'real' person to the students, sharing their own joys and disappointments, and not being a faceless embodiment of knowledge.

This teacher must also genuinely value, accept and empathically understand the students to allow a trusting relationship to develop. The role changes from that of a teacher and evaluator, to a facilitator of learning. The members of the class, including the teacher, become a community of learners.

The DNE was not quite convinced. 'I think some of my tutors would need a great deal of help to achieve that! It does sound interesting though, if not perhaps a touch idealistic. How do I know this approach will work in nursing education?'

Bob then reached for the work of Burnard, who has written extensively on the value of experiential methods and the facilitation of learning in nursing. Burnard (3) suggested that experiential knowledge is gained through direct encounter. Students learn either by direct experience in the present, or by reflecting on past experience in order to make sense of the present.

Students enter nursing as adults, bringing with them a wealth of valuable life experience. Many of the skills of nursing do not have to be taught, as they are already grounded in personal experience. A skilled facilitator is able to make use of these experiences, as well as providing new experiences. Burnard (4) believed that this is particularly relevant for the development of interpersonal skills.

'I accept that it is useful, but doesn't the facilitation of all these experiences take up much more time than the traditional methods?'

Bob then explained that much propositional knowledge — concepts, theories, models and propositions — may be gained from reading books and articles. This leaves more classroom time for experiential learning.

Referring to Burnard (4), Bob quickly added that, if teachers control the learners' educational experiences too much, they limit the amount of personal growth that can occur. Nursing education will then churn out clones of the profession, who do not question what they see, and who neither trust nor know themselves.

'Yes, well that's certainly worth thinking about, but I do think there are times when learners need specific and structured teaching, for example, just before their final exams. Do you have anything else to offer?'

The candidate continued. Knowles (5) developed the theory of andragogy, the art and science of teaching adults. He acknowledges that adults have a vast range of experience, which forms a basis for new learning. Therefore, pedagogical methods of teaching were not appropriate in adult education.

Burnard (3) summarises the major differences of androgogical learning:

- Adults need to be able to apply what they have learned

- Adults have a wealth of personal and life experiences that should be used in education

- Adult learning involves an investment of self and any new learning will affect that self-concept

- Adults are mostly self-directed and their education should accommodate this.

The relationship between teacher and student should be one of mutual respect. Eduard Lindeman highlighted this in 1926 by stating: 'None but the humble become good teachers of adults. The student's experience counts for as much as the teacher's knowledge' (5).

Knowles (5) suggests that as adults, students should help formulate the curricula, rather than adapt themselves to what is offered. Burnard (3) says that, in nursing education, even though the national boards set out a syllabus, students still have considerable scope to decide how and when various topics were learned.

The DNE nodded: 'Yes, I agree that we must acknowledge that student nurses are adults, and treat them appropriately. Thank you Bob for such an interesting and illuminating discussion. I shall be in touch to let you know of my decision.'

References

1. Maslow A (1971) *The Farther Reaches of Human Nature*. Penguin, Harmondsworth.

2. Rogers C R (1983) *Freedom to Learn for the 80's*. Merrill, Ohio.

3. Burnard P (1987) Teaching the teachers. *Nursing Times*, 83, 9, 63–65.

4. Burnard P (1988) Building on experience. *Senior Nurse*, 8, 5, 12–13.

5. Knowles M (1978) *The Adult Learner: A Neglected Species*, 2nd edn. Gulf Publishing, Houston, TX.

12. Humanist Ideology and Nurse Education: Humanist Educational Theory

Michael Purdy

Nurse education is dominated by the humanist perspective and the educational theory that it generates. Following a brief description of the perspective's phenomenological foundations and definition of humanist ideology, humanist educational theory is illustrated in an outline of the key contributions of John Dewey, Carl Rogers, Malcolm Knowles and Paulo Freire. The article concludes by noting Freire's sociological challenge to the individualism of the humanist perspective. This challenge recognizes the ideological and social control role of education in securing the reproduction of power relations and leads to questioning the function of individualism and the interests that humanist ideology may serve.

Introduction

The humanist perspective dominates the field of nurse education. Its significance has grown as the preparation of nurses for practice has become regarded less as a course of training and more as an educational process.

This article seeks to contribute to the debate concerning the status of the humanist approach in nurse education. The task will be to outline key philosophical assumptions that inform the perspective, identify a body of humanist educational theory that nurse educationalists draw on extensively and begin to question the social function that humanist ideology may perform. The question of the limitations of humanist educational theory in nurse education is taken up in a second article.

Phenomenological foundations

It is impossible to assess the humanist perspective without first appreciating its phenomenological foundations. It is from these foundations that the humanists derive their assumptions about the nature of the social world and about knowledge of this world.

The key distinguishing characteristic of all phenomenology is its overriding concern with the subjective dimension of personal experience. The approach is grounded in a particular ontology (theory of being), which claims that the social world is qualitatively different to the natural material world. What distinguishes the social from the natural world is human consciousness. The social world is a world full of meaning, a world in which the individual organizes his/her environment, and in consciously acting upon

Michael Purdy: 'Humanist Ideology and Nurse Education. 1. Humanist Educational Theory' in *NURSE EDUCATION TODAY* (1997), 17, pp. 192-195. Reprinted by permission of the publisher Churchill Livingstone.

the world transcends the limitations that it imposes upon him/her. It is this active subjectivity of the social actor that is the focus of the phenomenological approach.

This ontology generates a specific epistemology (theory of knowledge), in which knowledge of the social world is seen to be the product of individual subjective experience rather than of theory. Since meaning is not considered to be an effect of the social world, but rather of individuals' intentions and interpretations established through their actions, then in order to understand this world one must do more than merely observe it, one must interpret it and understand its significance to the 'actors' involved. 'Interpretation is taken to mean the active commitment . . . to the symbolic reconstruction of the "actor's world"' (Brittan, 1973, p. 25).

Humanist ideology

Humanist ideology is taken here to refer to a series of ideas and beliefs, broadly informed by the ontological and epistemological assumptions of phenomenology, which are responsible for a particular view of the educational process. This ideology will be seen to have social and political effects, principally through its individualism.

An essential feature of the humanist perspective is its rejection of *reductionist* accounts of psychological and social processes. It advances a concern for the humanity of man rather than concern for an aspect of psychological processing or sociological context. For example, humanists insist that the educational process should address the affective as well as the intellectual (cognitive) dimensions of learning. This demand for a more holistic approach to understanding education and learning leads it to reject both behaviourist and cognitive positions in psychology; the former for failing to take account of individuals' consciousness and interpretive faculties and the latter for its avoidance of the affective dimension. It also rejects sociological approaches for their social determinism which, it is alleged, reduces the individual to a passive product of the social system. Humanist ideology can, therefore, be seen to exist in a space outside of reductionist and over-deterministic theories.

Humanist educational theory

In educational theory the humanist perspective is exemplified in the work of, amongst others, John Dewey (1915), Carl Rogers (1951, 1961, 1983), Malcolm Knowles (1975, 1980), Knowles *et al.* (1984), Paulo Freire (1972, 1985) and Freire & Shor (1987).

John Dewey

Dewey's contribution to the humanist view lies in his conception of education as growth and in his belief that education can provide a catalyst for both personal and social change and development.

According to Dewey, education is growth, it has no other purpose:

> 'Since growth is the characteristic of life, education is all one with growing, it has no end beyond itself . . . Education is thus a fostering, a nurturing, a cultivating process. All of these words means that it implies attention to the conditions of growth.'

> (Dewey, 1915, pp. 52-53, 10)

The role of the educator is, therefore, to facilitate the process of growth by which individuals personally develop. This process is seen to ensure 'a healthy evolving life adjustment process leading to further development and growth' (Archambault, 1966, p. 165) in which individual freedom is enhanced and autonomy developed.

Insofar as education allows for each and every individual to grow and develop, it facilitates democracy. Dewey's views clearly call for a philosophy of liberalism to pervade society and, in pointing to the potential for *social* change which education could facilitate, he is straining at the reins of the humanist perspective.

Carl Rogers

In Rogers' humanist psychology, Dewey's notion of education as growth is endorsed, but from within a strictly phenomenological perspective. His approach generates a view of 'client-centred therapy' which, Rogers argues, is transferable to the field of education insofar as both are learning processes, the aim of which is 'the constructive development of persons' (Rogers, 1983, p. 284).

The guiding assumption in Rogers' work is the optimistic belief that humans are essentially positive, growth-orientated organisms: 'The organism has one basic tendency and striving — to actualize, maintain and enhance the experiencing organism' (Rogers, 1951, p. 487). This potential for self-actualization may be realized under certain conditions, those permitting free and open development according to individual inclination.

Like therapy, education can, according to Rogers, pursue the principles of acceptance and respect for the individual's views and beliefs and the facilitating of an open learning climate in which students can feel free to express and choose their own direction for learning.

An important feature of Rogers' view of student-centred learning is that from the point of view of the teacher it is 'non-directive' (Rogers, 1951). It is not the teacher who sets the agenda but the student. Therefore:

> 'Teaching should be characterized by a deep respect for the idiosyncratic potential of each individual. Its focus should be enabling the student to free himself from environmental and emotional inhibitors that prevent him from learning and fully functioning.'
>
> (Pine & Boy, 1977, p. 111)

Like Dewey before him, Rogers sees the purpose of education as individual growth, to enable the development of the 'fully functioning person'. However, modern society, with its authoritarian and hierarchical institutions, frustrates this potential and Rogers regards society and its institutions as 'too restrictive and static' (Nye, 1975), as suffocating the individual. Nevertheless, certain features of the modern condition demand a humanist educational process. Specifically, the pace and extent of 'change' require the cultivation of adaptability on the part of the learner, which the humanist model is capable of achieving.

In many ways Rogers' humanist position offers a means whereby individuals may accommodate and adapt themselves to such conditions, but it fails to offer a basis for challenging and changing the conditions.

Malcolm Knowles

The view of changing social conditions demanding a different educational process to the tradition of education as transmission of knowledge is, together with Rogers' notion of student-centred learning, taken up and developed by Knowles through his conception of adult learning as 'andragogy'.

According to Knowles, self-directed learning has been called for by social conditions. The change that Knowles refers to is that of the 'rate' of social change itself:

> 'The simple truth is that we are entering into a strange new world in which rapid change will be the only stable characteristic. And this simple truth has several radical implications for education and learning. For one thing, this implies that it is no longer realistic to define the purpose of education as transmitting what is known . . . the main purpose of education must now be to develop the skills of enquiry.'

> (Knowles, 1975, p. 15)

The fact that one can no longer learn for life, but is continuously faced with the challenge of new learning experiences, means 'that it is no longer appropriate to equate education with youth' (Knowles, 1975, p. 16). This fact leads Knowles to develop his concept of 'andragogy' as the style of learning which characterizes adult education: 'Andragogy is defined . . . as the art and science of helping adults (or, even better, maturing human beings) learn' (Knowles, 1975, p. 19). Distinct from the traditional model of pedagogy, andragogy forms the basis for self-directed learning.

Knowles' concept of andragogy embraces the humanist emphasis on the individual as growth-orientated, an emphasis present in both Dewey and Rogers' work. In the case of Knowles this growth is interpreted as a process of maturation (Knowles, 1980), which incorporates many dimensions, including the transition from dependence to autonomy and from passivity to activity.

Paulo Freire

The possibility of education 'liberating' the individual and facilitating the transition from passivity to activity, is the fundamental theme of Freire's work. That education has an emancipatory potential is due to the fact that, according to Freire, it can never be a neutral process:

> 'I do not want to fall into a false and nonexistent nondirectivity of education. For me, education is always directive, always. The question is to know towards what and with whom it is directive?'

> (Freire & Shor, 1987, p. 109)

Education is always a *social* process, either constraining and controlling individuals and social groups or offering them a means to understand their lives and transform their situations. For Freire, the opportunity the educational process can offer for individuals to reflect on their (social) situation is the essential basis which enables them to take some degree of control over their lives and transform their situation.

Freire's view of the educational process is clearly humanistic: 'For Freire . . . education is "the practice of freedom" in which the learner discovers himself and achieves his humanity by acting upon the world to transform it' (Jarvis, 1983, p. 92). However, unlike Dewey, Rogers and Knowles, Freire is situated at the 'edge' of the humanist paradigm, insofar as phenomenological and individualistic values are replaced by structural and political ones. What distinguishes Freire is his concern for the social dimension of the educational process, a concern that takes him beyond simply endorsing the humanist perspective. Thus, whilst education may indeed lead to individual emancipation through critical reflection on one's 'situation' generating action to change the conditions of one's life, it may also prevent such reflection insofar as it performs an ideological function, the aim of which is to produce acceptance of one's situation and thereby reproduce the same sociopolitical structures.

Conclusions

A sociological perspective

It is the reproductive function of educational processes that Althusser alerts us to in his notion of the educational system as a 'state ideological apparatus' (Althusser, 1969). The institutionalization of education has also been seen to involve both individuals becoming increasingly dependent on institutions to satisfy their learning needs, and thereby relinquishing personal power and control, and to self-reliance being viewed as unreliable. In short, 'reliance on institutional treatment renders independent accomplishment suspect' (Illich, 1971, p. 3).

The sociological perspective challenges the humanist emphasis on human agency; that is, on the fundamental ability of individuals to change and control their lives and situations. It does this by identifying structural constraints within which human agency may, or may not, operate. This is not to suggest a conspiratorial model, according to which a dominant ruling class possesses absolute power and control via various institutions (including educational systems) and other groups are merely passive pawns. Power is never that one-sided, and resistance and struggle are always the rule rather than the exception (Foucault, 1980). Human agency is able to have influence, but the humanist ideal can only be realized through social rather than individual action. Liberation and empowerment are social not individual processes. Freire recognizes this: 'I don't believe in self-liberation. Liberation is a social act. Liberating education is a social process of illumination' (Freire & Shor, 1987, p. 109). Thus:

> 'The pursuit of full humanity . . . cannot be carried out in isolation or individualism, but only in fellowship and solidarity . . . No one can be authentically human while he prevents others from being so. The attempt *to be more* human, individualistically, leads to *having more*, egotistically: a form of dehumanization.'

> (Freire, 1972, p. 58)

117

Freire, therefore, challenges the individualism of a purely humanist perspective. Moreover, he suggests, albeit implicitly, a possible interest which humanist ideology may serve; this is, the individual competitiveness of the capitalist marketplace!

Awareness of the socio-political and ideological dimensions of any institutionalized educational process raises questions as to the nature, purpose and extent of 'self-directed' learning and student-centredness as envisaged by the humanists. This is not to deny its reality, but to recognize that such 'individualism' exists within, and is tolerated and valued by, specific institutional structures that may themselves endorse the interests of particular social groups. [The question of which interests humanist ideology — and its promotion in nurse education — may serve, is raised in part 2 of this article.]

References

Althusser L (1969) Ideology and ideological state apparatuses: (notes towards an investigation). In: L Althusser (ed) 1971 *Lenin and Philosophy and Other Essays*. NLB, London.

Archambault R D (1956) The philosophical bases of the experience curriculum. In: R D Archambault (ed) 1966 *Dewey on Education: Appraisals*. Random House, New York, pp. 160–181.

Brittan A (1973) *Meanings and Situations*. Routledge and Kegan Paul, London.

Dewey J (1915) *Democracy and Education*. The Free Press, New York.

Foucault M (1980) *Power/Knowledge: Selected Interviews and Other Writings 1972–1977*, edited by Colin Gordon. The Harvester Press, London.

Freire P (1972) *Pedagogy of the Oppressed*. Penguin, Harmondsworth.

Freire P (1985) *The Politics of Education: Culture, Power and Liberation*. Macmillan, London

Freire P, Shor I (1987) *A Pedagogy For Liberation: Dialogues On Transforming Education*. Macmillan, London.

Illich I D (1971) *Deschooling Society*. Calder & Boyers, London.

Jarvis P (1983) *Adult and Continuing Education: Theory and Practice*. Croom Helm, London.

Knowles M (1975) *Self-Directed Learning: A Guide For Learners and Teachers*. The Adult Education Company, New York.

Knowles M (1980) *The Modern Practice of Adult Education: From Pedagogy to Andragogy*. The Adult Education Company, New York.

Knowles M *et al* (1984) *Andragogy in Action: Applying Modern Principles of Adult Education*. Jossey-Bass, San Franciso.

Nye R D (1975) *Three Views of Man: Perspectives from Sigmund Freud, BF Skinner and Carl Rogers*. Brooks/Cole Publishing, Monterey, CA.

Pine G J, Boy A V (1977) *Learner-Centered Teaching: A Humanist View*. Love Publishing, Denver, CO.

Rogers C R (1951) *Client-Centered Therapy: Its Current Practice, Implications and Theory*. Constable, London.

Rogers C R (1961) *On Becoming a Person: A Therapist's View of Psychotherapy*. Constable, London.

Rogers C R (1983) *Freedom To Learn for the 80s*. Charles E Merrill Publishing, Columbus OH.

13. A Review of Two Theories of Learning and their Application in the Practice of Nurse Education

Margaret A. Coulter

From the range of learning theories which may be applied in the practice of nurse education, two contrasting theories have been selected. The 'conditions of learning and theory of instruction' (Gagné, 1985) derives from the behaviourist perspective in psychology, and Rogers' (1983) description of learning has evolved from the Humanistic School. This discussion initially focuses on Gagné's work beginning with a review of his 'conditions of learning', and is followed by a consideration of Rogers' approach through the 'facilitation of learning' (Rogers, 1983). The respective strengths and limitations of the two theories as applied in nurse education are then compared.

Introduction

At a time of great change in nurse education with developments such as Project 2000 in basic nurse preparation and the recently commenced Post Registration Education and Practice Project (PREPP) investigating post registration education, it is appropriate to review various approaches to learning so that the most suitable is adopted for a given situation. The two approaches considered in this paper are the behaviourist perspective of Gagné and Rogers' humanistic approach.

A behaviourist approach to learning

In 'essentials of learning for instruction' and 'the conditions of learning and theory of instruction' (Gagné, 1975; 1985) a behaviourist approach to learning is presented. Learning is defined as:

> 'a change in human disposition or capability that persists over a period of time and is not simply ascribable to processes of growth.' (Gagné, 1985)

To determine whether or not learning has taken place, Gagné (1975) states that the individual's behaviour before and after the learning incident should be compared. Pre- and post testing which are used quite frequently in nurse education may have derived from Gagné's work.

The behaviourist perspective is evident when learning is described as a process which is 'formally comparable to other human organic processes such as digestion and respiration' (Gagné, 1975). Bigge (1982) contends that Gagné regards aspects of the individual such as his motives, goals, intentions, and expectations as being of only secondary importance.

Margaret A. Coulter: 'A Review of Two Theories of Learning and their Application in the Practice of Nurse Education' in *NURSE EDUCATION TODAY* (1990), 10, pp. 333–338. Reprinted by permission of the publisher Churchill Livingstone.

The teacher's role

Gagné presents a teacher-centred approach to learning, stating that:

> 'Teachers carry out the task of promoting learning by providing instruction.' (Gagné 1975)

'Instruction' is comprised of the planning and controlling of events external to the learner. Gagné (1975) views the teacher as the 'designer of instruction', the 'manager of instruction', and the 'evaluator of student learning'. Joyce and Weil (1986) however contend that Gagné does not regard the learner as completely passive, suggesting that it is the learner's activity, or making the appropriate 'connections' which results in learning, with the instructor only providing the conditions.

The learning process

In the 'information-processing model' Gagné (1985) describes the learning process. Stimuli from the environment are detected by receptors which send this information to the 'sensory register' and from there it is transferred to the short-term memory and later to the long-term memory. Encoding of information takes place. Through the process of 'retrieval' information is recalled and the 'response generator' sorts out an appropriate action or performance. The action is carried out by effectors.

In the 'conditions of learning' Gagné (1985) differentiates between 'external' conditions of learning, and 'internal' ones. According to Gagné each learner has 'capabilities' which are internal to him, whereas the stimulus situation is outside the learner (Gagné, 1985).

Gagné describes eight conditions of learning, or learning types. These form a 'learning hierarchy' (Gagné, 1985). At the basic level is 'signal learning', or 'classical conditioning' after Watson and Pavlov. Next, is 'stimulus-response learning', followed by 'chaining', 'verbal association', 'discrimination learning', 'concept learning', 'rule learning' and finally, 'problem-solving'. Acquisition of any new skill or capability depends upon the successful learning of the subordinate ones.

Joyce and Weil (1986) describe the teacher's function in a teaching session using Gagné's model of instruction. The learner would be informed of the objectives for the session. The stimuli are then presented to the class. Attempts are made to increase the learner's attention. The learner is urged to recall earlier material. The teacher aims to construct the conditions under which the appropriate response (performance) will occur. The teacher decides on the sequences of learning, and subsequently prompts and guides learning. Events are thus firmly in the control of the teacher.

Psychomotor skills learning

An area of nurse education in which Gagné's work is highly regarded is psychomotor skills learning. The ability to perform psychomotor skills smoothly and efficiently is suggested as one dimension of the 'art' of nursing (de Tornyay & Thompson, 1982). Benner (1984) contends that skill performance is an area where the expert and the novice can readily be identified. The 'expert' functions at a much higher level than the 'novice', and interestingly she states that the term 'novice' does not just apply to new recruits to nursing, but also to any nurse who is unfamiliar with a particular speciality.

Gagné's description of 'chaining' has relevance for skills acquisition in nurse education. Conditions for chaining have been identified by Gagné and are cited by de Tornyay and Thompson (1982). Firstly, each stimulus-response connection needs to have been learned already. Secondly, the steps or links in the chain must be carried out in a set sequence. Thirdly, all of the elements in the chain need to be carried out close together to encourage formation of the chain. Fourthly, through repetition the performance becomes smoother. Fifthly, the final step in the chain needs to have its own intrinsic reward as this provides reinforcement. Lastly, having learned the skill under certain conditions the learner should then be able to apply it in other situations, discriminating where it is appropriate to do so.

Thus the teacher of psychomotor skills in nursing analyses each skill and divides it into parts which make up the overall skill. The parts are then placed in order. The whole skill is demonstrated, then the parts are identified and demonstrated again. Following the demonstration phase the learner has the opportunity to practice the skill, and the teacher may provide guidance and reinforcement. Throughout, the teacher attempts to identify factors in the external environment that could interfere with learning (de Tornyay & Thompson, 1982).

A humanistic approach to learning

Rogers' contribution to education theory has arisen out of his work in non-directive counselling. A core theme in Rogers' view on psychotherapy is that through positive relationships individuals grow, which he considered was a valuable idea to translate into education (Rogers, 1983). The goal of education is a 'fully functioning person'. He is critical of traditional schools which he describes as 'conservative, rigid, bureaucratic, resistant to change' (Rogers, 1983), and instead he presents his ideal; a system in which schools assist students 'to learn how to learn'. For nurse education this would mean that nurses would develop their own abilities to be self-directed in their learning both during preparation for the professional 'register', and in their subsequent careers.

The teacher/facilitator's role

Rogers departs from traditional thinking when he discusses the characteristics of the teacher. Rather than being the 'teacher and evaluator', the teacher becomes a 'facilitator of learning' (Rogers, 1983). The teacher is urged to be himself, to be 'real' to the students. Through promotion of the concept of 'responsible freedom' students are encouraged to be responsible for their own learning. Aware that a possible criticism of an unstructured approach could be that students would find it bewildering, he advocates building in enough limits and requirements to reassure students.

Rogers (1983) states that teaching is a 'vastly over-rated function'. The argument presented is that knowledge imparted now is soon out of date. We live in a time of great change. He comments on the role of education in periods of upheaval that:

> 'The only man who is educated is the man who has learned how to learn;
> the man who has learned how to adapt to change; the man who has
> realised that no knowledge is secure, that only the process of seeking
> knowledge gives a basis for security.' (Rogers, 1983)

Much of Rogers' discussion on the teacher–student relationship has direct parallels
with Freire's writing on education in 'pedagogy of the oppressed' (1972). Freire
comments that education is suffering from 'narration sickness'. A 'banking' concept of
education in which teachers tend to 'deposit' information in students is presented as
the traditional view of education (Freire, 1972). The traditional approach contrasts
sharply with Libertarian education:

> 'The teacher is no longer merely the one who teaches, but one who is
> himself taught in dialogue with the students, who in their turn while
> being taught also teach.' (Freire, 1972)

In such an exchange the growth of both teacher and student is stimulated, a dimension
which Rogers also discusses (Rogers, 1983).

The learning process

Rogers (1983) differentiates between 'learning' which consists of absorbing facts,
regurgitating them, soon after which they are forgotten, a 'meaningless' exercise; and
'learning' characterised by boundless curiosity and student initiated learning which is
'meaningful'. Rogers compares learning which involves the 'mind only', and learning
which is 'significant, meaningful, experiential learning'.

> 'Significant learning combines the logical and the intuitive, the intellect
> and the feelings, that concept and the experience, the idea and the
> meaning.' (Rogers, 1983)

The learning environment

According to Rogers (1983) the teacher can exhibit three 'attitudes' which facilitate
learning: realness in the facilitator of learning; prizing, acceptance, trust; and,
empathic understanding. The learning environment in his terms is one which nurtures
rather than controls.

Four stages are highlighted in the 'non-directive interview', a favoured teaching
strategy, in which the student should experience: A release of feeling or catharsis;
insight or reorganisation followed by; action, and finally; integration that leads to a
new orientation. Thus there is a great concentration on the emotional elements in this
approach to learning sessions which may be particularly valuable in nurse education
in the development of interpersonal skills, and self-awareness. During these sessions
the 'emotional attitudes' of students may be of even greater relevance than the
'content' of their accounts (Joyce & Weil, 1986).

Discussion

In the two learning theories described there are significant differences. The way in
which learning is defined in each reflects either a behaviourist orientation (Gagné,
1985), or a humanistic one (Rogers, 1983). The teacher's role is defined differently by

each theorist. Gagné's (1975) description of the teacher as 'instructor', contrasts with Rogers' (1983) 'teacher as facilitator'. Gagné's overall approach is a teacher-centred one, whereas Rogers aims for progression towards student-centred learning. Learner initiated enquiry is not evident in Gagné's approach, whereas Rogers emphasises the activity of the learner, to a great extent, even recommending students self-evaluation. Rogers also places much greater emphasis on the internal capabilities of the individual than Gagné.

The types of teaching methods employed are influenced by the predominant learning theory. Gagné for example, is wary of the discussion group method believing that little real learning would take place (Joyce & Weil, 1986). In contrast, Rogers' approach would probably draw on this method in preference to a lecture.

Bigge (1982) suggests that Gestalt-field theorists would find Gagné's model of instruction too limited for 'reflective teaching and learning'. The format is quite rigid and does not appear to encourage exploration of issues. In contrast Rogers' methods may afford the student greater freedom to explore. Bigge points out that Gagné makes no claims in his approach for learning conditions pertaining to complex human performance as might occur in the inventor or very creative individual. This perhaps underlines the limitations of using only one learning theory in nurse education.

However the strengths of Gagné's approach should also be recognised. The logical way in which large number of facts may be transferred to learners using Gagné's theory of learning remains a valuable property. Undoubtedly nursing students still require a significant body of knowledge to guide practice. Nurses require a satisfactory knowledge base from which to develop problem-solving and care planning skills but students may be unable to identify specific learning needs, especially at the novice stage. Through Gagné's 'learning hierarchy' students have the opportunity to build up their knowledge.

Gagné's model is also particularly useful in the areas of psychomotor skills acquisition. However important aspects of skill learning are less well described by Gagné, such as mental rehearsal before performance, and the learner's perception of the environment in which the skill is to be performed (de Tornyay & Thompson, 1982).

A nursing curriculum that is too heavily biased in favour of one approach may restrict the educational development of students. Sweeney (1986) cautions that a teacher-centred orientation in nurse education may result in students failing to develop skills in critical thinking, research awareness, ability to deal with change, or self-direction in continuing education. All of these attributes are vital in the proposed new role of 'specialist practitioner' described in the United Kingdom Central Council (UKCC)'s Project 2000 document (UKCC, 1986). In a rapidly changing society where developments in health care are continuous, greater flexibility and openness to change is crucial in all practitioners. Thus any reform of post registration education will also need to address how such characteristics can be enhanced.

In helping nurses 'learn how to learn' as Rogers would advocate, it is much more likely that individuals will be able to cope with change, and perhaps be more effective change agents. Cooper (1983) comments that in the field of continuing education in nursing, nurses are now encouraged to be more self-directing in their learning. Teachers in this area may take on more of a facilitator's role and thus 'help the individual learn how to learn' (Cooper, 1983). Moran (1980) has indicated that the role of the staff development officer in nursing could be more effective if the focus was on facilitating self-directed learning rather than having formal sessions. There are also resource implications as any scheme of mandatory updating would be very costly and investing in the promotion of self-directed learning could be more economical.

The vision of a group of nurses being transformed to a 'community of learners' (Rogers, 1983), is a particularly exciting notion, for example in a group of qualified nurses undertaking a course where the ideas generated by the group may be transferred into their working environment leading to improvements in the quality of care.

This contrasts with the learning environment engendered in Gagné's approach, where the aspect of 'control', a hallmark of behaviourist thinking is evident. By developing greater equality in teacher–student relationships such as would occur using Rogers' approach it has been argued that this fits in more with the ethos of a systematic approach to nursing. For example there is no room for authoritarian attitudes in the nurse–patient relationship (Sweeney, 1986). Jones (1981) also indicates that nurses may experience greater difficulty in establishing significant 'therapeutic relationships' with their patients if they have not been given the opportunity to experience such relationships in their own education.

Initially those who were sceptical of Rogers' ideas on learning criticised the approach because there had been little evaluative research of the method (Rogers, 1983). However, in 'Freedom to Learn for the 80's' (Rogers, 1983), there are references to completed studies which indicate situations in which the method has been effective. A number of nursing education research studies have also been undertaken (Richardson, 1988; Jones, 1981), and these would appear to demonstrate the potential for nurse education of self-directed learning techniques. 'Learning how to learn' therefore has major significance for the future professional development of all nurses.

It has been suggested that experiential methods as might be employed in a Rogerian rather than a behaviourist approach may be perceived as stressful by some teachers and students (Burnard, 1989a; Jones, 1988). Prior to incorporating such methods into the curriculum, teachers need to be adequately prepared in the use of new techniques (Burnard, 1988). Also, Burnard (1989b) argues that too many experiential learning exercises take on the characteristics of children's games, which seems contradictory in adult education where the aim is to facilitate adult learning.

The current major changes in nurse education will have implications for resources in colleges of nursing. The size of student groups undertaking Project 2000 preparation are large and there may be a temptation to return to widespread use of the lecture method, as this may appear to be an economical way to use both teachers and available classrooms. It is crucial that nurse educators identify areas of the curriculum which should be approached using other teaching methods. Gagné's method of teaching may appear much more economical of resources in the short term. However this should also be counter-balanced by the long-term rewards of Rogers' approach, which would hopefully produce a more self-directed learner.

There is a strong case for employing a combination of approaches to learning in a nurse education programme. They need not be in total conflict as suggested in this paper. For example Rogers' ideas could be used to develop the interpersonal skills and research elements of the curriculum, and provided that the students are treated as responsible adult learners, selected aspects of the curriculum such as psychomotor skills learning could draw on Gagné's work.

References

Benner P (1984) *From Novice to Expert*. Addison-Wesley Publishing Company, Menlo Park.

Bigge M L (1982) *Learning Theories for Teachers* (4th ed). Harper and Row, New York.

Burnard P (1988) Building on experience. *Senior Nurse* 8, 5: 12–13.

Burnard P (1989a) Exploring nurse-educators' views of experiential learning: a pilot study. *Nurse Education Today* 9: 39–45.

Burnard P (1989b) Playschool. *Nursing Times* 85, 17: 36–37.

Cooper S S (1983) *The Practice of Continuing Education in Nursing*. Aspen Publishing, London.

Friere P (1972) *Pedagogy of The Oppressed*. Penguin Books, Harmondsworth.

Gagné R M (1975) *Essentials of Learning For Instruction*. (expanded ed.) The Dryden Press, Hinsdale, Illinois.

Gagné R M (1985) *The Conditions of Learning and Theory of Instruction*. Holt, Rinehart and Winston, London.

Jones S (1988) A painful experience. *Senior Nurse* 8, 6: 23.

Jones W J (1981) Self-directed learning and student selected goals in nurse education. *Journal of Advanced Nursing* 6: 56–59.

Joyce B, Weil W (1986) *Models of Teaching* (3rd ed). Prentice-Hall Inc, Englewood Cliffs.

Moran V (1980) Facilitating self-directed learning: the role of the staff development director. In: S. S. Cooper (ed) *Self Directed Learning in Nursing*. Nursing Resources, Wakefield, Ma.

Richardson M (1988) Innovating androgogy in a basic nursing course: an evaluation of the self-directed independent study contract with basic nursing students. *Nurse Education Today* 8: 315–324.

Rogers C (1983) *Freedom To Learn For The 80's*. Charles E Merrill Publishing Company, London.

Sweeney J (1986) Nurse education: learner-centred or teacher-centred? *Nurse Education Today* 6: 257–262.

de Tornyay R, Thompson M A (1982) *Strategies For Teaching Nursing*. (2nd ed). John Wiley and Sons, New York.

UKCC (1986) *Project 2000*. United Kingdom Central Council for Nursing, Midwifery and Health Visiting, London.

UKCC (1990) Discussion paper on Post-Registration Education and Practice. United Kingdom Central Council for Nursing, Midwifery and Health Visiting, London.

14.   The Nature of Learning
What is it . . . ?
Alan Rogers

Introduction

Some readers may understandably be tempted to give this chapter a miss. The world of educational psychology is full of division and uncertainty, and it is not always clear how a consideration of the various learning theories can help us as teachers of adults in the practice of our craft.

Nevertheless, it is always useful to stand back from what we are doing and look at it in terms of general principles. On the one hand, it is surely necessary that the overall theories should be pressed into service to assist concretely the teaching process; there is otherwise little point in all the speculation. This is beginning to happen: although relatively few of those who research into learning processes have devoted time and space to considering the relevance of their studies to the activity of teaching, there is a small but growing interest in the application of this type of theory to practice.

From the point of view of the teacher of adults, then, an examination of theory is important. For how we view learning affects how we teach. Teaching is concerned with the promotion of learning, and we therefore need to understand what it is that we are promoting. In particular, part of our task is to help our adult student participants to 'learn how to learn', or rather to learn how to learn more effectively. To be able to do this properly, we need to be aware of what is involved in the process of learning.

The distinctiveness of adult learning

And here we run immediately into an issue which has been debated widely among educators particularly. For the first question that needs to be addressed is whether the differences which characterise adult learning are so great that they call for a different view of learning from that applicable to younger age groups. The issue is whether the learning — and thus the education built upon it — that occurs throughout the whole of life in both youth and adulthood is essentially the same or whether adult learning — and thus the education of adults — is distinctive. Is there any justification for discussing *adult* education at all or are we just talking about education in general and 'good' (i.e. effective) education in particular?

In many ways this is the most crucial question facing teachers of adults. We have to decide whether we believe that teaching adults is different from teaching children or younger persons or not; whether the same strategies by which we were taught as young people, and which we may already be using in other settings, are appropriate for the groups of adults now under our supervision. It is not just a question as to whether the adult student participant — the mother, the worker on the farm or in the factory,

Alan Rogers: 'The Nature of Learning: What is it . . .?' from *TEACHING ADULTS* (Open University Press, 1996; 2nd edn), pp. 74–93.

shop or office, the trainee or manager, the churchgoer, the local resident, the interested member of the public, the keen sportsman or -woman — whether they all *expect* all education to be the same, whether they expect or wish to be taught in the same way they were taught at school or college. The question is rather how we as teachers of adults see our student participants.

Those who teach adults are divided in their approach to this question. Many — indeed, I think an increasing number — argue that there is only one activity, 'education', and that adult education is essentially the same as teaching younger persons. The education of adults is for them merely one branch of the whole field. But others point out that within this field of education, we already draw distinctions; we distinguish between the various branches in one way or another. The education of primary children, of secondary pupils and of students in further, advanced or higher education all call upon different teaching–learning processes. We may at times use similar methods with all of these groups, but the basic approach in each case is varied. We cannot teach an 18-year-old in the same way as an 8-year-old. We assume that each level of student can cope with distinct learning tasks and that they are motivated to learn most efficiently through the adoption of teaching–learning styles appropriate to the stage of development they have reached.

We have in part then answered the question. Even if there is only one general activity, education, there are variations between groups of learners. The question thus becomes: in what ways does the teaching of adults differ from the teaching of younger students? It is the difference in degree that is at issue.

At the same time, by concentrating on various strategies appropriate to different levels of student learners, taking into account their motivations, their experience, skills of learning and the development of their capabilities, we have immediately created another problem. For we have noticed that adults are enormously varied, far more varied than any school class or college year. Some have much wider ranges of (relevant and irrelevant) experience to draw upon than others; and among those with a wide range of experience, some are apparently more willing and more able to learn from this experience than others (some studies of soldiers returning from active campaigning have shown this). The range of motivations will be very wide indeed. And some adults have been away from education for a long time and in some cases have never developed the range of their formal educational skills greatly, while others have continued to use on a regular basis and in a structured way the talents for learning they have acquired. Do we treat the former like primary and/or secondary pupils and the latter in a more 'advanced' way, using sophisticated techniques of learning and more complex conceptual materials? Or is there a common way in which all adults learn that can form the basis for our adult teaching?

Both of these seem to be true. It is necessary to adapt our methods of teaching adults to the range of educational skills they possess. Those with the least developed skills, either because they never fully mastered them during their initial education or because the formal learning skills they once possessed have fallen into disarray, will need to be helped in building up these skills as well as coping with the task of the moment. Those who are accustomed to learning may often be left with the activity to work at on their own. Both formal and non-formal strategies may be appropriate at different times, with different groups and at different stages of each learning task. But at the same time, there are ways in which the learning processes of adults in general are distinctive, and we will best serve our student participants if we can understand these processes and build our educational programmes upon them.

This is a huge field, fraught with dangers and complexities. Whole books have been written about learning theories or about small parts of one particular theory. The language is often abstruse, and there is no agreement as to the 'true' models; polemics fly. Particularly there is a call by some writers today for a complete transformation of the relations between teacher and taught, and between all members of the learning group (including the teacher) and knowledge, authority and expertise. There is no general consensus yet among adult educationalists, although there are signs of some growing together. To attempt to sum all this up within the compass of two chapters may seem to be courting disaster.

To assist you with finding your way through this section, it may be helpful to set out here its structure. It will look in turn at the following topics:

- what do we mean by 'learning'?
- when do we learn?
- adult learning: the natural 'learning episode';
- why do we learn?
- how do we learn?
- learning styles;
- and finally, the implications of this discussion for the teacher of adults.

What is learning?

In common parlance the word 'learning' carries at least two meanings. There is first a general one of some kind of change, often in knowledge but also in behaviour. 'I met Mr X today and learned that he had lost his job.' 'Today a new bus timetable was introduced. A spokesman for the council said that he believed the public would soon learn to use the new routes.' But there is also a more intense sense of the verb 'to learn' meaning to memorise, learn by heart: 'Take this poem home and learn it.'

We may leave on one side the meaning of the word as 'memorising' and concentrate instead on the 'learning as change' meaning. To say that 'learning is change' is too simple. First, not all change is learning. The changes brought about by ageing or other physical processes can hardly be described as 'learning changes', though they may in their turn bring about learning changes. Secondly, some forms of learning are confirmation rather than changes of existing patterns of knowledge and behaviour. Since the knowledge is more strongly held or the behaviour more intensely engaged in after the learning has taken place, it can still perhaps be said that learning is change, but on these occasions the changes are directed more towards reinforcement than to alteration of patterns of knowledge and behaviour.

Learning as change takes two main forms. There are those more or less automatic responses to new information, perceptions or experiences that result in change; and secondly there are those structured purposeful changes aimed at achieving mastery. There is a difference in meaning between the use of the word in contexts such as: 'He burned his fingers. He learned not to do that again', and 'I had some trouble with the machine but I learned how to manage it.' The second implies both purpose and effort which the first, being unintended and involuntary, lacks.

What we usually mean by 'learning' are those more or less permanent changes brought about voluntarily in one's patterns of acting, thinking and/or feeling. There is a widely held (and even more widely practised) view of learning which says that it is the receipt of knowledge and skills from outside. But recent work on learning indicates that

- learning is active, not the passive receipt of knowledge and skills;

- learning is personal, individual: we can learn from and in association with others, but in the end, all learning changes are made individually;

- learning is voluntary, we do it ourselves; it is not compulsory.

There are then two models of learning, traditional and modern:

Traditional/input	*Modern/action*
passive	active
receipt	search
fill a deficit	seek for satisfaction
responsive to outside stimulus	initiated by inner drive
keywords: 'give, impart'	keywords: 'discover, create'
transfer of knowledge/skills	problem-solving
need for teacher	self-learning

Areas of change (learning domains)

There have been several attempts to describe the different areas of learning change. Many of these are overlaid with philosophical assumptions about human nature and the nature of knowledge that are difficult to test. Sometimes they are seen to be hierarchical — that is, some areas of learning are viewed as being of a higher order than others, though not necessarily dependent on prior learning.

The main and traditional distinction has of course been between learning knowledge and learning skills; but others have elaborated on this. Several have pointed to the need to include the learning of attitudes as a third area of learning. In the field of learning objectives, knowledge, skills and attitudes (KSA) is a well-worn path. Bloom (1965) drew a clear distinction between learning in the cognitive domain and learning in the affective domain. Kurt Lewin (1935) suggested that learning changes occur in skills, in cognitive patterns (knowledge and understanding), in motivation and interest, and in ideology (fundamental beliefs). Gagné (1972) identified five 'domains' of learning:

- *motor skills* which require practice;

- *verbal information* — facts, principles and generalisations which, when organised into larger bodies of information, become knowledge: 'the major requirement for learning and retaining verbal information appears to be its presentation within an organised, meaningful context';

- *intellectual skills* — the skills of using knowledge; those 'discriminations, concepts and rules' that characterise both elementary and more advanced cognitive learning in a way that motor skills and verbal information do not;

- *cognitive strategies* — the way knowledge is used; the way the individual learns, remembers and thinks; the self-managed skills needed to define and solve problems. These require practice and are constantly being refined;

- and *attitudes*.

Learning then takes place in a number of different spheres. We may categorise these using the mnemonic KUSAB:

1. We may learn new *knowledge* as we collect information that is largely memorised.

2. Such knowledge may be held uncomprehendingly. We thus need to learn to relate our new material in ways that lead to new *understanding*, that process of organising and reorganising knowledge to create new patterns of relationships.

3. We may learn new *skills* or develop existing skills further; not just physical skills, our ability to do certain things, but also skills of thinking and of learning, skills of coping and solving problems and survival strategies.

4. Further, since we can learn new knowledge, new understanding and new skills without necessarily changing our attitudes, the learning of *attitudes* is a distinct sphere of learning.

5. Finally, it is possible for learning changes to be brought about in all four of these areas without accompanying alterations in our way of life, our pattern of behaviour. It is therefore necessary to learn to apply our newly learned material to what we do and how we live, to carry out our new learning into changed ways of *behaving*: what some people would call to learn 'wisdom', in short.

The way these five areas of learning change relate to each other is complex. Changes in attitude rely to a large extent on changes in knowledge and understanding, and behavioural changes can hardly take place without accompanying changes in one or more of the other areas. But the relationship between changes in knowledge and attitude or between new knowledge and changed behaviour is idiosyncratic and uncertain. When new knowledge (e.g. 'smoking can damage your health') meets contrary behaviour (the habit of smoking), one of a number of different reactions may occur. The information may be decried, ignored or rejected ('It's all very exaggerated', or 'I know but I don't care'); the new knowledge may be accepted but rationalised away by other knowledge ('Less than 30 per cent of smokers die of cancer caused by smoking and I'll be one of the lucky ones', or 'It is more dangerous to cross the roads than to smoke'); or the new knowledge can be accepted and the way of life adapted to fit in with it. The way any individual reacts to learning changes in any one domain seems to depend on personality and situational factors.

From the teacher's point of view, it is useful to keep the distinctions between these different areas of learning in mind during the preparation of the learning programme. We will find it helpful to ask ourselves whether our teaching is *primarily* in the area of skills or knowledge or understanding or attitudes or behaviour. For this will influence the practices we adopt in the programme of learning. Most of our teaching will cover several different areas of learning, probably all of them. It is doubtful whether they can be kept apart. Nevertheless, while bearing in mind that teaching which concentrates primarily on one of these areas (e.g. skills) inevitably involves learning in other areas (knowledge, understanding, attitudes and behaviour) as well, we need to ask ourselves precisely what sort of learning change we and our student participants are attempting to deal with at this particular stage of the learning programme.

When do we learn?

Learning is not of course confined to the classroom.

It is strange how many people who know a lot about adult education and lifelong learning use language very loosely. They talk about 'motivating people to learn', they urge that we need 'to get people into learning' — by which they mean that they wish to persuade people to come to classes, thereby implying that there is no learning going on outside of the classes. They use the word 'learners' to mean those people who are in the classes, as if those who are not inside their classes are not learners. 'Learning' and 'education' thus very frequently get mixed up. Even experienced adult educators use the term 'lifelong learning' and speak about adult education as existing 'to provide opportunities for lifelong learning' when they really mean 'lifelong education', that the function of adult education is to provide structured programmes of directed learning, often classes, which are open to people of any age. They do not realise that 'lifelong learning' is simply that, learning which goes on more or less all the time without any help from adult educators, that 'opportunities for lifelong learning' exist around us every day and in everything we do. But as we have already seen, there is a distinction to be drawn between learning and education. All education must involve learning; but not all learning is education.

We do therefore need to stress very clearly that learning is quite independent of the classroom. People are learning all the time, whatever they are doing.

Learning is part of living

Learning comes from experience. It is closely related to the way in which individuals develop in relation to their social and physical environment. And since experience is continuous, so too learning is continuous. It occurs throughout life, from start to finish. Nearly everything we do has been learned and is constantly being relearned.

And this means that learning is individual. It is not a collective activity. 'Each individual is processing the experience uniquely for personal use. . . . In learning, the individual is the agent, even though the agent may be subject to the social pressures of the group' (Brookfield, 1983: 1–4). Learning is affected and may even to some extent be controlled by society or other collectives, but the learning activity itself — introducing learning changes — is personal.

Learning desires

Learning, then, is natural, as natural as breathing. It is the continual process of adapting to the various changes which we all face, changes in our social and cultural contexts, changes in our own social roles, the daily tasks we perform, our own personal growth and development.

But it goes deeper than this. Within every individual there is a bundle of learning desires. In part they spring from the drive towards adulthood which we have already seen, the urge towards more maturity, the search for meaning, the drive towards more responsibility and autonomy. In part they spring from half-finished earlier learning activities. In part they spring from our own interests and experiences, an earlier spoken or written word or a glimpse of something having aroused unsatisfied curiosity.

Some of these learning desires are very pressing, arising from or reinforced by urgent matters. But most of them lie dormant, overlaid by more immediate concerns, awaiting either a suitable learning opportunity or an increased sense of need to bring them to life (this is the 'I've always wanted to learn something about this or that' syndrome). For some people, these desires for more learning have been damaged or buried deep by other experiences (often by formal education, especially at secondary levels where discovery learning methods are sometimes less frequently used than at primary level), but they still exist and can in appropriate circumstances be awakened.

Intentional and unintentional learning

Much of our learning — perhaps most of it — is unintended. A good deal is very casual: it comes from chance happenings (roadside posters, snatches of overheard conversation, newspaper reading or television watching, meeting people: 'adventitious learning [which] springs from accidental encounters with unintentional sources' (Lucas, 1983: 2–3). There are however some 'sources of learning' [who] intend learning to take place — through mass campaigns, advertisements, political persuasion, social propaganda, etc. — even though the learner has no intention of engaging in learning.

But beyond this, there are occasions when we engage in some more purposeful learning activity, some structured process of mastering a situation — learning to deal with a new piece of equipment, for instance, or to adjust to new bus timetables or to cope with a new baby. At certain times throughout their lives, all adults will bend their energies and attention to achieving some learning task directed towards a set goal. Some of these occasions may call for formal methods of learning (learning to drive a car is probably the biggest formal programme of teaching adults in many countries) but with most of them we cope more informally (see Figure 1).

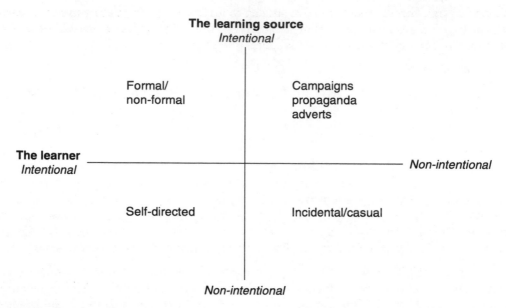

Figure 1   Learning matrix

Learning episodes

Such 'learning episodes', as we may call these intended purposeful learning activities, are usually voluntary and are always purposeful. Some of course come from external requirements: a new task set for us by our employers for, example, or changes in legislation which call for changes in our working practices; learning called for by some of the welcome or unwelcome changes that may come in our personal circumstances, and so on. Many an adult has had to learn about new financial matters through divorce or separation. But the majority are undertaken voluntarily and with some measure of enthusiasm and commitment. And they are always purposeful: they are designed to achieve a particular goal which the learners set for themselves. Learning episodes are therefore distinct from the incidental and unintended learning which characterises the majority of our learning experiences.

Such learning episodes arise from a perceived need or challenge — from those changes in our social relationships, in our occupations (however widely defined that term may be used), in our personal development or in preparation for further learning which we wish to pursue. It is therefore clear that such learning episodes are closely related to the lifespan development of each one of us, however that lifespan development is defined.

Learning objectives or 'clearing up messes'?

These learning episodes are voluntary, intentional, purposeful; the adult learner is seen to be active, struggling with reality, rather than responsive to stimuli. And this would seem to suggest that they are directed by clearly perceived learning objectives.

To some extent, this is true. When we set out to learn to meet some need or to increase our expertise in some field of interest, there will be occasions when we will be able to focus our efforts on defined learning objectives, when we can see what it is that we are trying to achieve. When deciding to learn to drive a car, for example, we can set for ourselves a clear goal, and we can see relatively plainly whether we are making progress towards the achievement of this goal. We can clear our mind of all that will block the way and set out to achieve the mastery we require of ourselves.

But in other cases, the situation is not so clear. Ackoff (1978) (talking about managers) has pointed out that we are often in a more confused situation: we

> 'are not confronted with problems that are independent of each other but with dynamic situations that consist of complex systems of changing problems that interact with each other. I call such situations 'messes'. Problems are extracted from 'messes' by analysis; they are to messes as atoms are to tables and chairs . . . [We] do not solve problems, [we] manage messes.'

This would seem to be particularly true of many learning episodes which we undertake throughout our lives — for example, coping with a new baby. Our task in these cases is not straightforward, simply meeting a need. Rather, it is to unravel a tangle, to sort out a mess.

In these circumstances, how and what we learn depends on how we define the situation we are facing. We analyse the issue, determine what the problem looks like so far as we can see it, and try to solve it. How we do that depends on how much and what kind of experience we can bring to the 'mess'. That will determine the way we look at the problem and the language in which we express it. Learning is a haphazard process of trial and error and we often get it wrong. As Donald Schön puts it in regard to his chosen professionals:

> 'Problems must be constructed from the materials of problematic situations which are puzzling, troubling and uncertain . . . [We] are frequently embroiled in conflicts of values, goals, purposes and interests . . . the effective use of specialised knowledge to well-defined tasks depends on a prior structuring of situations that are complex and uncertain.'

(Schön, 1983)

Learning episodes and the teaching of adults

These structured and purposeful learning episodes may be undertaken by the learners on their own or they may invoke the assistance of some helper. And it is here that they can be seen to be of considerable significance for teachers of adults. For our purpose is to create one or a number of such learning episodes for our adult student participants.

Not only this but, since they are intended and purposeful, these natural learning episodes reveal more about the sort of learning opportunity that we as teachers of adults seek to construct than do the more ubiquitous, haphazard and largely unintentional learning activities that spring from the constant interaction of the individual with the environment. The way adults learn purposefully on their own will tell us much about the way they will learn in our programmes.

Some adult educators are hesitant about using these natural learning episodes as the basis for building a theory of adult learning. They point out that each of us engages with the environment in ways limited by our experience and existing learning abilities, and that this social environment itself controls our learning. They suggest that what is needed is to break free from such restraints. Nevertheless, these episodes show us something of the way adults learn and the special features of adult learning as distinct from the processes of schooling. They can form a guide as we construct learning opportunities for those who come to our programmes.

Characteristics of learning episodes

There are three characteristics about these self-directed learning activities that are relevant to our discussion.

First, *they are usually episodic in character, not continuous*. They come in short bursts of relatively intensive activity, absorbing the attention, and they usually come to an end as soon as the immediate purpose has been felt to be achieved. There are some, particularly in the self-fulfilment area, that spring from long-term interests (gardening, for instance, or following trends in modern or classical music); but even within these overall patterns of persistent learning, there come more intensive short-term episodes of learning directed towards the achievement of some immediate goal. We cannot keep this sort of pressure up for long; we need to be motivated by an achievable purpose; and when that is over, there may come a rest or a slower pace of learning before the next episode occurs. (How far this episodic character is part of our way of life in a modern Western society rather than an inherent adult process is not clear, but it would seem to be of more general application than confined to just one form of social structure and culture.)

Secondly, *the goal that is set is usually some concrete task, some immediate problem that seems important*. Such learning episodes, self-directed or otherwise, are in general aimed at the solution of a particular problem. The situations they are designed to meet are concrete rather than theoretical. We need to decorate this room, to master the relationship between these stamps, to cope with this particular change in the family circle, to understand a new procedure at home or at work, and so on. Even when the learning is part of a long-term and developing interest (chess, say, or cooking), the individual episode of learning is directed towards a particular goal to be achieved.

There are several implications flowing from this:

* We do not on the whole approach any situation academically. To decorate a room, we do not study design as such. To cope with a family issue, we do not take a course on interpersonal relations or psychology — although we might well consult books on the subject. We are not concerned so much with a subject as to resolve a one-off concrete situation.

* This means that the learning task is rarely pursued in a systematic way. It is limited learning, limited to the task in hand. Adult learners do not often pull down

a textbook and start at the beginning, with a general introduction to the field of study, nor do they pursue it from A to Z in sequence to the end. It is only with those who have had extensive experience of formal education, who have developed and maintained advanced study skills, that a systematic exploration of a field of knowledge becomes at all common. This is a replication in private of the formal systems of learning that characterise schooling and is thus confined to relatively few, and to a few occasions in their lives. They too will also engage in the more limited goal-oriented episodes of learning at other times. Most of us most of the time use only those parts of any subject that help us to meet our immediate task.

- The learners do not start with the simple and move on to the more difficult. They tackle the problem with which they have to deal at the level at which it occurs in their lives. They cope with quite difficult language and terms from the start so long as these are of direct relevance to the learning process.

- The learners do not on the whole draw on compartmentalised knowledge such as was learned at school, history separated from geography or maths from physics. They bring all that they know from all sorts of fields to bear upon the particular instance. Such an academic compartmentalised approach may occur on occasion, especially in the self-directed learning activities [noted above]; but even here there is often a particular need to be met that leads to the use of knowledge from different fields of study rather than a restricted compartmentalised approach to knowledge.

- Such episodes are aimed at immediate rather than future application. There are, it is true, some learning episodes which are intended as a preparation before embarking on a course of action: religious preparation classes, pre-marriage groups, holiday language courses, pre-retirement programmes are examples of these. But on the whole, most learning episodes are undertaken in the process of doing a particular task or meeting a situation. The material, as it is mastered, is applied at once. We learn how to use a new washing machine by using it; we learn a new bus timetable as we use the service; we learn how to cope with a baby by coping with a baby.

Thirdly, since most of these learning episodes are directed towards specific goals, *there is relatively little interest in overall principles.* Few attempts are made by the learner to draw general conclusions from the particular instance being learned. Once the immediate situation has been resolved, the goal attained or the problem solved, the adult learner normally brings the process of investigation to a close, storing away the learning gained for another day. What is stored is the way to cope with the particular situation, not general principles. Learning to use a new washing machine will be concentrated on the specific instrument in hand, not on washing machines in general. The learning needed to cope with a new bus timetable will deal not with the entire transport system but with the one or two routes needed to make a particular journey. Learning a new craft or industrial technique will be confined to what is needed for the moment, not to wider applications. All of these situations may arouse in our minds wider issues of obsolescence and modern technology, or public and private transport provision or the demands of new processes as a whole; but these will occur mainly as spasmodic thoughts and grumbles, usually quickly pushed away and forgotten. The efforts are centred on the immediate and the particular, not on the long-term and the general.

Why do we engage in these learning episodes?

There is a very large literature which suggests that all learning (certainly all purposeful learning) comes from a sense of need.

> 'Learning is something which takes place within the learner and is personal to him [*sic*]; it is an essential part of his development, for it is always the whole person who is learning. Learning takes place when an individual feels a need, puts forth an effort to meet that need, and experiences satisfaction with the result of his effort.'
>
> (Leagans, 1971)

There is much truth in this, and the awakening of a sense of need has been identified by most writers on adult learning as a precondition of effective learning. But we have to tread carefully here. Not all purposeful learning comes from a sense of need; some for example comes from an increased interest.

'Needs', then, is a dangerous concept in adult education. It often leads to an assumption that 'I know what you need to learn even though you don't know what you need.' 'Needs' are externally identified; 'wants' are internally identified. Purposeful adult learning, the kind of voluntary learning episodes we have been talking about above, come from identified wants rather than externally set needs. It is a search for satisfaction in some sense or other.

Motivation and learning

Much has been written about motivation in relation to the education and training of adults. In many forms of adult education and extension in developing countries, it forms the keystone of the training programme. But in the West, rather less consideration has been given to it in practice. In most forms of adult education (except perhaps those industrial and professional development programmes where some of the participants may be seen to be reluctant participants), we tend to rely on the fact that adult student learners come to us of their own free will, that they are already interested in the subject, that they are already motivated to learn. We forget that initial motivation to learn may be weak and can die; alternatively that it can be strengthened and directed into new channels. This is the task of the teacher of adults — and as such we need to understand motivation.

Motivation is usually defined as those factors that energise and direct behavioural patterns organised around a goal. It is frequently seen as a force within the individual that moves him or her to act in a certain way. Motivation in learning is that compulsion which keeps a person within the learning situation and encourages him or her to learn.

Motivation is seen as being dependent on either *intrinsic* or *extrinsic* factors. Extrinsic factors consist of those external incentives or pressures such as attendance requirements, external punishments or examinations to which many learners in formal settings are subjected. These, if internalised, create an intention to engage in the learning programme. Intrinsic factors consist of that series of inner pressures and/or rational decisions which create a desire for learning changes.

Most adult learning episodes are already dependent on intrinsic motivational factors; but not all of them are. It has been argued that intrinsic factors are stronger and more enduring than extrinsic factors. But even within intrinsic motivation, there is a hierarchy of factors. For example, a desire to please some other person or loyalty to a group which may keep a person within a learning programme even when bored with the subject are seen as intrinsic motives of a lower order than a desire to complete a particular task in itself.

There are three main groups of ideas behind the development of a theory of motivation. The first says that motivation is an inner drive to fulfil various needs. The second says that motivation can be learned. And the third claims that motivation relates to goals set or accepted by oneself.

Needs-related motivation

Many people see motivation as internal urges and drives based on needs. All individuals vary in the composition of these needs and their intensity. At their simplest instinctual level, they may be the avoidance of pain and the search for pleasure, or the Freudian drives related to life, death, sex and aggression; but all such instincts can be modified by learning.

Most theorists see a motive as a learned drive directed towards a goal, often regarded as a search for the reduction of tension or conflict. Boshier (1989) and others see this as having two main dimensions: the reduction in inner conflicts between different parts of the self and different experiences (intra-resolution); and the reduction of conflicts and tensions between the self and the external social and physical environment (extra-resolution). The individual is seeking for harmony, for peace. Such directed drives may be aroused and sustained, as we have seen, by incentives (external factors) and by goals set or accepted by the individual (internal factors).

Some writers have distinguished between needs (seen to be physical) and drives (psychological). More often however the distinction is drawn between primary needs (viscerogenic, related to bodily functions) and secondary needs (psychogenic). The latter come into play only when primary needs are to a large extent met.

Two major writers, Carl Rogers (1974) and Abraham Maslow (1968), have helped us to see learning as the main process of meeting the compulsions of inner urges and drives rather than responding to stimuli or meeting the demands of new knowledge. Whether viewed as goal-seeking (based on limited and specific goals set by themselves) or ideal-seeking (related to objectives set by the value system the learners have come to accept and hold), both argue that the learner is impelled to seek out learning changes from within rather than by outside imperatives. Rogers viewed this as a series of drives towards adulthood — autonomy, responsibility, self-direction — though it is now clear that the precise forms which such drives take are culturally bound, varying from society to society. Maslow concentrated on the urge to satisfy in part or in whole a hierarchy of needs.

Abraham Maslow is recognised as the apostle of the 'needs' school of thought. He distinguished basic drives from temporary needs, and established a hierarchy which is often quoted (Figure 2); and he developed a theory of 'pre-potency' — that one need must be largely satisfied before the next need can come into full play.

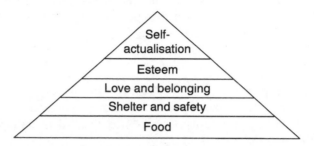

Figure 2   Maslow's hierarchy of needs

Maslow argued that all people are driven through the first four stages of basic needs. As each lower need is in part met, the next higher level of need is triggered. Several levels of need can be in operation at the same time. The highest level of need, self-actualisation, may not be reached by some individuals on more than an occasional basis. This level consists of a need to create, to appreciate, to know and to understand. (Maslow indicated in his teaching a further level of need above self-actualisation: self-transcendence, a need to express tangibly concern for others, but this hardly appears in his writings.)

Maslow's concern for self-actualisation accounts for the increasing popularity of the many adult education programmes of today designed to enhance the students' understanding of the 'self' — programmes like learner-generated 'life histories' or autobiographies, and the programmes of creative writing aimed at increasing self-confidence and self-expression.

From the point of view of the teacher of adults, Maslow's work will be a reminder that within any group of adult learners there will be a wide variety of needs, and within each individual student participant there will be a different mixture of needs. This mixture will be constantly changing as the learning proceeds and as the individual's life situation changes. This is why predetermined and uniform learning outcomes can never be achieved in adult learning programmes, why each adult learner will take away from any learning situation what he or she will require, why adult learning is unique to each learner and uncertain.

But Maslow's hierarchy of needs fails us as adult educators precisely at the point we need it most. It offers us an analysis of the *preconditions* to the type of learning we are most interested in: the self-evident truth that the prior personal and social needs (food, security, personal relationships and a sense of esteem) must be satisfied, at least in part, before motivation for the more creative, evaluative and self-fulfilling kinds of learning will be aroused. But it also reminds us that when some of our student participants come to our programmes from a desire for social relationships or to gain some sense of esteem, as many do, they are being driven by needs that must be met at least partially before further learning can take place.

Maslow also suggests that if the lower levels of needs are satisfied in part, the motivation to self-actualisation will be automatically triggered because it is inherent within each person. If it is not so triggered, this is because one of the lower levels of need has been inadequately met. This is by no means certain: and in any case, it does not explain the motivation towards different forms of self-actualisation which occurs between individuals.

To explain this, we need to turn to other work on motivation. We have already noted Carl Rogers's view of the drive towards adulthood — towards maturity and autonomy. Houle (1961) sees motivation as more complex, as being related to the goal-orientation or process-orientation or subject-orientation that comprises the inherent learning drives of the individual. A different picture is that of a spectrum consisting at one end of those who are 'high-achievement oriented' (not just ambitious, though it includes them: this group embraces those who seek to play chess or do crosswords or make bread or breed pigeons better than their neighbours) and at the other end those who are anxious about failure. The former experience has been called an 'approach motivation', a drive towards engaging in some activity or other, while the latter experience an 'avoidance motivation'. Success encourages the former, and failure does not put them off easily, it can become a further challenge; whereas both success (generally regarded as a 'flash in a pan' that will not necessarily be repeated) and failure alike encourage the latter to withdraw.

The danger with this — as with so many such schemes of categorisation — is that of assigning individual student learners to particular categories; for such 'personality types' can themselves become a hindrance to learning, a demotivaton. The very designation itself may prescribe the way in which people will behave and will certainly determine the way we view other people. There is some value in knowing that such factors are at work; but they are not determinants but explanations of what is happening.

Learned motivation

Such achievement orientation suggests that motivation can be learned. It is thus seen by some as the fruit of the reward-and-punishment systems that people have been exposed to during the course of their prior development. If this is true, then perhaps motivation may be altered by a new system of approvals and disapprovals, by specific training activities accompanied by a change of the learning environment to emphasise achievement rather than failure. Exactly what the factors are that lead to motivation being learned is not clear. Stimulus–response theories may help here; success and pleasure in early educational experiences seem to play a part. It is pointed out, for example, how many of those who liked their schooling and were a success in educational environments return to participate in adult education activities of both a formal and non-formal kind, while although others use the lack of education to rationalise their lack of success, relatively few are motivated by this lack to return to education. But the issues remain unclear.

Motivation and goals

The third group of ideas centre themselves round the concept that motivation is related to the goals set and accepted by the participants for themselves. It has been noted that motivation is highest among those who are most concerned with the process involved, who are satisfying their goals in each task, whereas those who have their sights set on goals which are further away (to pass an examination or to get a better job after the course is over) have a lower level of motivation. Motivation then seems to be related to the nearness of achieving the desired goal.

The importance of this to the teacher is that the student participants need to see clearly the immediate goals, to accept them for themselves, to believe them to be achievable and to be able to see some progress towards their attainment, if their motivation to learn is to be kept at the highest possible level. But there is a further factor here: confidence. Individuals will be more positively motivated if they are confident that they can not only cope with the learning situation but alter it to meet their own needs.

The learning situation

For it is important for us to realise that motivation relates as much to the situation in which the learning episode is taking place as to the individual. So far most of the theories of motivation have regarded the learner as a person divorced from any particular setting. But all learning is located within a particular time and place; and we know from the work of Herzberg (1972) and others that this setting influences motivation as much as the internal drives and avoidances.

Herzberg's work related to industrial activities; but it is of direct relevance to learning. He developed the concept of 'motivators' and what he called 'hygiene' factors (demotivators). He saw 'motivators' as those factors which make the participants 'feel good' about their work — a sense of achievement, recognition, responsibility, advancement and personal growth. Most of these are internal factors; and when they are present, the participants have a positive attitude towards their tasks. These feelings however are not on the whole long-lasting, they need to be continually reinforced. But they spring directly from the work in hand.

In contrast, the 'hygiene' factors that create a sense of dissatisfaction normally spring from external factors in the context of the activity — from inappropnate direction or methods, inadequate working conditions, unsatisfactory relationships within the group and so on. These tend to be longer-lasting in their nature.

These two sets of factors are not the plus and minus of the motivational situation. The presence of motivators and the reduction of hygiene factors are both necessary to achieve positive motivation. Removing the hygiene factors alone without increasing the presence of motivators will not help the task, and similarly strengthening the motivators without removing the demotivators will not increase effectiveness.

It is thus clear that motivation factors in learning lie as much within the learning situation as within the individual student participants themselves. In this context, the teacher of adults plays a vital role. Motivation is as often in the eye of the beholder as is beauty. We need to be reminded of McGregor's Theory X and Theory Y: that the teacher may assume that all learners have an inherent dislike of work and will avoid it if they can (Theory X), that they wish to escape from responsibility, that they have a static range of abilities that nothing within the learning situation will improve, that it is the function of the teacher to direct them to the work of learning (McGregor, 1960).

Theory X	*Theory Y*
The average human being has an inherent dislike of work and will avoid it if he/she can.	The expenditure of physical and mental effort in work is as natural as play and rest.
Because of this, most people need to be coerced, controlled, directed and threatened with punishment to get them to put enough effort to contribute to organisational goals.	External control and threats of punishment are not the only means to encourage them to make an effort to contribute to organisational goals. People will engage in self-direction and self-control to achieve objectives to which they are committed through the rewards which the achievement itself brings.
The average person prefers to be directed, wishes to avoid any responsibility, has relatively little ambition, and wants security above all.	The average person, under the right conditions, learns not only to accept but to seek responsibility. The capacity to exercise a fairly high degree of imagination, ingenuity and creativity in the solution of organisational problems is widely, not narrowly, distributed. In most societies, the intellectual potential of the average person is not fully utilised.

In this case, in the way of all self-fulfilling prophecies, we as teachers become part of the extrinsic factors influencing motivation; we become a hygiene factor ourselves, a demotivator. Or (Theory Y) we can assume that learning changes are natural to all human beings and certainly are the expressed desire of our student-learners; that they are willing to accept responsibility for their own learning; that it is external factors such as the educational system itself and the existing patterns of work in society rather than internal factors that are inhibiting the student participants from exercising their imagination, creativity and ingenuity; that all students are capable of breaking out. In this case, the teacher will become a 'motivator' in the learning environment.

Motivation then depends as much on the attitudes of the teacher as on the attitudes of the students.

The implication of all of this for the teacher of adults is varied. Although it is useful to look at needs and at other views of initial motivation, it is probably best for the teacher not to rely solely on this original impetus but to seek to build up new kinds of drive in relation to the subject-matter itself. An emphasis on the extrinsic factors of motivation rather than the intrinsic will not lead to a durable level of motivation towards achieving the learning task. Although many adults are motivated by such concerns, it would seem that, particularly for adults, a stress on attendance, examinations and discipline is not an appropriate way to heighten or build new forms of motivation, although other forms of incentive may be helpful in some circumstances.

Further reading

Belbin E, Belbin R M (1972) *Problems in Adult Retraining*. Heinemann, London.

Bloom B S (1965) *Taxonomy of Educational Objectives*. Longman, London.

Gagné R M (1972) Domains of Learning, *Interchange* 3(1): 1–8.

Gagné R M (1975) *The Conditions of Learning*. Holt, Rinehart and Winston, New York.

Habermas, J. (1978) *Knowledge and Human Interest*. Heinemann, London.

Lenz E (1982) *The Art of Teaching Adults*. Holt, Rinehart and Winston, New York.

Lovell R B (1980) *Adult Learning*. Croom Helm, Beckenham.

Maslow A H (1968) *Towards a Psychology of Being*. Van Nostrand, New York.

Rogers A (1992) *Adults Learning for Development*. Cassell, London, and Education for Development, Reading.

Rogers A (1993) Adult learning maps and the teaching process. *Studies in the Education of Adults*, 22(2): 199–220.

Schön D A (1983) *The Reflective Practitioner: How Professionals Think in Action*. Basic Books, New York.

Smith R M (1983) *Helping Adults Learn How to Learn*. Jossey Bass, San Francisco, CA.

Smith R M (1984) *Learning How to Learn: Applied Theory For Adults*. Open University Press, Milton Keynes.

Squires G (1987) *The Curriculum Beyond School*. Hodder and Stoughton, London.

15. Recent Cognitive Perspectives on Learning — Implications for Nurse Education

Janelle Cust

Nurse educators must keep abreast of contemporary learning theory so that their teaching reflects current ideas of best practice. In view of this, it is important to report on recent developments in the field of learning. Of particular significance is the fact that behaviouristic explanations of learning have largely been replaced with cognitive perspectives which emphasise the complexity of the learning process. Memory, learning, problem solving and expertise have all been investigated from a cognitive stance. The highlights of this work include, firstly, the portrayal of learning as an active, constructivist, cumulative and self-regulated process leading to the development of understanding and complex, skilled performance. Secondly, the highly important role played by knowledge in learning has been identified and described. Lastly, novice–expert differences in problem solving and academic and practical performance more generally are well understood as a result of investigations of expertise in many domains. In this paper, these three significant perspectives from cognitive psychology will be examined and their implications for the education of undergraduate nurses described. Developements in the field of nursing that reflect or challenge a cognitive outlook are also identified.

Introduction

Contemporary cognitive psychologists are a diverse group of researchers whose wide-ranging interests include memory, learning, problem solving and expertise and, increasingly, the instructional process (Gagné, 1985; Resnick, 1989; Thomas, 1988). Many adopt an information processing framework. Here, the computer is a metaphor for the mind and the focus is on the way information is acquired, stored, retrieved and used (Siegler, 1983). Computer models of learning have been developed by some (Clancy, 1988). Insights from cognitive psychology are important among those that inform current learning theory (Prosser & Trigwell, 1993).

The shift from behaviourism to a cognitive framework occurred gradually but was particularly marked in the 1960s and 1970s (Shuell, 1986). Behaviourists disregard mental activity and view learning as a response to the external environment in which behaviours are built up through contiguity, repetition and reinforcement. Although cognitive theorists acknowledge the role of these mechanisms in relation to simple forms of learning, they stress the part that thinking processes play in complex human performance. Much of their work, therefore, has examined the complicated mental events that characterise the process of learning. Learning is depicted as an active,

Janelle Cust: 'Recent Cognitive Perspectives on Learning — Implications for Nurse Education' in *NURSE EDUCATION TODAY* (1995), 15(4), pp. 280–290. Reprinted by permission of the publisher Churchill Livingstone.

constructivist process in which learners strive for understanding and competence on the basis of their personal experience. Moreover, cognitive theorists have demonstrated that successful learning is dependent on the interaction of learning and knowledge, including the knowledge that constitutes the task as well as the student's background knowledge (Glaser, 1984). Finally, in contrast to the behaviourists who equate successful learning with behavioural change, cognitive theorists regard the outcomes of successful learning as understanding and skilful performance.

In this paper, three significant themes from the literature on cognitive psychology are examined and the implications for the education of nurses outlined. The themes explored are the nature of constructivist learning, the role of knowledge in learning and the characteristics of expertise. Viewpoints from the nursing literature that reflect or challenge the cognitive perspectives are also identified.

The nature of constructivist learning

Cognitive psychologists and educators regard learning as a constructivist process in which the learner actively seeks and constructs information on the basis of past knowledge and experience (Shuell, 1986). It is based on the premise that human beings act upon the environment rather than simply respond to it, as the behaviourists would have it. The conventional view of the learner passively receiving and recording transmitted information, therefore, has been replaced with an image of the learner as a purposeful agent extracting and imposing meaning. Such a view of learning is not new, stemming as it does from various traditions. Among these were the Gestalt theories of perception, the British psychologist Bartlett's pioneering work in the 1930s on memory, and theories of cognitive development like Piaget's innovative work (Paris & Byrnes, 1989). In this section, what successful learners do when they construct knowledge in their search for understanding will be identified in terms of interdependent cognitive, motivational and metacognitive factors.

Cognition

The cognitive component of constructivist learning has been described in terms of overlapping 'active', 'constructive' and 'cumulative' features (Shuell, 1986). Thus information cannot be absorbed from the teacher or from textbooks, rather, the learner must encounter knowledge in *active* and effortful ways. Deeply processing ideas ensures that they are well remembered (Craik & Lockhart, 1979). As well as being depicted as mentally vigorous, cognitive theorists describe learning as *constructivist* since old knowledge is always revised, reorganised and even reinterpreted in order to reconcile it with new input (cf. Piaget's (1952) assimilation and accommodation processes) (Spiro, 1977). Making such links guarantees that learning will be meaningful and not simply rote. Furthermore, since new knowledge always builds on and makes use of previous information, the learning process is described as highly *cumulative*. Those, then, with substantial background knowledge in relation to a task, will learn more rapidly and efficiently.

Weinstein & Mayer (1985) have developed a useful taxonomy of learning strategies that typify the active processing of information as described above. Included in the taxonomy are rehearsal (copying, underlining), organisation (outlining, drawing a mind map), elaboration (generating examples, finding an analogy, linking ideas), comprehension monitoring (checking for understanding, self-questioning) and affective strategies (relaxing, reducing distractions). Apparently many students do not adopt these strategies when learning. For example, research on adult reading and studying of textbooks, an activity of major importance in professional education, has demonstrated how in efficient adults are in monitoring their reading (Pressley & Ghatala, 1990). Is it feasible, then, to attempt to teach nursing students learning strategies? Where study skills programs incorporating learning strategies have been offered as adjuncts to the student's academic program, the results in terms of long-term impact and transferability to relevant subject matter have been inconclusive (Dansereau, 1985; Gibbs, 1977; Martin & Ramsden, 1987). There is even evidence of training programs being counter-productive (Ramsden *et al.* 1987).

There does seem to be a case, however, for teaching and cueing learning strategies in relation to specific nursing content (Segal *et al.* 1985). While effective teachers typically employ many of the strategies outlined as instructional tools (they evoke an apt metaphor when a difficult concept is introduced, ask for implications arising from an issue and refer to time management skills when an assignment is given), here the emphasis is on teaching students themselves to adopt appropriate strategies as they learn. They can be prompted to think of an analogy, relate material in one course to another, create a topic network and develop questions from their reading, all in conjunction with relevant subject matter. They may also benefit from structured learning activities incorporating note-taking, textbook reading and essay writing at appropriate junctures (Gibbs, 1977).

Modelling is a powerful technique for illustrating strategic learning. For example, teachers can make overt or 'visible' thought and skill processes while solving a problem, constructing an argument, wrestling with disciplinary dilemmas and performing clinical behaviours. Another modelling format involves supplying completed examples of work which demonstrate and annotate correct strategy use such as a problem solved, a nursing care plan or a completed essay (Chi & Bassok, 1989; Dansereau, 1985). These exemplars can be beneficial aids in providing explicit, expert guidance for students prior to undertaking tasks. They can also be made available to students once they have completed a task in order to offer feedback by comparison with their own performance.

Motivation

Important as the cognitive processes are to constructivist learning, it is inconceivable that students will encounter ideas actively, process them deeply and sustain their academic endeavour unless they are motivated to do so. There are numerous theoretical explanations of the complex motivation process (Weiner, 1990). Classical constructivist theorists, Piaget (1952) for example, have asserted that motivation is intrinsic to human learning, requiring no special formulations to account for it. Humans have an innate propensity to seek knowledge about their world; learning naturally incorporates motivation.

Other cognitive psychologists have proposed special constructs to account for motivation. Bandura (1986, 1989), for example, has described two mechanisms, self-efficacy (perceptions of competence) and personal agency (perceptions of control), that reciprocally influence one another. Self-efficacy belief, or judgements about one's competence in particular tasks, influence what academic tasks students attempt, the kind and amount of studying they do and the proficiencies they acquire. In turn, exercising personal control in studying and learning strengthens beliefs about one's capabilities. Weiner's (1979) attribution theory has also been influential. This theory assumes that what motivates student behaviour are the attributions or explanations students give for their successes and failures. These attributions, which include luck, ability, effort and task difficulty, differentially influence students' motivation and performance. In terms of self-efficacy and attribution theories, successful students will be those who regard themselves as competent and in control and who generally attribute their successes and failures to their own efforts. Although difficult to engender, appropriate academic motivation appears to be influenced by the following: subject matter that is relevant and appropriately challenging; teaching that is enthusiastic and supportive; frequent informative and encouraging feedback; grading that is non-competitive and criterion-referenced and opportunities for self-management and a degree of ownership of work (Watkins, 1984; Fransson, 1977; Thomas, 1988).

Metacognition

A third characteristic of constructivist learning has been referred to as metacognition. An imprecise term, it is usually regarded as an executive capacity with two components: knowledge of cognition and regulation of cognition (Brown, Bransford, Ferrara & Campione, 1983). Various sub-processes are thought to be involved in metacognition including what one knows, predicting the outcome of one's performance, planning ahead, efficiently scheduling time and cognitive resources, and monitoring and revising one's efforts to learn (Brown, 1978). Capable students take charge of their learning by reflecting on and controlling what they do. They are intellectually curious and resourceful, they analyse their thinking and learn from their errors, and they persist in the face of difficulties. There has been growing recognition that metacognition is an important factor in academic achievement including higher order intellectual behaviour such as problem solving, decision making and critical thinking (Resnick, 1987; Swanson, 1990).

While metacognitive awareness and self-regulation seem to be spontaneously adopted by skilful students, less able students appear to lack self-awareness and fail to monitor their progress (Chi & Bassok, 1989; Pressley & Ghatala, 1990). Metacognitive awareness involving reflection on activities that are usually performed mindlessly enables students to learn from experience and to apply the learning in new situations. A range of metacognitive awareness activities have been implemented in course and clinical work for nursing and other tertiary students to expose and examine what students know and feel about ideas and learning experiences. Examples of these activities include keeping journals and other writing tasks, discussing work with a partner, group dialogue in which ideas are explained and views defended, reflective partnerships during clinical practice and teaching others (Boud *et al.* 1985; Emden, 1991). As students articulate their thoughts through these activities, ideas and feelings are clarified, gaps and discrepancies in knowledge become evident and knowledge develops and changes.

The twin aspect of metacognition, control of cognition or self-regulation, is the ability to plan, organise, monitor, evaluate and modify one's own performance. In traditional adult education programs the expectation has been that students will develop self-regulation as they apply themselves to academic study and to assignments. However, many educators, including nurse educators, have recognised that self-direction is more likely when students are involved in activities such as learning contracts, problem-based learning, collaborative tasks and self-assessment (Barrows & Tamblyn, 1980; Heron, 1988; Thompkins & McGraw, 1988). By structuring the learning environment in these ways, educators have attempted to promote a purposeful and high level of cognitive engagement in learning. There is some evidence of the success of these activities (Caffarella, 1983; Dart & Clarke, 1991; Newble & Clarke, 1987). For example, in their investigation of students' reports of their approaches to studying in problem-based and conventional medical curricula, Newble & Clarke (1987) found deep processing was strongly linked to the problem-based program. It is a fact, nevertheless, that some students respond passively even when opportunities are provided for self-direction, which serves to highlight the complexity of this behaviour (Dart & Clarke, 1991).

But what is understanding?

For cognitive theorists, understanding is regarded as the outcome of constructivist learning. However, while cognitive theorists have paid much attention to mental structures and processes, they have failed to address, in any direct way, what it is to understand (Unger *et al.* 1993). A conception of understanding that has emerged proposes a 'performance' view of understanding. Here, understanding consists of performing (as an academic, nurse, teacher, athlete) flexibly and creatively in new situations. Thus, in academic learning, understanding is evident when students operate on knowledge in various ways such as explaining, giving examples, drawing out implications, developing an argument, gathering and weighing evidence, solving a problem, considering alternative viewpoints and critiquing ideas (Unger *et al.* 1993). In other words, understanding in relation to academic learning is manifested whenever learners engage in 'thought performances' that extend the information given. Merely reproducing information provides no evidence of understanding. Understanding can be promoted and demonstrated then, when students engage in a range of 'understanding performances' in relation to each topic (or problem).

The role of knowledge in learning

The critical role played by knowledge in the learning process has been elucidated by the cognitive theorists. Both the student's background knowledge and the knowledge that characterises the learning task are implicated.

Prior knowledge

In constructivist explanations of learning, new knowledge is always built on the basis of previous experience and ideas. Prior knowledge, therefore, plays a crucial role in learning, for events are comprehended not simply in relation to incoming information

149

from the environment, but also in terms of information stored in long-term memory. Many studies have revealed the impact of existing knowledge on learning (Bransford & Johnson, 1972; Dooling & Lachman, 1971; Glaser, 1984).

The construct of 'schema' has been a useful one to conceptualise prior knowledge. Schemata are coherent knowledge structures that are stored in the memory. They arise from, and mentally represent, frequently experienced situations such as those pertaining to recognising people, executing a tennis stroke, visiting the doctor, remembering the route to work, understanding the nature of a theory and reading a textbook. These contextually-based mental entities profoundly influence all aspects of learning including perception, comprehension, memory, reasoning and problem solving (Rumelhart & Ortony, 1977). Consider, for example, the sentence 'The notes were sour because the seam split' (Bransford & McCarrell, 1974, p. 222). Without the clue 'bagpipe' and therefore a schema for 'bagpipe playing', the sentence is likely to be meaningless. In other words, the absence of relevant prior knowledge impedes comprehension. Conversely, the presence of schemata create automatic expectations regarding what events to anticipate when entering hospital, attending an academic meeting, or going to the theatre. Similarly, the schemata that nursing students possess of self, nursing, knowledge, learning and teaching will strongly influence their interpretation and experience of the curriculum.

Prior knowledge not only facilitates learning by allowing the learner to make sense of ideas and events, it also accounts for misconception effects when information is screened through schemata that are incomplete or incorrect. Studies in science and many other theoretical fields have revealed the prevalence of misconceptions and the difficulty of eradicating them (Chinn & Brewer, 1993). An example of a misconception held by nursing students entering their undergraduate program was documented by Higgins (1989). The students were found to possess a narrow, medically focussed conception of nursing which was likely to undermine the achievement of the program's wider aims and objectives.

Other misconceptions which have an impact on the way students interpret and tackle generic academic learning tasks have been identified including faulty notions of knowledge, learning and essay-writing. Here the concept of knowledge has been understood as facts which are objective and indisputable rather than as useful, constructed information which is subject to revision. Perry (1970) suggests that a limited view of knowledge is often responsible for student learning difficulties. The idea of learning has been conceptualised not as a process of developing understanding and interpreting reality, but as a process of memorising information (Marton & Saljo, 1984). When a limited understanding of the idea of learning is held, a surface approach is adopted and superficial outcomes result (Van Rossum & Schenk, 1984). The schema of an essay held by some students is of a descriptive, knowledge-telling narrative rather than an account concerned with knowledge-transformation in which development of a viewpoint or construction of an argument are featured (Flower, 1979; Hounsell, 1984). These frequent misconceptions related to academic learning as well as ones that are common in the nursing domain seem worthy of being addressed in undergraduate nursing programs.

There are several teaching principles suggested by the studies of schemata and misconceptions. The first imperative when teaching is to identify what students know about topics, concepts and issues as well as discovering how that knowledge is organised. Existing knowledge can then be built upon. Various techniques have been developed to tap students' preconceptions as well as to capture the overall organisation of a body of knowledge (Bihl-Hulme, 1985; Naveh-Benjamin *et al.* 1986; West & Pines, 1985). Secondly, new knowledge must be linked to past ideas and experiences, for example, by means of advance organisers or by revising, comparing and contrasting relevant older ideas (Ausubel, 1960; Alverman & Hynd, 1989). Thirdly, teachers can provide schemata that act as higher-level organising structures to aid learning, including schemata for essay writing (Hayes & Flower, 1980), scientific research (journal) reports (Barnett, 1984), scientific theories (Brooks & Dansereau, 1983) and scientific text (Cook & Mayer, 1988) (cf. nursing models). Finally, identified misconceptions must be challenged by encouraging the airing and full discussion of alternative viewpoints, and in the case of stubbornly held convictions, confronting students with convincing anomalous information since misconceptions can be very resistant to change (Champagne *et al.* 1985; Roth & Anderson, 1988; Svensson & Hogfors, 1988).

Task knowledge: declarative, procedural and conditional knowledge

Influenced by the work of computer scientists who had to consider knowledge in the form of both data bases and operations required to access those bases, information processing theorists adopted the distinction between declarative and procedural knowledge (Anderson, 1976). This distinction is a helpful one for teachers since the learning conditions for each type of knowledge differ considerably (Gagné, 1985). However, replacement of this global categorisation with a precise analysis of fundamental nursing tasks in terms of constituent knowledge and skills could be a most useful undertaking.

Declarative knowledge

Declarative or propositional knowledge (knowing that) consists of concepts, facts, propositions and theories which are acquired, not through direct action with the world, but through comprehension of verbal and written material. It has been proposed that such knowledge, once abstracted, resides in mental structures called semantic networks — organised webs consisting of ideas and their relationships (Tulving & Donaldson, 1979). Propositional knowledge has long dominated educational curricula. By means of lectures, demonstrations and textbooks this symbolic and codified information is conveyed with the intention that students will acquire and apply the theoretical ideas in order to extend their understanding of issues and to solve problems in the real world.

The concepts, principles and theories that constitute declarative knowledge provide knowledge that would otherwise have to be acquired through prolonged experience. However, because it is not directly experienced, this abstract information can be difficult to learn. To make complex academic information more meaningful, cognitive psychologists have advocated the use of representations such as metaphors, analogies and mental models. Metaphors, for example, provide vivid depictions that link familiar and unfamiliar ideas. The heart has been represented as a pump, the immune system as an army defending territory and nurses as angels, handmaidens and sergeant majors. Mental models, of complex scientific material, for instance, enable students to construct their own coherent representations of difficult subject matter resulting in improved retention and transferability (Mayer, 1989). Methodologies for transforming knowledge to make it more accessible are widely used by experienced teachers and include ones that are verbal (narration, examples, case studies, humour), visual (slides, videos, illustrations, charts, diagrams) and physical (models, demonstrations) (Wilson *et al.* 1987). While representing or transforming knowledge is one means of facilitating the learning of declarative information, learning theorists from other lines of inquiry have also stressed the importance of providing well-organised courses (Eizenberg, 1988), focussing on key understandings and avoiding over-loading (Marton & Ramsden, 1988).

Procedural knowledge

While declarative knowledge is information about things, procedural knowledge (knowing how) is the ability to do things. It is the information involved in performing cognitive and psychomotor skills such as solving a problem, writing an essay, typing, caring for a patient or teaching a class (Ryle, 1949). Anderson's (1983) theory of skill acquisition proposes that procedures are derived initially from declarative information. (An example would be when a teacher or student verbalises the guidelines for preparing a sterile field prior to implementing the asepsis process.) Procedural knowledge is said to reside in the memory in the form of condition-action rules or productions which specify actions that can be taken when the right conditions are present. There are two types of productions, pattern-recognition and action-sequences, with the former often prompting the latter. Both pattern-recognition and action-sequences develop gradually over time, the former through processes such as generalisation and discrimination and the latter by means of practice and feedback in three phases which match those identified by Fitts (Fitts & Posner, 1967; Gagné, 1985). Expertise in all fields of endeavour is characterised by extensive procedural knowledge. It has been estimated that top-level experts possess between 50 000 and 100 000 units of procedural information in their knowledge base! (Simon & Kaplan, 1989)

In the explanation of procedural knowledge described above, professional practice consists of applied propositional knowledge. For other than the acquisition of relatively simple skills, this positivist interpretation of performance adopted by the cognitive psychologists has been rejected by various scholars writing about performance in the practice professions. Schön (1983, p. 18), for example, contends that professional practice situations are characterised by '. . . complexity, uncertainty, instability, uniqueness, and value conflict . . .' and cannot be resolved by recourse to neat, simple theoretical propositions that are an outcome of positivist research. This view is shared by a number of nurse theorists, including Bender & Rubella (1982), Lawler (1991) and Street (1990). In fact, notions about the complexity and primacy of practice and the consequent need for practice theory made an early appearance in the nursing literature with the work of Wald & Leonard (1964). For such scholars, complex procedural knowledge is acquired as one interacts with the world by means of inventing actions and copying the actions of others. Rather than remaining in the head and controlling action, knowledge is actually embodied in the action. Because such knowledge is likely to remain implicit unless it is deliberately invoked and studied, an important contribution to the advancement of professions such as nursing is thought to involve deriving theory from practice by documenting, analysing, interpreting and codifying this practical knowledge (Benner & Wrubel, 1982).

Research in a range of academic and professional fields has depicted highly skilled performance as smooth, fast and seemingly effortless with reduced cognitive demands that leave the expert free to attend to other novel aspects in the situation (Shiffrin & Dumais, 1981). It has been suggested that this level of automated skilled action, comparable with the fifth and final stage of nursing competence identified by Benner (1984), is the result of thousands of hours of practice accumulated over at least 10 years (Simon & Kaplan, 1989). These unsurprising findings simply highlight what has always been a problem for professions, like nursing, that have a practical focus. That problem concerns the extensive practice required to develop professional competence and the implications that follow in terms of reasonable expectations for the skill level of the beginning practitioner. Naturally, nurse educators have responded to this dilemma. For instance, the rationale for diversified clinical experience in preference to specialisation in the undergraduate program has been questioned since the former is likely to delay the development of a high level of proficiency (Benner, 1984). Moreover, the identification of a limited number of essential clinical skills that can be well-learned by undergraduate nurses has been undertaken (Mulquiney *et al.* 1991).

Conditional knowledge

The failure of academic knowledge and skills to influence future problem solving and practical action is well known (Wong, 1979). To overcome this problem of inertness, an awareness of when and why to use declarative and procedural knowledge, that is conditional knowledge, is required (Glaser, 1984). Such knowledge is evident when a nurse assisting a patient readily recognises that the situation calls for the application of relevant declarative knowledge about such things as the patient's illness and treatment as well as appropriate procedural skills relating to assessment and other nursing care activities. Case studies, simulations, problem-based learning, role-plays, video-based episodes are popular learning formats for conditionalising knowledge by embedding it in contexts that simulate reality (Bransford *et al.* 1990). However, although these activities assist students to appreciate conditions under which certain knowledge is relevant, that knowledge is likely to remain context-bound unless skilful teaching fosters the mindful abstraction of important principles or elements from the situation and the application of these in new situations (Salomon & Perkins, 1989). In some recent writing on this perennial and intractable issue of transfer, a more radical stance has been taken in stressing the unavoidably 'situated' or context-bound nature of learning. In this view, learning is regarded as enculturation making it essential that students are involved in authentic activities of the (nursing) community with teachers acting as practitioners (Brown *et al.* 1989).

The characteristics of expertise

One of the most important contributions of the cognitive theorists has been their analysis of skilled performance in a variety of domains. This work has led to the identification of characteristics that experts in many fields of endeavour typically exemplify. There is every reason to suppose that expert nurses also manifest these same characteristics.

Expertise

Extensive studies of novice–expert differences have provided a clear picture of the nature of academic and practical expertise. Thus, experts have highly specialised knowledge and skills pertaining to their own field. This knowledge is well organised into clusters that permit them to recognise meaningful patterns and principles in their domain. They know when to use their knowledge. Both short-term and long-term memory functions are excellent. Familiar mental and physical tasks are performed quickly and effortlessly, requiring little conscious control. Difficult problems are carefully analysed and a schema built that constrains the problem and suggests solutions. Finally, when appropriate, experts monitor their performance by testing for understanding and checking for errors (Glaser & Chi, 1988).

Perhaps the most striking finding from the investigations of expertise is that highly competent performance is characterised, not by powerful thinking and reasoning skills, but by the extent and quality of the background knowledge possessed. It was studies of chess players that first demonstrated the impact of knowledge on complex, skilled performance. Experienced players do not think of more moves, nor do they think further ahead. Their advantage lies in their knowledge base which contains a large number of familiar game configurations providing templates for future reference (Chase & Simon, 1973; Chi, 1978). Similar findings have been replicated in research related to medical and radiological diagnosis, physics, social science thinking and many other areas (Chi *et al.* 1981; Johnson *et al.* 1981; Lesgold *et al.* 1988; Voss *et al.* 1983).

This knowledge-based conception of proficiency in learning and performance has led to a revised view of intelligence in which the defining feature of intelligent behaviour is its abundant store of domain knowledge which can be drawn upon to advance new learning as opposed to efficient general underlying intellectual or reasoning abilities (Curtis & Glaser, 1981). Hence, what a traditional IQ test score actually represents, in large measure, is an individual's accumulated verbal and mathematical knowledge (Yates & Chandler, 1991). This being the case, it can also be assumed that academic marks and grades reflect, to a considerable extent, how knowledgeable students are.

Problem solving

The work on expertise has often been undertaken within a framework of problem solving. A problem is said to exist when one has a goal but no readily available means of reaching that goal (Newell & Simon, 1972). Most work has been done on relatively well-defined problems; problems in maths and physics, for instance, in which the problem components such as the initial state and the goal state, are clearly designated. Nursing problems, like teaching and most everyday problems, however, are often ambiguous or ill-structured (Voss & Post, 1988). Thus, in nursing care the goal may be concerned with responding to the patient's illness in terms of improvement of the situation rather than problem resolution in the form of a clear-cut diagnosis. The problem solving process has received considerable attention in the nursing literature (Tanner, 1987).

The long-held view was that problems are solved, bottom-up, by applying general reasoning or logical thinking strategies in a step-by-step fashion so that several possible solutions are generated and then tested systematically (hypothetico-deductive reasoning). These strategies were considered to be independent of the problem solver's existing knowledge and the type of problem involved. Current research findings suggest an alternative, top-down, knowledge-based explanation accounts for the marked differences in novice and expert problem solvers (Chi *et al.* 1982).

When they encounter familiar problems, experts carefully assess the problem, taking more time to do so than novices. Then, rather than trying out several possible solutions as novices do, a schema is selected which, once adapted to the problem, is likely to effectively represent the problem as well as suggesting a solution procedure to execute. Employing these processes, experts typically solve problems more quickly and accurately than novices (Chi *et al.* 1982; Lesgold *et al.* 1988). Although Benner & Tanner (1987) are unsympathetic to the information processing view of problem solving, the above depiction of the competent problem solver does bear similarities to Benner's (1984, p. 32) description of the final stage of proficiency in which 'the expert nurse, with an enormous background of experience, now has an intuitive grasp of each situation and zeroes in on the accurate region of the problem without wasteful consideration of a large range of unfruitful, alternative diagnoses and solutions'. The 'intuitive grasp' mentioned by the author appears consistent with the picture from cognitive psychology of a skilled problem solver automatically processing routine problems by drawing on a huge bank of schemata that facilitates the classification of problems and suggests solutions to implement.

The solving of ill-structured and unfamiliar problems may not be so straightforward, even for experts. Such problems may require a combination of schema-guided thinking and reasoning skills. For example, in medical diagnosis when faced with a patient's symptoms, the selection and testing of more than one schema or hypothesis may be required (Johnson *et al.* 1981). However, when reasoning processes are used in these circumstances, they do not appear to account for novice–expert differences. It is the knowledge brought to bear on the diagnostic task that provides the advantage for medical experts. They possess precise disease knowledge which includes a detailed understanding of the symptoms associated with common and less common diseases. Further, their medical knowledge is well organised, often into hierarchies and cross referenced, which greatly facilitates problem solving in the situations they encounter (Feltovich *et al.* 1984; Johnson *et al.* 1981).

Given the findings that competent problem solving is related to the possession of extensive propositional and schemata knowledge in a specific domain, heuristic strategies like the nursing process may offer a helpful framework for novice nurses, but they are no substitute for a well developed network of information associated with much experience in solving real nursing problems (Benner, 1984; Henderson, 1982).

How to help students make the transition from novice to expert status, which is normally achieved through extensive experience, is not well understood. However, what the studies of expertise have highlighted is the need to establish curriculum goals, content and assessment that mirror the complexity of highly competent performance.

Fostering expertise: new forms of assessment

New forms of assessment have emerged in response to the cognitive theorists' emphasis on complex human performance (including high levels of understanding, problem solving and practical competence) as the goal of learning. For example, tasks have been fashioned that evoke complicated, integrated abilities, ones that are representative of real workplace tasks or important problems and issues in the disciplinary field. Known as 'performance assessment', individually and in groups, involving short and long-term projects, students are asked to display their abilities; to actually do meaningful things such as solve ill-defined problems, observe and collect data, experiment and invent, read and write, and perform competently in practical spheres (Wolf et al. 1991). Another assessment tool that taps student multidimensional abilities is the portfolio. It is a collection of samples of the students' work that are typical of the domain such as maths problems representing different topics, writing in different genres and documentary evidence of teaching competence (Wolf et al. 1991).

This new kind of assessment is well illustrated in the way clinical nursing competencies are currently being assessed using the Objective, Structured Clinical Examination (OSCE) (Ross et al. 1988). In the case of theoretical course work, assignments and examinations that rely on recognition and recall of basic facts (e.g. multiple choice, short answer) would be replaced with tasks that require students to understand, integrate, apply and critically examine important ideas. These new forms of qualitative assessment not only require careful specification of the abilities to be assessed, they also raise questions about the role of measurement and judgement in assessment (Biggs, 1992; Ewell, 1991).

Summary

Recent research in cognitive psychology has attempted to unravel the complicated events that characterise complex learning. Three significant themes from this field of study have been examined in this paper. Firstly, learning has been described as a constructivist process in which students actively construct knowledge on the basis of personal experience with the implication that teachers must help students become active participants in their own learning. Next, the role of knowledge in learning has been emphasised alerting teachers to the fact that the knowledge the student brings to the learning situation is an important consideration as well as the knowledge that is involved in the learning task. Finally, the studies of expertise indicate the importance of providing educational experiences that are likely to foster understanding and practical competence. These propositions suggest a critical role for the nurse educator in designing, initiating, monitoring and evaluating learning. In particular, nurse educators can assist student learning by:

- Designing courses in which goals, content and assessment reflect the complex understanding and performance that a professional education seeks to attain.

- Providing significant opportunities for self-regulated and collaborative learning.

- Exposing what students know and building on it, helping them to see connections, and challenging misconceptions.

- Organising and transforming complex material in ways that make it more meaningful.

- Encouraging students to articulate their ideas and reflect on their knowledge and ways of learning.

- Modelling understanding and practical competence.

References

Alverman D E, Hynd C R (1989) Effects of prior knowledge activation modes and text structure on nonscience majors' comprehension of physics. *Journal of Educational Research* 83 (2): 97–102.

Anderson J R (1976) *Language, memory, and thought.* Lawrence Erlbaum Associates, Hillsdale, New Jersey.

Anderson J R (1983) *The architecture of cognition.* Harvard University Press, Cambridge, Massachusetts.

Ausubel D P (1960) The use of advance organisers in the learning and retention of meaningful verbal material. *Journal of Educational Psychology* 51 (5): 267–272.

Bandura A (1986) The explanatory and predictive scope of self-efficacy theory. *Journal of Social and Clinical Psychology* 4 (3): 359–373.

Bandura A (1989) Human agency in social cognitive theory. *American Psychologist* 44 (9): 1175–1184.

Barnett J E (1984) Facilitating retention through instruction about text structure. *Journal of Reading Behaviour* 16 (1): 1–13.

Barrows H S, Tamblyn R (1980) *Problem-based learning: an approach to medical education.* Springer, New York.

Benner P E (1984) *From novice to expert: excellence and power in clinical practice.* Addison-Wesley, Menlo Park, California.

Benner P, Tanner C (1987) How expert nurses use intuition. *American Journal of Nursing* 87 (1): 23–31.

Benner P, Wrubel (1982) Skilled clinical knowledge: the value of perceptual awareness, Parts I and 2. *Journal of Nursing Administration* 12 (5): 11–14, 12 (6): 28–33.

Biggs J (1992) A qualitative approach to grading students. *Herdsa News* 14 (3): 3–6.

Bihl-Hulme J (1985) Creative thinking in problem-based learning. In: D Boud (ed) *Problem-based learning in education for the professions.* pp. 177–183. Higher Education Research and Development Society of Australasia, Sydney.

Boud D, Keogh R. Walker D (1985) *Reflection: turning experience into learning.* Kogan Page, London.

Bransford J D, Johnson M K (1972) Contextual prerequisites for understanding: some investigations of comprehension and recall. *Journal of Verbal Learning and Verbal Behavior* 11 (6): 717–726.

Bransford J D, McCarrell N S (1974) A sketch of a cognitive approach to comprehension: some thoughts about understanding what it means to comprehend. In: W B Weimer, S Palermo (eds) *Cognition and symbolic processes.* Lawrence Erlbaum Associates, Hillsdale, New Jersey.

Bransford J D, Vye N, Kinzer C, Risko V (eds) (1990) Teaching thinking and content knowledge: toward an integrated approach. In: B F Jones, L Idol (eds) Dimensions of thinking and cognitive instruction, pp. 391–379. NCREL/Erlbaum, Hillsdale, New Jersey.

Brooks L W, Dansereau D F (1983) Effects of structural schema training and text organization on expository prose processing. *Journal of Educational Psychology* 75 (6): 811–820.

Brown A L (1978) Knowing when, where, and how to remember: a problem of metacognition. In: R Glaser (ed) *Advances in Instructional Psychology*, Vol. 1. pp. 77–165. Lawrence Erlbaum Associates. Hillsdale, New Jersey.

Brown A L, Bransford J D, Ferrara R A, Campione J C (1983) Learning, remembering and understanding. In: J H Flavell, E M Markman (eds) *Cognitive development*, Vol. III. P H Mussen (ed) *Handbook of Child Psychology*, 4th edn. pp. 77–166. Wiley, New York.

Brown J S, Collins A, Duguid P (1989) Situated cognition and the culture of learning. *Educational Researcher* 18 (1): 32–42.

Caffarella R (1983) Fostering self-directed learning in post secondary education: the use of gaming contracts. *Lifelong Learning* 7 (3): 7–10, 25–26.

Champagne A B, Gunstone R F, Klopfer L E (1985) Instructional consequences of students' knowledge about physical phenomena. In: L H T West, A L Pines (eds) *Cognitive structure and conceptual change*, pp. 61–90. Academic Press, Orlando.

Chase W G, Simon H A (1973) The mind's eye in chess. In: W G Chase (ed) *Visual information processing*, pp. 215–281. Academic Press, New York.

Chi M T H (1978) Knowledge structures and memory development. In: R S Siegler (ed) Children's thinking: what develops, knowledge structures and memory development, pp. 73–96. Lawrence Erlbaum Associates, New Jersey.

Chi M T H, Bassok M (1989) Learning from examples via self-explanation. In: L Resnick (ed) *Knowing, learning and instruction*, pp. 251-282. Lawrence Erlbaum Associates, Hillsdale, New Jersey.

Chi M T H, Feltovich P J, Glaser R (1981) Categorisation and representation of physics problems by experts and novices. *Cognitive Science* 5 (2): 121–152.

Chi M T H, Glaser R, Rees E (1982) Expertise in problem solving. In: R J Sternberg (ed) *Advances in the psychology of human intelligence*. Vol. 1, pp. 7–75. Lawrence Erlbaum Associates, Hillsdale, New Jersey.

Chinn C A, Brewer W F (1993) The role of anomalous data in knowledge acquisition: a theoretical framework and implications for science teaching. *Review of Educational Research* 63 (1): 1–49.

Clancey W J (1988) Acquiring, representing, and evaluating a competence model of diagnostic strategy. In: M T H Chi, R Glaser, M J Farr (eds) *The nature of expertise*, pp. 343-418. Lawrence Erlbaum Associates, Hillsdale, New Jersey.

Cook L K, Mayer R E (1988) Teaching readers about the structure of scientific text. *Journal of Educational Psychology* 80 (4): 448–456.

Craik F, Lockhart R S (1972) Levels of processing: a framework for memory research. *Journal of Verbal Learning and Verbal Behavior* 11 (6): 671–684.

Curtis M E, Glaser R (1981) Changing conceptions of intelligence. American Educational Research Association, *Review of Research in Education* 9: 111–148.

Dansereau D F (1985) Learning strategy research. In: W Segal, S F Chipman, R Glaser (eds) *Thinking and learning skills, Vol. 1. Relating instruction to research*, pp. 209–239. Lawrence Erlbaum Associates, London.

Dart B C, Clarke J A (1991) Helping students become better learners: a case study in teacher education. *Higher Education* 22 (3): 317–335.

Dooling D J, Lachman R (1971) Effects of comprehension on retention of prose. *Journal of Experimental Psychology* 88 (2): 216–222.

Eizenborg N (1988) Approaches to learning anatomy: developing a programme for preclinical medical students. In: P Ramsden (ed) *Improving learning*, pp. 178–198. Kogan Page, London.

Emden C (1991) Becoming a reflective practitioner. In: G Gray, R Part (eds) *Towards a discipline of nursing*. Churchill Livingstone, Edinburgh.

Ewell P T (1991) To capture the ineffable: new forms of assessment in higher education. American Educational Research Association, *Review of Research in Education* 17: 75–125.

Feltovich P J, Johnson P E, Moller J H, Swanson D B (1984) The role and development of medical knowledge in diagnostic expertise. In: W Clancey, E H Shortliffe (eds) *Readings in medical artificial intelligence: the first decade*, pp. 275–319. Addison-Wesley, New York.

Fitts P M, Posner M I (1967) *Human performance*. Cooks/Cole, Belmont, California.

Flower L (1979) Writer-based prose: a cognitive basis for problems in writing. *College English* 41 (1): 19–37.

Fransson A (1977) On qualitative differences in learning: iv — Effects of intrinsic motivation and extrinsic text anxiety in process and outcome. *British Journal of Educational Psychology* 47 (3): 244–257.

Gagné E D (1985) *The cognitive psychology of school learning*. Little Brown, Boston.

Glaser R (1984) Education and thinking. The role of knowledge. *American Psychologist* 39 (2): 93–104.

Glaser R, Chi M T H (1988) Overview. In: M T H Chi, R Glaser, M J Farr (eds) *The nature of expertise*, pp. xv–xxviii. Lawrence Erlbaum Associates, Hillsdale. New Jersey.

Gibbs G (1977) Can students be taught to study? *Higher Education Bulletin* 5 (2): 107–118.

Hayes J R, Flower L S (1980) Writing as problem solving. *Visible Language* 14 (4): 388–399.

Heron J (1988) Assessment revisited. In: D Boud (ed) *Developing student autonomy*, 2nd edn, pp. 77–90. Kogan Page, London.

Henderson V (1982) The nursing process — is the title right? *Journal of Advanced Nursing* 7 (2): 103–109.

Higgins L (1989) Students' perceptions of priorities in nurse education: research findings and their curriculum implications. *Higher Education Research and Development* 8 (2): 117–127.

Hounsell D (1984) Learning and essay writing. In: F Marton, D Hounsell, N Entwistle (eds) *The experience of learning*. Scottish Academic Press, Edinburgh.

Johnson P E, Duran A S, Hassebrock F *et al.* (1981) Experience and error in diagnostic reasoning. *Cognitive Science* 5 (3): 235–283.

Lawler J (1991) *Behind the screens: nursing, somology, and the problem of the body*. Churchill Livingstone, Melbourne.

Lesgold A, Rubinson H. Feltovich P, Glaser R, Klopfer D, Wang Y (1988) Experience in a complex skill: diagnosing X-ray pictures. In: M T H Chi, R Glaser, M J Farr (eds) *The nature of expertise*, pp. 311–342. Lawrence Erlbaum Associates, Hillsdale, New Jersey.

Martin E, Ramsden P (1987) Learning skills, or skill in learning? In: J T E Richardson, M W Eysenck, D W Piper (eds) *Student learning, research in education and cognitive psychology*, pp. 155-167. The Society for Research into Higher Education and Open University Press, Milton Keynes.

Marton F, Ramsden P (1988) What does it take to improve learning? In: P Ramsden (ed) *Improving learning, new perspectives*, pp. 268–286. Kogan Page, London.

Marton F, Saljo R (1984) Approaches to learning. In: F Marton, D Hounsell, N Entwistle (eds) *The experience of learning*, pp. 36–55. Scottish Academic Press, Edinburgh.

Mayer R E (1989) Models for understanding. *Review of Educational Research* 59 (1): 43–64.

Mulquiney J, Finn T, Dean M, Janovsky V, Denmead E, Green J (1991) The development of a Psychomotor Skills Profile for the beginning nurse practitioner graduating from the Institute of Nursing Studies 1990: the implications for curriculum change. Unpublished research study. Faculty of Nursing, University of Sydney.

Naveh-Benjamin M, McKeachie W J, Lin Y, Tucker D G (1986) Inferring students' cognitive structures and their development using the 'ordered tree technique'. *Journal of Educational Psychology* 78 (2): 130–140.

Newble D, Clarke R (1987) Approaches to learning in a traditional and innovative medical school. In: J T E Richardson, M W Eysenck, D W Piper (eds) *Student learning, research education and cognitive psychology*, pp. 39–46. The Society for Research into Higher Education and Open University Press, Milton Keynes.

Newell A, Simon H A (1972) *Human problem solving*. Prentice-Hall, Englewood Cliffs, New Jersey.

Paris S G, Byres J (1989) The constructivist approach to self-regulation and learning in the classroom. In: B J Zimmerman, D H Schunk (eds) *Self-regulated learning and academic achievement: theory, research, and practice*, pp. 169–200. Springer-Verlag, New York.

Perry W G (1970) *Forms of intellectual and ethical development in the college years: a scheme*. Holt, Rinehart and Winston, New York.

Piaget J (1952) *The origins of intelligence in children* (Translated by M. Cook). International Universities Press, New York.

Pressley M, Ghatala E S (1990) Self-regulated learning: monitoring learning from text. *Educational Psychologist* 25 (1): 19–33.

Prosser M, Trigwell K (eds) (1993) *Higher Education Research & Development (Special issue on learning: theories in practice)* 12 (1).

Ramsden P, Beswick D, Bowden J (1987) Learning processes and learning skills. In: J T E Richardson, M W Eysenck, D W Piper (eds) *Student learning. Research in education and cognitive psychology*, pp. 168–176. The Society for Research into Higher Education and Open University Press, Milton Keynes.

Resnick L B (1987) *Education and learning to think*. National Academy Press, Washington.

Resnick L B (ed) (1989) *Knowing, learning and instruction. Essays in honor of Robert Glaser*. Lawrence Erlbaum Associates, Hillsdale, New Jersey.

Ross M, Carroll G, Knight J, Chamberlain M, Fothergill-Bourbonnais F, Linton J (1988) Using the OSCE to measure clinical skills performance in nursing. *Journal of Advanced Nursing* 13 (1): 45–56.

Roth K, Anderson C (1988) Promoting conceptual change, learning from science textbooks. In: P Ramsden (ed) *Improving learning, new perspectives*, pp. 109–141. Kogan Page, London.

Rumelhart D E, Ortony A (1977) The representation of knowledge in memory. In: R C Anderson, R J Spiro, W E Montague (eds) *Schooling and the acquisition of knowledge*, pp. 99–135. Lawrence Erlbaum Associates, Hillsdale, New Jersey.

Ryle G (1949) *The concept of mind*. Penguin, Harmondsworth.

Salomon G, Perkins D N (1989) Rocky roads to transfer. *Educational Psychologist* 24 (2): 113–142.

Schön D A (1983) *The reflective practitioner: how professionals think in action*. Basic Books, New York.

Segal J W, Chipman S F, Glaser R (eds) (1985) *Thinking and learning skills. Vol. 1. Relating instruction to research*. Lawrence Erlbaum Associates, London.

Shiffrin R M, Dumais S T (1981) The development of automatism. In: J R Anderson (ed) *Cognitive skills and their acquisition*, pp. 111–140. Lawrence Erlbaum Associates, Hillsdale, New Jersey.

Shuell T J (1986) Cognitive conceptions of learning. *Review of Educational Research* 56 (4): 411–436.

Siegler R S (1983) Information processing approaches to development. In: W Kessen (ed) *History, theory and methods. Vol. I.* P H Mussen (ed) *Handbook of child psychology*, 4th edn, pp. 129–211. Wiley, New York.

Simon H A, Kaplan C A (1989) Foundations of cognitive science. In: M Posner (ed) *Foundations of cognitive science*, p. 41. Institute of Technology Press, Cambridge, Massachusetts.

Spiro R J (1977) Remembering information from text: 'the state of schema approach'. In: R C Anderson, R J Spiro, W E Montague (eds) *Schooling and the acquisition of knowledge*, pp. 137–165. Wiley, New York.

Street A (1990) *Nursing practice, high hard ground, messy swamps and pathways in between*. Deakin University, Geelong, Victoria.

Svensson L, Hogfors C (1988) Conceptions as the content of teaching: improving education in mechanics. In: P Ramsden (ed) *Improving learning, new perspectives*, pp. 162–177. Kogan Page, London.

Swanson H L (1990) Influence of metacognitive knowledge and aptitude on problem solving. *Journal of Educational Psychology* 82 (2): 306–314.

Tanner C A (1987) Teaching clinical judgment. In: J Fitzpatrick, R Taunton (eds) *Annual Review of Nursing Research*, Vol. 5, pp. 153–173. Springer, New York.

Thomas J W (1988) Proficiency at academic studying. *Contemporary Educational Psychology* 13 (3): 265–275.

Thompkins C, McGraw M (1988) The negotiated curriculum. In: D Boud (ed) *Developing student autonomy*, 2nd edn, pp. 172–192. Kogan Page, London.

Tulvin E, Donaldson W (eds) (1972) *Organization of memory*. Academic Press, New York.

Unger C, Wiske S, Simmons R, Perkins D (1993) *Toward a pedagogy of understanding*, American Educational Research Association, Atlanta, Georgia.

Van Rossum E J, Schenk S M (1984) The relationship between learning conception, study strategy and learning outcome. *British Journal of Educational Psychology* 54 (1): 73–83.

Voss J F, Greene T A, Penner B C (1983) Problem-solving skill in the social sciences. In: G H Bower (ed) *The psychology of learning and motivation: advances in research theory*, Vol. 17, pp. 165–213. Academic Press, New York.

Voss J F, Post T A (1988) On the solving of ill-structured problems. In: M T H Chi, R Glaser, M J Farr (eds) *The nature of expertise*, pp. 261–285. Lawrence Erlbaum Associates, Hillsdale, New Jersey.

Wald F S, Leonard R C (1964) Towards development of nursing practice theory. *Nursing Research* 13 (4): 309–313.

Watkins D (1984) Student perceptions of factors influencing tertiary education. *Higher Education Research and Development* 3 (1): 33–35.

Weiner B (1979) A theory of motivation. *Journal of Educational Psychology* 71 (1): 3–25.

Weiner B (1990) History of motivational research in education. *Journal of Educational Psychology* 82 (4): 616–622.

West L H T, Pines A L (1985) *Cognitive structure and conceptual change*. Academic Press, Orlando.

Weinstein C E, Mayer R E (1985) The teaching of learning strategies. In: M C Wittrock (ed) *Handbook of research on teaching*, 3rd edn, pp. 315–327. Macmillan, New York.

Wilson S M, Shulman L S, Richert A E (1987) 150 different ways of knowing: representations of knowledge in teaching. In: J Calderhead (ed) *Exploring teachers' thinking*, pp. 60–83. Cassell, London.

Wolf D, Bixby J, Glenn J, Garner H (1991) To use their minds well: investigating new forms of student assessment. American Educational Research Association, *Review of Research in Education* 17: 31–74.

Wong J (1979) The inability to transfer classroom learning to clinical nursing practice: a learning problem and its remedial plan. *Journal of Advanced Nursing* 4 (2): 161–168.

Yates G C R, Chandler M (1991) The cognitive psychology of knowledge: basic research findings and educational implications. *Australian Journal of Education* 35 (2): 131–153.

16. How Nurses Learn and How to Improve the Learning Environment

Bryn D. Davis

This paper considers some of the evidence that can help nurse teachers more effectively prepare nurses for practice. In particular it is concerned with how students learn and how teachers can improve the learning environment.

There are four main sections to the paper. The first looks at learning styles and considers the importance of matching teaching style to the learning style of the student. The second section considers the research into the process of integrating theory and practice in nursing education and the relationship between theory, the classroom and the clinical area.

The next section of the paper looks at factors influencing the process of becoming a nurse. Socialising agents such as people and techniques are reviewed in the light of research evidence from nursing and similar professions. Finally the paper represents a series of ways in which it is possible to assess and improve the learning environment for the student nurse, including human aspects, equipment and information.

Introduction

> 'To do is to be' J J Rousseau
> 'To be is to do' J P Sartre
> 'Do be do be do' F Sinatra

When any process or activity is going well, achieving its goals, being efficient and satisfying, it can be seen as 'going like a song', and the process of concern here involves doing (nursing), being (a nurse), and becoming. The process of becoming a nurse has been subjected to extensive research over the last 3 decades at least. Much of this research has been undertaken in the USA, although latterly an increasing amount has been done in the UK.

In the light of the changes now being imposed on nursing education, particularly those that are the result of Project 2000, this paper is an attempt to draw on some of the relevant research in order to inform the development of curricula which will facilitate this process.

How do nurses learn?

Student nurses have to learn how to do things, how to explain things and also they have to acquire and develop a particular self image involving attitudes, values and beliefs. With particular reference to the first two of these; manual and interpersonal

Bryn D. Davis: 'How Nurses Learn and How to Improve the Learning Environment' in *NURSE EDUCATION TODAY* (1990), 10(6), pp. 405–409. Reprinted by permission of the publisher Churchill Livingstone.

skills; and academic skills and knowledge, research into learning styles may be of relevance.

When students enter a nurse education programme they bring with them a particular personal view of the world, of people, how it all works and what it all means; and also they bring with them a personal way of learning.

The study of learning styles has become of increasing importance in nursing education over the last few years. Tomlinson (1981) has presented a review of research findings which offer guidance as to how learners might approach new information or experiences. He identifies such styles as:

a)   'operation and comprehension learning';

b)   'field dependent and field independent learning';

c)   'deep and surface learning'.

These styles have been reviewed and considered in the manual 'Managing Change in Nursing Education' (ENB, 1987). There the conclusion was that there is no single style that encompasses all nurse learners.

Using a model of learning styles developed by Kolb (1976), Ramprogus assessed the styles of a group of first year nurse learners (1988). The styles proposed included 'assimilators', 'accommodators', 'convergers' and 'divergers'. He found that the majority of students fell into a new category 'allrounder', (52%), because they did not emphasise any one particular style.

Ramprogus also produced evidence to suggest that students offered a 'Learning How to Learn' course would perform better on nursing related tests. Other results (relating to trained nurses) have indicated that particular styles can be identified for different nurse learners and also that students can acquire or modify learning styles (such as those of Pask & Scott, 1972; Gott, 1982).

In an American study using the same Kolb model Hodges, (1988), found a wide variety of styles being used, but that there seemed to be a predominance of a concrete cognitive style; a sensing, feeling, judging, feminine personality and a subjective perceptual mode which emphasises non-visual sensory experience, and kinaesthetic or tactile imagery.

The authors of the ENB Manual, (ENB, 1987), argue that it is important that nurse teachers attempt to match up their teaching styles with the learners' learning styles. This would seem to demand an ability to assess the individual learner's learning style as well as the teaching style of the individual tutor.

Integration of theory and practice

This has been identified as a problem in nurse education for some time now, and again much research and development has been undertaken. The importance of teachers who are also seen practising has been demonstrated by Davis (1983). The relationship between teaching/learning in the classroom and in the clinical setting is one that has been addressed by Alexander (1983) and further contributions have been offered by

Wong and Wong (1987). The role of the clinical teacher and in particular the setting up of joint appointments between clinic teachers and ward sisters has been an exciting development although it has its advocates and its critics, some of whom suggest the role of lecturer practitioner as a more viable alternative (see Wright, 1985; Durgahee, 1990; Vaughan, 1987, 1990).

The automatic assumption is that theory means classroom has been holding back nurse education for decades. This has been influenced to a certain extent by the regulations that require pre-registration courses to provide a minimum number of hours of theory and a minimum number of hours of practice. This has perhaps been important in the light of the apprenticeship nature of nurse education in the UK, where it has been important to ensure that there was time for theory and to prevent the overexploitation of the student as a worker. In the future with supernumerary learners this may not be such a problem unless regulations from the EEC continue this practice. It is going to be important that the EEC is lobbied to ensure that such regulations are not used restrictively in the way in which learners learn their nursing (theory and practice).

Socialisation

Much nursing education research has been concerned with the process by which newcomers to the profession 'become' nurses. This process has also been extensively studied with respect to other professions and occupations as well, and many nurse researchers have been influenced in their approach by such research.

The medical profession, the military professions, the church, the police and managers in industry have all had a variety of approaches applied but the one that seems to have stirred the most interest has been the qualitative approach of Becker *et al.* (1961) with the medical profession, and van Maanen (1973) with the police. Other approaches still used however involve some survey techniques to achieve similar goals.

From these and other similar studies a range of common socialisation factors have been identified:

1. Reference groups and significant others:

    a) anticipatory socialisation — influences from other people prior to undertaking training;

    b) influences from others during training;

    c) influences from others regarding the development of professional self-image;

    d) peer group support.

2. Special socialising techniques:

    a) 'homogenising' — reducing individuality, for example by the use of uniforms, standard hairstyles and cuts;

    b) 'hazing' — submissive and degrading work under time and accuracy pressures with severe punishments for failure. These could be physical and brutal but are often subtle, and intellectual-emotional.

Early studies in the USA confirmed many of these factors as applying to nursing, and recent studies in the UK have demonstrated similar processes at work here. For example that of Melia (1987), who identified six factors or processes at work, learning the rules; getting the work done; learning and working; nursing in the dark; just passing through; and doing nursing and being professional.

Another approach in this country has been to look at the attributes and characteristics of significant others as agents of socialisation. Research such as that by Davis (1983), Fretwell (1982), Ogier (1982) and Orton (1981) has demonstrated the kind of professional skills and personal attributes required of significant others as seen by the learners themselves.

Davis looked at the process of professional socialisation and identified from the literature the importance of significant others in that process, (1983). Using the students' own words and constructs the characteristics of the people the students would go to with a variety of problems, and also the characteristics of those they modelled themselves on, were described. Generally the students' preferred the ward staff to the teaching staff as resources and models, and among those, they tended to prefer those who they saw more as people than as professionals. The constructs used by the students to describe their significant others emphasised the importance of working with them, liking them, seeing them participating in the care of patients, and being accessible.

Orton identified the importance of the recognition of the student's needs and a commitment to teaching on the part of the ward sister as being characteristic of a high student orientation ward and a learning situation valued by the student, (1981). Ogier (1982), identified approachability, nurse learner orientation, and directiveness as being characteristics of the ward sister's leadership style which influenced her relationship with the nurse learners coming under her supervision.

A very complex pattern of interrelating factors was identified by Fretwell, (1982), including ward sister's orientation (doctor, patient or administration); leadership style (autocratic; democratic or laissez-faire); and teaching role (active or passive).

In conclusion to this discussion of how student nurses learn, it would seem that students bring with them a particular learning style, derived from a variety of previous learning experiences, but which can be modified with suitable interventions and guidance by the teachers. Also, and in particular, the ward staff seem to be significant others in the socialisation process of becoming a nurse and that they too bring with them a personal style, depending on their own training and their personal attributes. It would seem that there is room for the development of attributes and skills in the ward staff that would support the development of more effective learning styles in the student. The preparation of the ward staff as mentors for nurse learners, especially with respect to the implementation of supernumerary status for learners under Project 2000, must take into account the findings of research such as that described here.

Nurse teachers themselves can also take a leaf out of this book to consider how significant they are, or could be, to student nurses. The same attributes should apply to them also. Perhaps development along the lines of lecturer-practitioner roles may make a difference here.

The clinical learning environment

As well as the people in the learning environment there are other aspects that can be considered in the study of how nurses learn.

One of these is the kind of nursing that is practised in the clinical setting. Aspects of this include the model(s) of nursing being implemented, the staffing mix, and management strategies for the delivery of care.

Over 10 years ago now Grant (1979) and Pembrey (1980) reported on investigations into the implementation of the nursing process and patterns of ward management. A major criterion arising from these studies is that of the importance of an individualised approach to patient care as a basis for the nurse learner experience. Student nurses who can see the whole process of an individual patient's care as documented in a care plan has a much clearer picture than one who has only participated in a series of disconnected tasks. The integration of theory and practice is also much more likely under the nursing process and with the supportive documentation of the care plan (always provided that this is carried out properly). Recent attempts to evaluate the quality of careplanning hint that this is not always to be relied on (e.g. Kitson, 1986; Billings, 1989).

Another approach has been the study of a style of nursing known as primary nursing. Experiments in a variety of settings have been reviewed in Pearson (1988). This development has recently been receiving a high profile in the nursing journals and through the establishment of the UK Primary Nursing Network under the aegis of the King's Fund Centre and hosted by the School of Nursing Studies at the University of Wales College of Medicine, Cardiff. It is claimed that this strategy achieves an even better experience of continuity of care and thus a much more meaningful learning opportunity for the student nurse.

Other researchers have looked quite intensively at the learning opportunities available in a particular setting as a major factor in the way in which students' learn. The kind of interventions (involving psycho-social as well as psycho-physical skills) that are available for observation and for practice have a powerful influence on the development of competency, (e.g. Lewin and Jacka, 1987; Reid, 1985). Thus the choice of placements for the learner and the timing of placements in relation to theoretical aspects of study is crucial.

As well as the opportunities for observation and practice of nursing activities in good relationship with classroom work (and as mentioned above it should be possible for some of the theoretical teaching/learning to occur in the clinical setting too) it is important that the clinical learning environment is also supported with adequate and suitable equipment for the student to use and on which to practice. Information resources are also important in the clinical setting, human and documentary (and perhaps even computer based).

These resources are of course also important in the school/college of nursing setting. This is a major strand in the argument for the establishment of links with higher education under the proposals of the UKCC and Project 2000. Teachers who are well qualified in the subjects to be studied, access to suitable learning areas such as workshops and laboratories and the opportunity to mix with students from other disciplines are important aspects of education for adults. A useful summary of the factors and processes involved in establishing or identifying suitable learning environments has been made available by the ENB (1987).

In conclusion, there are many factors involved in the process of becoming a nurse and many influences on the way in which student nurses learn. The students themselves contribute much as do the teachers and nurses with whom they study and work. The social and physical structures existing between and within the classroom and the clinical setting are potent influences as is the nature, accessibility and availability of information about nursing and its informing disciplines.

If the knowledgeable doer, or the reflective practitioner is the goal of nurse education then a complex, and sophisticated system is required to facilitate it. The outcome is related to the structure and the process of nurse education. This paper has attempted to identify and consider those aspects that research suggest would be the most likely to bring about the desired result.

Essentially we are concerned with helping a group of human beings to develop and add to attributes, information and skills already possessed to a level of competency and expertise that will ensure that the quality of care they provide is of the highest standard, and is capable of modification in the light of continuing experience.

References

Alexander M F (1983) *Learning to nurse; integrating theory and practice.* Churchill Livingstone, Edinburgh.

Becker H S, Hughes E C, Greer B, Strauss A L (1961) *Boys in White.* University of Chicago Press, Chicago.

Billings J (1989) Evaluation of Nursing Process Documentation. Eastbourne Health Authority, Eastbourne.

Davis B D (1983) Student nurses perception of their significant others. In: B D Davis (ed) *Research into Nurse Education.* Croom Helm, Beckenham, Kent.

Durgahee T (1990) Joint appointments in nursing education. Unpublished PhD thesis. Sussex University, Falmer, Brighton.

ENB (1987) *Managing change in nursing education; section 2: the teacher's role.* English National Board, London.

Fretwell J E (1982) *Ward teaching and learning.* Royal College of Nursing, London.

Gott M (1982) *Learning nursing.* Royal College of Nursing, London.

Grant N (1979) *Time to care.* Royal College of Nursing, London.

Hodges L C (1988) Students entering professional nursing: learning styles, personality type and sex-role identification. *Nurse Education Today*: 868–876.

Kitson A (1986) Indicators of quality in nursing care: an alternative approach. *Journal of Advanced Nursing* 11: 133–144.

Kolb D A (1976) *Learning Style Inventory: Technical Manual*. McBer & Co, Boston, USA.

Lewin D C, Jacka K (1987) Classroom instruction and clinical opportunity in student nurses training: integration and measurement. In: B D Davis (ed) *Nursing Education: Research and Developments*. Croom Helm, Beckenham Kent.

Melia K (1987) *Learning and working: the occupational socialization of nurses*. Tavistock, London.

Ogier M (1982) *An ideal sister*. Royal College of Nursing, London.

Orton H D (1981) *Ward Learning Climate*. Royal College of Nursing, London.

Pask C, Scott B C E (1972) Learning strategies and individual competence. *International Journal of Man Machine Studies* 4, 3: 217–253.

Pearson A, (ed) (1988) *Primary Nursing*. Croom Helm, London.

Pembrey S (1980) *Ward sister: key to nursing*. Royal College of Nursing, London.

Ramprogus V K (1988) Learning how to learn nursing. *Nurse Education Today* 8: 59–67.

Reid N C (1985) *Wards in Chancery*. Royal College of Nursing, London.

Tomlinson P (1981) *Understanding Teaching*. McGraw Hill, Toronto, Canada.

Van Maanan J (1973) Observations on the making of policemen. *Human Organisations* 32: 407–418.

Vaughan B (1987) Bridging the gap. *Senior Nurse* Vol. 6, May.

Vaughan B (1990) Knowing that and knowing how: the role of the lecturer practitioner. In: J Salvage, B Kershaw (eds) *Models for Nursing 2*. Scutari Press, London.

Wong J, Wong S (1987) Towards effective clinical teaching in nursing. *Journal of Advanced Nursing* 12: 505–513.

Wright S (1985) Reflecting on joint appointments. *Senior Nurse* Vol 3, Dec.

Facilitating Clinical Learning

The concept of facilitation is being used increasingly in nursing and midwifery education, with many involved in the education process advocating a change from the traditional, formal teacher/student relationship to that of a more dynamic and interactive partnership between facilitator and student. The more traditional approach is based on a hierarchical model with the teacher having the position of power because of his/her knowledge and experience, and is still very prevalent in both academic and clinical learning environments.

Facilitation, on the other hand, promotes the ideals of sharing and partnership in the learning process where both student and facilitator are working together on a relatively equal basis to maximise the learning experience. Carl Rogers (1969) is recognised as one of the principal proponents of the concept of facilitation. Rogers sees anyone involved in promoting learning as a facilitator, a provider of resources for learning and someone who shares his/her feelings as well as knowledge with students. Thus the prerequisites for an effective facilitator are awareness of self, being oneself in the learning environment, accepting and trusting students, and empathy (Quinn, 1995).

Facilitating learning in a formal classroom setting is somewhat different to doing so in a clinical learning environment. The basic qualities of genuineness, trust and empathic understanding suggested by Rogers are required whatever the environment, but the learning experiences are bound to be less structured and more opportunistic than those involved in a formally designed programme of study.

Nicklin and Kenworthy (1995) suggest that the challenge to practice-based facilitation of learning is to *"enthral the student with the quality of practice demonstrated by skilled practitioners who have themselves reached the level of discrimination."* In this context dissemination means that the individual has reached the stage in their own development where they are in a position to influence others (Steinaker and Bell, 1979). Clearly, in order for facilitators to reach this stage they require a sound knowledge base in relation to teaching and learning strategies and must have developed the practical skills to be able to implement these strategies appropriately and effectively. Each clinical area is a unique, ever changing and dynamic learning environment for both students and trained staff alike. It is important that as facilitators of learning you are aware of this environmental uniqueness.

If you also take into consideration the uniqueness of each individual student in relation to such things as learning skills, learning style and past experiences, you may then start to realise the importance of the role of planning for the facilitator.

The focus of the extracts in this section is therefore on the facilitation of learning in the clinical environment, and a range of strategies is explored and their application to practice explained and analysed.

References

Quinn F M (1996) *The principles and practice of nurse education*. Chapman and Hall, London.

Rogers C (1994) *Freedom to learn*. 3rd edn. Merrill, Columbus, Ohio.

Nicklin P, Kenworthy N (1995) *Teaching and assessing in nursing practice*. 2nd edn. Scutari Press, London.

Steinaker N, Bell M (1979) *The experiential taxonomy: A new approach to teaching and learning*. Academic Press.

17. Teaching and Learning in Practice Placements

Francis M. Quinn

The placement of students in practice settings, under appropriate professional supervision, is a fundamental educational strategy in nursing and midwifery education. Most students, and many professionals, would argue that learning gained from placement experience is much more meaningful and relevant than that gained in the lecture room, and theoretical support for this can be found in the writings of learning theorists such as Carl Rogers, Malcolm Knowles, David Kolb and Donald Schon. The term 'practice placement' covers a wide variety of settings, including hospital wards and departments, community health centres, GP surgeries, schools, nurseries, day centres, residential homes, and industry.

Although practice placement is much more common in pre-registration programmes, many post-registration courses or pathways contain requirements for professional practice. Fish and Purr (1991), however, argue that the profession has not addressed the role and purpose of clinical practice in continuing education programmes. Their findings indicate that there is still a predominant view of practice as being 'application of theory', with little appreciation of the 'bottom-up' approach to theory generation; they also found an emphasis on narrow training outcomes such as attainment of competencies. They concluded that supernumerary status led to far more learning than if the student were a full member of the working team, as the former allowed greater opportunities for thinking and reflection on practice.

Practice placements may be undertaken in a new placement or in the case of continuing education programmes, in the student's own practice setting. An example of the latter is the enrolled nurse conversion programme, where the student's placement may be their own practice setting. In principle, there should be no difference between these, but in the latter example there is the danger that qualified staff will forget that the enrolled nurse is now a student as well as a colleague, and who therefore requires specific support in relation to their conversion course.

It is important at this point to differentiate between experience and learning in practice placements; it is sometimes assumed that exposure to an experience is synonymous with learning from that experience, and while some learning probably does happen in this way it is not the kind of professional learning that comes from systematic analysis and reflection upon experience. The latter requires an environment conducive to learning and appropriate support from skilled practitioners and educationalists.

This chapter explores the Benner adaptation of the Dreyfus model of skill acquisition in nursing, the requirements for a satisfactory learning environment in practice

Francis M. Quinn: 'Teaching and Learning in Practice Placements' from *THE PRINCIPLES AND PRACTICE OF NURSE EDUCATION* (Chapman & Hall, 1995), pp. 180–198.

placements, placement audit, concepts and roles of supervision, mentorship and preceptorship, staff development for support roles, and stress and burn-out.

Benner's model of skill acquisition in clinical nursing practice

Patricia Benner's book *From Novice to Expert* (1984) has become one of the most frequently quoted research studies in nurse education. Benner conducted paired interviews with beginners and experienced nurses about significant nursing situations they had experienced in common, in order to identify any characteristic differences between their descriptions of the same situation. Additionally, she carried out interviews, critical incident technique, and participant observation with a sample of experienced nurses, new graduates, and senior students, to ascertain the characteristics of performance at different stages of skill acquisition. Using an adaptation of the five-stage model of skill acquisition developed by Dreyfus and Dreyfus (1980), she described the characteristics of performance at five different levels of nursing skill: novice, advanced beginner, competent, proficient, and expert. During her passage through these stages, the student relies less upon abstract rules to govern practice, and more on past experience. Nursing situations begin to be seen as a unified whole within which only certain aspects are relevant, and the nurse becomes personally involved in situations rather than a detached observer. It is important to note that Benner uses the term skill in its widest sense to mean all aspects of nursing practice, and not simply psychomotor skill performance.

Stage 1: novice. This level is characterized by rule-governed behaviour, as the novice has no experience of the situation upon which to draw, and this applies to both students in training and to experienced nurses who move into an unfamiliar clinical area. Adherence to principles and rules, however, does not help the nurse to decide what is relevant in a nursing situation, and may thus lead to unsuccessful performance.

Stage 2: advanced beginner. Unlike principles and rules, aspects are overall characteristics of a situation that can only be identified by experience of that situation. For example, the skills of interviewing a patient are developed by experience of interviewing previous patients, and the advanced beginner is one who has had sufficient prior experience of a situation to deliver marginally acceptable performance. Advanced beginners need adequate support from supervisors, mentors and colleagues in the practice setting.

Stage 3: competent. This stage is characterized by conscious, deliberate planning based upon analysis and careful deliberation of situations. The competent nurse is able to identify priorities and manage their own work, and Benner suggests that the competent nurse can benefit at this stage from learning activities that centre on decision-making, planning and co-ordinating patient care.

Stage 4: proficient. Unlike the competent nurse, the proficient nurse is able to perceive situations holistically and therefore can home in directly on the most relevant aspects of a problem. According to Benner, proficient performance is based upon the use of maxims, and is normally found in nurses who have worked within a specific area of nursing for several years. Inductive teaching strategies, such as case-studies, are most useful for nurses at this stage.

Stage 5: expert. This stage is characterized by a deep understanding and intuitive grasp of the total situation; the expert nurse develops a feel for situations and a vision of the possibilities in a given situation. Benner suggests that critical incident technique is a useful way of attempting to evaluate expert practice, but considers that not all nurses are capable of becoming experts.

The learning environment in hospital placements

The qualified staff are a key factor influencing the learning environment in hospital placements, the role of ward manager being particularly influential. Not only do they have control of the management of the area, but also serve as role-models for nursing practice. The leadership style and personality of the ward manager are important determinants of an effective learning environment (Orton, 1981; Fretwell, 1983; Ogier, 1982, 1986; Pembrey, 1980).

Characteristics of a good clinical learning environment

The following summarizes the main perceptions of students in these research studies with regard to the characteristics of a good clinical learning environment.

A humanistic approach to students

Qualified staff should ensure that students are treated with kindness and understanding and should try to show interest in them as people. They should be approachable and helpful to students, providing support as necessary, and be very much aware that they are students rather than simply pairs of extra hands. They should foster the students' self-esteem.

Team spirit

Qualified staff should work as a team and strive to make the student feel a part of that team. They should create a good atmosphere by their relationships within the team.

Management style

This should be efficient and yet flexible in order to produce good quality care. Teaching should have its place in the overall organization and students should be given responsibility and encouraged to use initiative. Nursing practice should be compatible with that taught in the College of Nursing and Midwifery.

Teaching and learning support

Qualified staff should be willing to act as supervisors, mentors, preceptors, assessors, and counsellors as appropriate, and these aspects are discussed later in this chapter. Opportunities should be given for students to ask questions, attend medical staff rounds, observe new procedures and have access to patients/clients records. Non-nursing professionals such as doctors, physiotherapists, dieticians and chaplains can also contribute to the learning environment provided they are made to feel part of the total team. It is important for the ward manager to spend a little time with new non-nursing colleagues in order to explain the ethos of the ward or department in relation to learning, thus encouraging them to see themselves as a resource for student learning.

It is not always appreciated that students themselves are very much a part of the learning environment and not merely the passive recipients of its influences. An effective environment will encourage the students to take responsibility for their own learning and to actively seek out opportunities for this. Critical thinking and judgement are fostered in an atmosphere where the student can question and dissent without feeling guilty or disloyal. An important part of the learning process is experimentation, in which the student can try to apply concepts and principles in different ways; this implies that the student will need to adopt different approaches to patients and to be innovative. There must of necessity be an element of calculated risk in this, and it is the responsibility of staff to ensure that the risk of danger to the patient is minimized. Reilly and Oermann (1985) suggest that teachers may set unrealistic demands on students by expecting them to do everything perfectly, whereas mistakes are an inseparable part of the learning process. Teachers and students should work together to examine the reasons for failures so as to learn by such mistakes.

There may be other students at different levels of training in a clinical area and this peer support can be invaluable. By planning for two students to work together, there can be substantial benefits for both, provided they take time to discuss approaches and decisions and their underlying rationale.

Helping the students to be self-directing in their learning is of the utmost importance. Knowles (1986) suggests that a learning need is the gap between where the student is now, and where he or she wants to be in regard to a particular set of competences. The student should be helped to become aware of his or her learning needs in order to become self-directing, and initial pre-placement discussions are invaluable as a way of establishing a preliminary learning contract.

The learning environment in community placements

So far we have discussed learning environments with reference to hospital settings, but the environment is equally important when students are in community placements. Prior preparation in advance of a student placement is vital to ensure that the student gains the most from it. It is good practice to establish empathy with the student many weeks before the actual placement, for example, by the mentor giving the student his or her work and home telephone numbers in order to discuss expectations, and also 'housekeeping' issues such as transport arrangements etc.

The physical environment is clearly very different from that of a hospital, particularly when it involves domiciliary visits to patients in their own homes. Nursing staff are guests in this situation, with no right of entry and consequently, much of the teaching will occur by observation, with discussion following later after leaving the patient's home. Much of this discussion takes place in the practitioner's car in a one-to-one setting, calling for very good interpersonal skills on the part of the teacher. The practitioner needs to put the student at ease and treat him or her as an equal. The effects of a strained relationship are much more difficult to cope with when there are only two people involved. Clinics and post-natal groups provide another community learning environment for students. When running a well-baby clinic the mentor can combine tutorials for both student and parent, since the information is common to both. In community placements, media resources are much more scarce than in hospital settings, and hence the mentor places greater reliance on discussion and role modelling strategies.

Practice placement audit

Auditing of practice placements forms a significant component of an institution's quality assurance system and helpful guidelines on educational audit have been produced by the English National Board for Nursing, Midwifery and Health Visiting (ENB, 1993). Practice placement audit focuses on six categories.

1. *Student learning experience/evaluation.* This includes provision for orientation, appropriate and accessible learning opportunities, adequate length of placement, ethos, appropriate care model, staff commitment, and mentorship system.

2. *Academic staff perspective.* This includes commitment to relationships with placement staff, maintenance of clinical competence, integration of theory and practice, monitoring of placement evaluation, and staff development of unit staff.

3. *Service provider unit staff perspective.* This includes a commitment to individualized care, team approach, multidisciplinary teamwork, communication with the College, commitment to PREPP by service managers, and appraisal system.

4. *RHA purchaser/other purchaser requirements.* This includes identifiable and agreed standards, and quality assurance mechanisms.

5. *Environment.* This includes adequate physical environment to deliver quality care, to facilitate development of competencies, to provide teaching and learning opportunities, space and equipment, and health and safety requirements.

6. *Quality assurance mechanisms.* This includes congruence of curriculum and placement, unit staff preparation, monitoring and annual review mechanisms, system for ensuring clinical knowledge base of academic staff, and adequate supervision of students.

Role of the lecturer-practitioner or link-teacher

Until quite recently there were two types of nurse teacher: the nurse tutor, whose primary responsibility lay in classroom teaching, and the clinical teacher, whose primary responsibility was teaching in practice placement settings. These roles have now been unified under the title of lecturer/practitioner, a qualified teacher who has retained clinical competence and whose responsibilities include teaching, supervision and assessment of students. The lecturer/practitioner role, however, requires a re-orientation of teaching staff towards practice, and this is not likely to happen in a short timescale. Many institutions are attempting to bridge the gap between education and service by the use of link-teachers, whose role is to establish relationships with a small number of clinical areas for the purposes of liaison, trouble-shooting and staff development. The latter is primarily aimed at qualified staff in clinical areas, who will be acting as supervisors, mentors and preceptors to students undertaking practice placements. The link-teacher model may be criticized on the grounds that it could be seen as an abdication of direct teaching and assessment responsibility by the College of Nursing and Midwifery. This is not to decry the important teaching and supervisory roles of practice-based staff, but to question whether they should be the sole providers of such support, given that practice placements may constitute up to one half of a student's programme of study. In the light of the dual impact of educational contracting and skill-mix, it is unlikely that service providers would be happy with a system in which they contract with colleges for educational provision, only to find that they are responsible for providing a considerable proportion of the teaching, supervision and assessment that forms part of the contract.

Teaching on a one-to-one basis demands skills quite different from those used in the classroom setting; both teacher and student are more exposed to each other and the encounter takes place in the presence of other staff, patients and visitors. The need to appear competent and credible to all these groups, including the student, can add considerable pressure on the teacher, making it more difficult to allow the student to make decisions or to try out new approaches. On the other hand, there can be great personal satisfaction in helping to provide good quality nursing care whilst at the same time facilitating the growth of nursing skills in the student. Gerrish (1992) identifies three key roles for teachers in practice settings:

1. *Educational support for practice-based staff.* This includes advice about dealing with supernumerary students on pre-registration programmes, and support for staff acting as mentors to students.

2. *Tutoring students.* This includes facilitating the development of students' autonomy as students, and their skills with regard to reflective practice.

3. *Facilitating good practice.* This includes awareness of current practice, providing a resource to unit staff, promotion of research-mindedness, and fostering a critical approach to practice.

Gerrish suggests that teaching in practice placements requires a commitment by the teacher, collaboration between education and service staff, and staff development for teachers on their new role in relation to practice.

Placement support systems for students and staff

There is a triad of terms used to describe practice placement support systems for students, supervision, mentorship and preceptorship. Within the literature, however, there is no consensus of opinion regarding definitions and some writers subsume all three concepts under umbrella terms such as 'practice facilitation'. For example, Butterworth and Faugier (1992) employ the term 'clinical supervision' to encompass mentorship, preceptorship, supervision of qualified practice, peer review, and maintenance of standards. Within the literature, the terms mentor and preceptor have been used largely to describe support systems for pre-registration nurses and midwives, but there is growing interest in the application of these in post-registration programmes. The UKCC Post-Registration Education and Practice (PREP) final proposals require all newly qualified nurses to complete a period of some four months under the guidance of a mentor, known as a preceptor, to ensure they do not assume too much responsibility, too soon or inappropriately.

Supervision

This is the least well-defined of the three terms and also the least developed in nursing, which has had to adapt models of supervision from other disciplines such as social work and psychotherapy (Faugier, 1992). In social work, supervision is defined as 'planned, regular periods of time that student and supervisor spend together discussing the student's work in the placement and reviewing the learning progress' (Ford and Jones, 1987). The English National Board for Nursing, Midwifery and Health Visiting (ENB, 1993) define a supervisor as 'an appropriately qualified and experienced first-level nurse/midwife/health visitor who has received preparation for ensuring that relevant experience is provided for students to enable learning outcomes to be achieved and for facilitating the students' developing competence in the practice of nursing/midwifery/health visiting by overseeing this practice. The role of the supervisor is a formal one and is normally included in the individual's managerial responsibilities.'

According to Faugier (1992), the role of the supervisor is to facilitate personal and professional growth in the supervisee, and to provide support for the latter's development of autonomy. She proposes a 'growth and support' model comprising the following elements:

1. Generosity of time and spirit

2. Rewarding supervisee's abilities

3. Openness

4. Willingness to learn

5. Being thoughtful and thought-provoking

6. Humanity

7. Sensitivity

8. Uncompromising rigour and standards

9. Awareness of personal supervisory style

10. Adoption of a practical focus

11. Awareness of differences in orientation between supervisor and supervisee

12. Maintenance of distinction between supervisory and therapeutic relationship

13. Trust

In their evaluation of practice-based learning in continuing professional education in nursing, midwifery and health visiting, Fish and Purr (1991) found that supervisors had heavy workloads and their role was not well-defined. They tended to lack status and demonstrated a striking lack of confidence about their teaching and facilitating roles.

Mentorship

Mentorship is perceived as an important concept by the nursing and midwifery professions, as evidenced by the considerable number of papers published in the area. These are not confined solely to journals, and significant papers on mentorship have been produced recently by the English, Welsh and Scottish National Boards for Nursing, Midwifery and Health Visiting. The English National Board (1993), for example, defines a mentor as 'an appropriately qualified and experienced first-level nurse/midwife/health visitor who, by example and facilitation, guides, assists and supports the student in learning new skills, adopting new behaviour and acquiring new attitudes'. Morle (1990) argues that the term mentorship is not defined sufficiently to be a useful concept, preferring to use the term preceptor to describe the assigning of a student to a role model and resource person in the clinical setting. Armitage and Burnard (1991) suggest that mentorship is primarily about a close, personal relationship with the student, whereas preceptorship is more concerned with the teaching, learning and role-modelling aspects of the relationship. Mentorship is seen by many writers as being a long-term relationship that extends throughout a student's programme, whereas others limit the concept to a relationship within a specific placement. In some systems, students are encouraged to choose their own mentors, and in others the mentor is assigned to the student. The former is preferable if possible, since it increases the likelihood of compatibility between mentor and student, an important factor in the relationship.

One of the controversial issues in mentoring is whether or not a mentor should also act as an assessor in relation to their students. Anforth (1992) argues that the role of mentor is incompatible with that of assessor, since it presents a moral dilemma between the guidance and counselling role and the judgmental assessment role. However, I find it difficult to understand why there should be a dilemma between these two aspects, since assessment should constitute an important teaching and learning strategy and not simply a punitive testing of achievement. If the mentor has an open, honest and friendly relationship with the student, assessment can provide a rich source of feedback and dialogue to further the student's development. At this point I should nail my colours to the mast with regard to mentorship: I use the term mentor to describe a qualified and experienced member of the practice-placement staff who enters into a formal arrangement to provide educational and personal support to a student throughout the period of the placement. This support may involve a range of functions including teaching, supervision, guidance, counselling, assessment and evaluation. However, the mentor is not the only member of the practice-placement staff who carries out these functions, and other staff will undertake these according to the needs of the student and the practice area.

Maggs (1994), in a discussion of research issues in relation to mentorship, acknowledges the need for more research, and also highlights the danger of researchers being compromised by associating too closely with the policies of funding bodies.

Preceptorship

From the foregoing discussion it is apparent that there is much overlap in the literature between the concepts of mentor and preceptor. Burke (1994) sees preceptors and students as having a short-lived, functional relationship for a specific purpose in a practice setting. Given my definition of mentorship above, I see preceptorship as a specific teaching and learning strategy rather than as a generic support system for students. My definition of a preceptor, therefore, is 'an experienced nurse, midwife or health visitor within a practice placement who acts as a role model and resource for a student who is attached to him or her for a specific time-span or experience'. Preceptorship utilizes the principle of learning by 'sitting next to Nelly' but in a more systematic and planned way. A student is attached to the preceptor for a relatively long period of time such as a day or a week, and 'shadows' the preceptor throughout. The student's role is to observe the various interactions and decisions that the preceptor is involved with in the course of his or her work, and then time is made available for the student and preceptor to meet privately to discuss the events that have occurred. During these meetings, there is two-way dialogue about the various approaches adopted and the decisions made by the preceptor; and the student can ascertain the basis for such decisions. Clearly the person chosen to be the preceptor needs to have the confidence and interpersonal skills to be questioned about why one course of action was taken rather than another, and the system needs an equally confident student who will not be overawed by the power differential. In management training, the preceptorship is often conducted in an institution other than the one in which the trainee works, and this has the advantage of avoiding a 'boss' relationship between preceptor and student.

Preceptorship offers not only benefits to the students, but also to the preceptors, since the system helps the preceptors to clarify their reasons for making particular decisions or taking certain courses of action.

Staff development for supervision, mentorship and preceptorship

The careful selection of practice-placement staff for these important roles is crucial, and Burke (1994) suggests that personal characteristics, clinical expertise, teaching skill, and motivation are important. Courses of preparation may take the form of recognized courses such as Teaching and Assessing in Clinical Practice (ENB 997 and 998), City and Guilds of London Course 7307, and the University of Greenwich/Nursing Times Open Learning unit Teaching and Learning in Practice. On the other hand, they may be specifically designed in-house courses of preparation, and these need careful joint planning between education and service, and also ongoing monitoring and quality assurance. Fish and Purr (1991) found that training for supervisors in post-registration education was infrequent and insufficient, lacking in current knowledge of theory and practice, and in debriefing and reflection from practice. The latter are quite new concepts in nursing and midwifery, and practice-placement staff will need preparation to help them approach students in a different way from that used in direct teaching. Encouraging student autonomy means a 'hands-off' approach which some experienced practitioners may find uncomfortable. There is also the potential for perceived threat on the part of practitioners who qualified some time ago, when supporting DipHE or undergraduate students. This may result in barriers arising between mentor and student, to the detriment of learning.

One very useful strategy for staff development is networking between practice-placement support staff. Networking can be formal or informal, and functions in much the same way as self-help groups by providing mutual support and sharing of experiences. Jinks and Williams (1994) describe a study of the effectiveness of an educational strategy for community nurses in relation to teaching, assessing and mentoring of Project 2000 students. They found that half the sample felt their preparation had been adequate and this correlated with the taking of a formal course of teaching and assessing.

Specific teaching and learning strategies in practice placements

Case-conferences

Ideally these should involve all members of the nursing team in discussion and evaluation of the nursing care of a particular patient. Medical staff have long used the case presentation method as a learning tool for students and qualified doctors, and the same principles apply to the use of nursing-care conferences. There is no standard format for such a conference, but it is usual for one nurse to present the patient's case and then for the whole team to be involved in the discussion. This helps the student to feel part of the nursing team as well as providing the skills in a public presentation of 'self'. Such conferences provide a useful holistic view of the patient and his or her problems, together with an opportunity to analyse critically the care that has been received, to the mutual benefit of both nurses and patients.

Ward report

Many trained nurses see the ward report as a valuable opportunity to do some teaching, since it involves the nursing team meeting together for a reasonable period of time during the day. If the report is made interactive, with each nurse explaining about their own patients, then it is more likely to be a useful learning experience. The ward manager or staff nurse often take time to ask questions about specific aspects of patients' conditions and care, and provided that the atmosphere is relaxed and informal, this can be a motivating way of learning. There are important trade-offs from a ward report in addition to the actual report itself, namely the fostering of team spirit and the development of public speaking ability and confidence in presenting information to peers.

Clinical rounds

Students can gain a great deal from accompanying a doctor or nurse on a clinical round. The former is useful for gaining insight into the role of the medical team in patient care, and it is interesting to listen to the discussion with regard to treatment. Students may find it valuable to accompany a nurse teacher on a similar round and to make comparisons of the needs of patients with similar conditions, and also to look at the difference in attitudes between such patients. Examples of pathology can be pointed out, for example oedema or inflammation, and the reasons discussed at the end of the round. Students should always carry a notebook to write down any queries or observations, but single sheets of paper must not be allowed as they can easily be lost and other patients may read the confidential details.

Reflective practice diary

Reflective diaries or records are one of the key strategies in experiential learning and consist of brief written descriptions of situations that can be used as the basis for reflection later. The following examples are from the reflective diary of a health visitor who is undergoing training as a mentor.

Situation 1: student's first day on community placement

The first day of the student's placement was spent in discussion and negotiation of her learning contract in the light of my case load requirements. Since child protection is a major facet of my work, I made it clear to the student that this aspect must by law take priority over all other matters. Before commencing their community placement students are required to complete a Community Profile so that they have insight into the area. However, the student in question arrived at my office having completed a Community Profile on a completely different area to the one in which I work. This meant that the student had no information whatsoever about the area, so we had to negotiate a series of sessions in which I could explain the key aspects of the placement community. I also contacted her personal tutor in the College of Nursing to emphasize how important it is for the student to undertake a Community Profile which relates to their placement.

Situation 2: student's first visit to a client's home

One of the items on my student's learning contract was to visit a family with a new baby. By accompanying me on the visit, the student was able to see and understand exactly what a health visitor does in such a visit. During a prior briefing discussion I explained the official standard for a new-birth visit, and asked the student to pay particular attention during the visit to how I taught the mother to look after the baby, and to compare my performance with that of the official standard. I wanted her to focus particularly on my use of verbal and non-verbal communication with the family, since interpersonal relationships are fundamental to the health visitor role.

On arriving back at the surgery following the visit, we had a debriefing session in which I challenged the student by asking her to evaluate my performance against the official standards, and how she would now approach her next new-birth visit in the light of what she had learned.

Situation 3: developmental assessment in the clinic

At age 18 months infants come to the clinic for assessment of physical and behavioural development, and this involves a variety of tests, e.g. hearing, speech, vision, motor movements etc. I acted as a role model for the student, in that she was asked to observe and record carefully my relationships and involvement with the clients, with particular emphasis in this case on the practical aspects of testing. One of the objectives in the student's learning contract was to develop the skills of developmental assessment of infants, so I planned the learning environment with this goal in mind. During the clinic, the student was asked to observe me performing the developmental assessment on a number of infants, and was then encouraged to participate in the assessment of a number of infants. Once I was satisfied that she had grasped the essential points, I allowed her to conduct an assessment in partnership with me, but she was asked to take the lead, and to treat me as her student, showing me what to do. This was a very effective way of teaching, as it showed the student aspects which she needed to study further.

Critical incident technique

Critical incident technique (CIT) is a useful tool for identifying aspects of practice which the student felt were particularly positive or negative (Flanagan, 1954). These critical incidents can then be reflected upon and analysed to give new insights into practice. Critical incident technique was used by Benner (1984) in her study of acquisition of nursing skill, and she identified critical incidents as any of the following:

- those in which the nurse's intervention really made a difference in patient outcome;

- those that went unusually well;

- those in which there was a breakdown;

- those that were ordinary and typical;

- those that captured the essence of nursing; and

- those that were particularly demanding.

Subjects were asked to include the following information in their description of critical incidents:

- the context;

- a detailed description;

- why the incident was critical to the subject;

- what the subject's concerns were at the time;

- what they were thinking about during the incident;

- what they felt about it afterwards; and

- what they found most demanding about it.

Learning contracts

Learning contracts are an effective tool for developing student autonomy in practice placements. It is useful to meet with students prior to the placement to begin the initial contract negotiation, and this can be modified as required once the placement has commenced. The theory and components of a learning contract are discussed in [Chapter 4].

Organizational stress and burn-out

One of the key psychological factors that is influenced by the type of learning environment is the concept of stress and anxiety; anxiety is an unpleasant emotion that occurs in anticipation of threat or harm and results in increased general arousal. Each individual has an optimal level of arousal at which they perform at their best; under-arousal or over-arousal results in a deterioration in performance of learning tasks, particularly complex ones. Figure 1 shows the relationship between arousal level and performance.

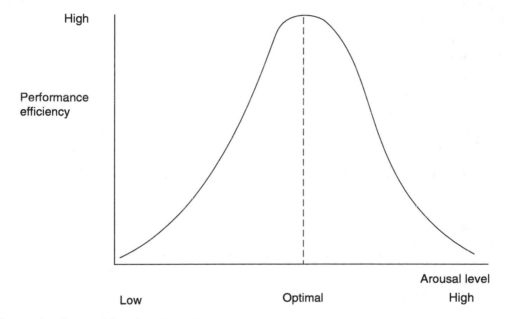

Figure 1 **Arousal level and performance**

It can be seen that arousal beyond the optimal level for a particular student will result in problems with learning and decision-making. It is quite likely that most practice placements are intrinsically stressful by nature of the human problems encountered there, such as patients in pain or dying. The pressure of work may also be stressful, particularly for student nurses who are still unsure of their practice, and there is a high element of risk involved in nursing patients in acute areas. All of these factors may combine to affect all but the most basic and well-learned responses, resulting in errors and negative experiences. Stress is a very difficult concept to define and one approach to stress is called 'person–environment fit theory' (Caplan, 1983), in which stress is defined as either demand exceeding the individual's capability, or capability exceeding the demand. Barnard (1985) points out that stress is a natural phenomenon that results in challenges of 'fight or flight', but that modern life-styles produce too much of the wrong sort of pressure. Duckworth (1985), on the other hand, finds the concept of organizational stress of little use, claiming that it distracts people from developing more useful theories and diverts attention away from awareness of the wide range of processes involved in psychological disturbance in organizations. He cites as examples of these disturbances such common behaviours as anger, jealousy and guilt, which would not be thought of as stress reactions. 'Burn-out' is another concept that is closely related to stress, and is characterized by emotional and physical exhaustion. It is a syndrome and as such, there will be wide variation in the range of symptoms that any individual will manifest.

Sources of organizational stress

Cooper and Marshall (1976) have identified five major sources of organizational stress:

1. factors intrinsic to the job — pressure of time and overload;

2. role-based stress — ambiguity, role-conflict, lack of clarity;

3. relationships — colleagues, subordinates, superiors;

4. career-development factors — fear of redundancy, promotion; and

5. organizational structure and climate — communication, politics, trust.

Another source of stress is the conflict between occupational and parental roles. Lewis and Cooper (1986), reviewing the literature, concluded that research is equivocal with regard to the stresses and benefits of employment versus home-making for women.

Hall (1976) suggests that there may be different job stressors at different stages in career development, as shown in Table 1.

Table 1   Job stressors in relation to career development (Hall, 1976)

Stage in career	*Needs*	*Stressors*
1. Establishment	Safety Recognition	Relations with superiors Role ambiguity
2. Advancement	Moving up the ladder Mastering the organization	Promotion Future development Work versus family
3. Maintenance	Levelling out Guiding others	Obsolescence Frustration about career

Effects of stress and burn-out

The reaction of the individual to stress occurs in three well-defined stages termed 'the general adaptation syndrome' (Selye, 1956).

1. *The alarm reaction.* This is a short-term reaction characterized by changes in physiology such as increased heart rate, respiration, endocrine activity and sympathetic-nervous-system activity.

2. *Resistance to stress.* In this stage the body processes return to normal and the individual adapts to the stress.

3. *Exhaustion.* This rarely occurs in psychological stress, although it is common in extreme physical conditions such as severe exposure. Here, the individual has used up all the resources for coping, and death may occur.

This adaptation syndrome is non-specific, in that it occurs when the person encounters any form of stress, of whatever severity. There is growing evidence of a link between stress and heart disease, and a number of tools have been devised to measure the extent to which individuals are prone to stress-related disease. Examples are 'the social readjustment scale' (Holmes and Rahe, 1967) and 'the job stress check' (Cooper, 1981).

Burn-out is characterized by both physical and psychological symptoms. Physical symptoms are typically fatigue, exhaustion, headaches and gut disturbances, sleeplessness, dyspnoea and inability to fight off minor infections (McConnell, 1982). Psychological problems occurring with burn-out are dislike of work, irritability, working harder to accomplish less and less, disenchantment, rigidity in interpreting policies and absenteeism.

Coping with stress and burn-out

One helpful way of coping is to embark upon an anti-stress programme such as that of Barnard (1985), which has three main parts.

1. *Know your own personality.* In order to best cope with stress, a degree of self-awareness is important; people with Type A personality tend to be hard-working, driving, competitive and aggressive, whereas Type B are more relaxed and placid and not very competitive. There is greater susceptibility to coronary heart disease in people with Type A personality, and although one cannot alter basic personality, it is important to realize this susceptibility and adjust the lifestyle accordingly.

2. *Choose an appropriate response to stress.* This involves general guidelines such as the avoidance of becoming overtired, ensuring adequate restful sleep, developing the ability to say no, acknowledging your limitations and being able to seek advice about stress.

3. *Your life in your hands.* This involves the use of time management and relaxation.

Barnard (1985) cites Cooper's advice on time management at work:

- arrange a period of time for organizing each day that cannot be interrupted;
- plan tasks in priority order;
- set realistic achievable deadlines;
- concentrate on one task at a time;
- avoid indecisiveness;
- consider each problem in depth;

- always take lunch outside of the office;

- do not neglect family time;

- develop a hobby that demands total concentration; and

- plan leisurely holidays.

There are a variety of relaxation techniques that can help reduce stress, such as physical-relaxation techniques and meditation. McConnell (1982) gives the following organizational strategies for helping staff to cope with stress:

- encourage staff to express feelings;

- support, encourage and reward risk-taking;

- provide recognition;

- work with knowledgeable and capable leaders;

- encourage sharing of needs and wants;

- invite staff to participate in decision-making;

- develop problem-solving skills; and

- include stress management in staff development programmes.

Social support from colleagues can help to reduce stress and there is some evidence that colleague support has a greater effect on stress reduction than family support (Glowinkowski and Cooper, 1985). It can be valuable if the ward, department or community group sets up peer-support groups to combat stress, where practitioners can discuss their reactions and feelings to organizational matters in a supportive atmosphere. A development of this is the notion of 'co-counselling', in which two people enter into a contract to give a stated amount of time to each other for the purpose of counselling.

References

Anforth P (1992) Mentors, not assessors, *Nurse Education Today*. 12: 299–302.

Armitage P, Burnard P (1991) Mentors or preceptors? Narrowing the theory-practice gap. *Nurse Education Today*, 11: 225–29.

Barnard C (1985) *Your Healthy Heart*. MacDonald, London.

Benner P (1984) *From Novice to Expert: Excellence and Power in Clinical Nursing Practice*. Addison-Wesley, London.

Burke L (1994) Preceptorship and post-registration nurse education. *Nurse Education Today*, 14: 60–6.

Butterworth T, Faugier J (1992) *Clinical Supervision and Mentorship in Nursing*. Chapman and Hall, London.

Caplan R (1983) Person–environment fit: past, present and future. In: C Cooper (ed) *Stress Research: Issues for the Eighties*. Wiley, Chichester.

Cooper C (1981) *The Stress Check*. Prentice-Hall, London.

Cooper C, Marshall J (1976) Occupational sources of stress. *Journal of Occupational Psychology*, 49: 11–28.

Darling L A (1984) What do nurses want in a mentor? *Journal of Nursing Administration*, Oct. 14(10): 42–4.

Dreyfus S, Dreyfus H (1980) A five-stage model of the mental activities involved in directed skill acquisition. Unpublished report supported by the Air Force Office of Scientific Research, University of California, Berkeley.

Duckworth D (1985) Is the 'organisational stress' construct a red herring? *Bulletin of the British Psychological Society*, 38: 401–404.

English National Board for Nursing, Midwifery and Health Visiting (1993) *Guidelines for Educational Audit*. ENB, London.

English National Board for Nursing, Midwifery and Health Visiting (1993) *Regulations and Guidelines for the Approval of Institutions and Courses*. ENB, London.

Faugier J (1992) in T Butterworth and J Faugier (1992) *Clinical Supervision and Mentorship in Nursing*. Chapman and Hall, London.

Fish D, Purr B (1991) An evaluation of practice-based learning in continuing professional education in nursing, midwifery and health visiting. *Project Paper 4*, ENB, London.

Flanagan J (1954) The critical incident technique. *Psychological Bulletin*, 51: 327–58.

Ford K, Jones A (1987) *Student Supervision*. Macmillan, London.

Fretwell J (1983) Creating a ward learning environment: the sister's role. *Nursing Times Occasional Papers*, 79 (21 and 22).

Gerrish K (1992) The nurse teacher's role in the practice setting. *Nurse Education Today*, 12: 227–32.

Glowinkowski S, Cooper C (1985) Current issues in organisational stress research. *Bulletin of the British Psychological Society*, 38: 401–404.

Hall D (1976) *Careers in Organisations*. Goodyear, New York.

Holmes T, Rahe R (1967) The social readjusment scale. *Journal of Psychosomatic Research*, 11.

Jinks A, Williams R (1994) Evaluation of a community staff preparation strategy for the teaching, assessing and mentorship of Project 2000 Diploma students. *Nurse Education Today*, 14: 44–51.

Knowles M (1986) *Contracting for Learning*. Jossey Bass, San Francisco.

Lewis S, Cooper C (1986) The stress of combining occupational and parental roles: a review of the literature. *Bulletin of the British Psychological Society*, 36: 341–5.

Maggs C (1994) Mentorship in nursing and midwifery education: issues for research. *Nurse Education Today*, 14: 22–9.

McConnell E (1982) *Burnout in the Nursing Profession*. Mosby, London.

Morle K (1990) Mentorship — is it a case of the emperor's new clothes or a rose by any other name? *Nurse Education Today*, 10: 66–9.

Ogier M (1982) *An Ideal Sister*. RCN, London.

Ogier M (1986) An 'ideal' sister — seven years on. *Nursing Times Occasional Papers*, 82 (2).

Orton H (1981) Ward learning climate and student nurse response. *Nursing Times Occasional Papers*, 77 (17).

Pembrey S (1980) *The Ward Sister — Key to Care*. RCN, London.

Reilly D, Oermann M (1985) *The Clinical Field: Its Use in Nursing Education*. Appleton Century Crofts, Norwalk.

Selye H (1956) *The Stress of Life*. McGraw Hill, New York.

18. An Analysis of the Concept *Facilitation*

Kathryn D. Cross

This paper is an analysis of the concept facilitation. *The analysis is based on a model suggested by Wilson (1969) cited in Walker & Avent (1988). The literature review shows the term used in physiological, educational, counselling/psychotherapy, social and theological contexts. The analysis leads to the compilation of the defining attributes of the concept* facilitation *which are: a process of enabling change; a climate for learning (mutual trust, acceptance and respect); and factors which relate to the nature of the process (student-centred, negotiated and collaborative). The antecedents relate to the facilitator qualities (realness, caring and empathy), access to a learning situation and the effects of motivation and social influences; the consequences of effective facilitation being reciprocal change (learning and understanding), reciprocal feedback and increased independence. To a limited extent the empirical referents have been discussed. Cases have been constructed to provide examples of the term facilitation used in a model, borderline, related and contrary situations. The analysis will be of particular interest to those in nurse education.*

Introduction

An analysis of the concept *facilitation* is important as it will help us define the attributes or characteristics of the concept. Concepts contain within them defining characteristics or attributes that enable us to decide which phenomena are good examples of the concept and which are not. Those which are not good examples are often called irrelevant attributes (Walker & Avant, 1988).

Concept analysis

The concept

The concept of facilitation is being used increasingly in nurse education, with many educationalists advocating a change from the traditional teacher role to that of facilitation. Brookfield (1986) has suggested that 'the facilitator of learning now exercises something of a conceptual stranglehold on our notions of correct educational practice, and to talk of the role of the teacher, or of teaching as a function, is unfashionable and distasteful to some educators of adults' (Brookfield, 1986, p.123).

The aims and purposes of the analysis

The writer aims to clarify the defining attributes of this concept in the hope that those who wish to adopt its principles and those who practice facilitation of learning may assume a greater understanding of its inherent principles and philosophy.

Kathryn D. Cross: 'An Analysis of the Concept *Facilitation*' in *NURSE EDUCATION TODAY* (1996), 16, pp. 350–355. Reprinted by permission of the publisher Churchill Livingstone.

All uses of the concept

A wide range of literature relating to the concept of facilitation was accessed in order that all uses of the term were considered. The sources included dictionaries and literature from general and nurse education, counselling and psychotherapy, theology and physiology.

'The concept of facilitation is relatively new in education, though the activities inherent to it have been discussed in educational writings over the last century or so' (Brookfield, 1986, p. 62). The term was applied to education explicitly from the 1960s, this resulting primarily from the work of the psychotherapist Carl R Rogers. Rogers developed a therapeutic counselling approach which he called client-centred therapy (Rogers, 1951). This involves the therapist in a non-directive role in which the client is encouraged to develop a deeper understanding of himself. The role of the therapist is to provide a non-critical atmosphere, in which there is no attempt to interpret for the client, but simply a reflecting back of his statements in order to assist him in developing self-awareness (Quinn, 1988). This concept of client-centred therapy led Rogers to formulate his student-centred approach to learning (Rogers, 1969). This approach places an emphasis on relevance, student participation and involvement, self-evaluation and the absence of threat in the classroom. Rogers sees the teacher as a facilitator of learning; a provider of resources for learning, and someone who shares his feelings as well as his knowledge with the students. Thus the prerequisites of an effective facilitator of learning are awareness of self, being oneself in the classroom, acceptance and trust of the students and understanding and empathy (Quinn, 1988). The term has now entered mainstream educational literature (Knowles, 1975; Brundage & Mackeracher, 1980; Cross, 1981; Knowles, 1984; Knowles *et al.* 1984). The term facilitation is also used in physiology and was recorded in the literature in 1895 (*Oxford English Dictionary*, 1989). The term is used to describe social facilitation, which is 'the stimulating effect on a person's behaviour of other people — even the mere presence of other people' (*Dictionary of Human Behaviour*, 1981, p. 117). Social facilitation was included as a valid use of the concept as it is relevant to teaching and learning. The term has theological origins, firstly in 1619 in relation to the action or process of facilitating or rendering easy . . . for the facilitation hereof, it (the Synod) doth renew some things decreed by the holy Canons' (*Oxford English Dictionary*, 1989, p. 649). Secondly in 1648 as 'a means of facilitating or helping forwards . . . a general habit of sincerity, which when it is referred to religious uses, proves a facilitation towards fidelity and the perseverance in them' (*Oxford English Dictionary*, 1989, p. 649). The term is used in a variety of contexts: all were considered relevant and were therefore included in the analysis.

Teaching, according to Rogers (1983, p. 119), 'is a highly over-rated function', in contrast to the facilitation of learning. Teaching by giving knowledge does not meet the requirements of today's rapidly changing world; what is required 'if we are to survive is the facilitation of change and learning', and this requires certain qualities in the facilitator (Rogers, 1983). Rogers suggests that 'the only man who is educated is the man who has learned how to learn; the man who has learned how to adapt and change; the man who has realised that no knowledge is secure, that only the process of seeking knowledge gives a basis for security. Changingness, a reliance on process rather than upon static knowledge, is the only thing that makes sense as a goal for education in the modern world' (Rogers, 1983, p. 120).

In 1969, Carl Rogers presented the freedom-to-learn notion and directed special attention to the personal qualities and behaviours of the teacher and the accomplishment of such student freedom. 'Real learning according to the phenomenological psychologists involves the total person rather than merely providing him with the facts to be memorised' (Burns, 1992, p. 264). However it was not until 1969 that Rogers published his proposals for education. Rogers sets for education, as he does for psychotherapy, the goal of enabling students to become fully functioning individuals and encouraging 'free curiosity' (Rogers, 1969 p. 105). He assumes that individuals have a natural potential for learning, but that they will only really learn that which is meaningful to them (Rogers, 1969, p. 157).

The translation of Rogers' humanistic approach into the process of teaching involves a total reappraisal of the role and function of the teacher. The humanists place a higher priority on learning than teaching. Maslow, in his definition of humanistic education, differentiates between intrinsic and extrinsic education by defining intrinsic education as that which changes the person and enables him to move toward his unique potential; and extrinsic education as education that is an end in itself (Maslow, 1968).

It is, however, 'naive to assume that simply because adults are under the direction of a teacher that learning is being facilitated. What is important to consider is the nature of the teaching–learning transaction itself and the extent to which mutual respect, negotiation, collaborativeness, and praxis are present' (Brookfield, 1986, p. 9). Brookfield outlines key principles to effective facilitation: these include the voluntary participation in learning, respect among participation for each other's self-worth, a collaborative relationship where there is continual renegotiation of activities and a general spirit of critical reflection. The ultimate goal is self-directed, empowered adults (Brookfield, 1986). Rogers also offers guidelines for the teacher-as-facilitator and requires that the teacher should have much to do with 'setting the initial mood or climate of the group or class experience', help elicit and clarify the purposes of the individuals in the class as well as the more general purposes of the group' and rely on 'the desire of each student to implement those purposes which have meaning for him, as the motivational force behind significant learning'. The teacher should look upon himself as a 'flexible resource to be utilized by the group' and attempt to organize and make available 'the widest range of resources for learning'. The teacher should, in responding to expressions from the class group, accept intellectual content and emotionalized personal feelings; be a participant learner and a member of the class group; remain alert to the expression of deep or strong feelings and endeavour to recognize and accept his or her own limitations (Rogers, 1969, p. 106–126).

Finally, facilitation is often discussed in relation to group facilitation skills. Group facilitation styles have been covered extensively elsewhere and will therefore not be further discussed in this paper (Heron, 1977; King, 1984; Burnard, 1989; Heron, 1989; Spinks & Clements, 1993; Bentley, 1994).

From the available literature, themes or common characteristics emerged. These were counted in an attempt to quantify the data. From the literature, 17 themes emerged.

A summary of the preliminary categories, their frequency and a definition are given in Box 1.

Box 1

Facilitation is an active process (19 occurrences). Facilitation is a 'means of facilitating or helping forwards' (*Oxford English Dictionary*, 1989, p. 649).

Facilitation lowers threshold or resistance (6 occurrences). 'The lowering of resistance in a neural pathway to an impulse, resulting from a previous or simultaneous stimulation' (*Random House Dictionary of the English Language*, 1966, 1967, p. 509).

Increase in responsiveness (6 occurrences). The 'increase in responsiveness of a nerve-cell of an effector cell produced by summation of impinging impulses' (*Penguin Dictionary of Biology*, 1980, p. 113).

The establishment of a preferred route or pathway (4 occurrences). 'The establishment of a preferred reflex pathway in the central nervous system by the repetition of the stimulus that excites the reflex response' (*Fontana Dictionary of Modern Thought*, 1988, p. 226).

Increased ease of transmission (17 occurrences). 'The increased ease of transmission of an impulse in a nerve fibre, caused by prior excitation' (*Collins English Dictionary*, 1991, p. 553). Also, 'the task of the facilitator is to speed up the learning process of the learner, guide him or her in the right direction and make sure he or she will end up in the right place' (Mak, 1992, p. 53).

Essential facilitator qualities (10 occurrences). These are firstly realness and genuineness, secondly non-possessive caring, trust and respect. Finally empathic understanding and sensitive listening (Rogers, 1969).

Collaborative, mutually beneficial relationship (17 occurrences). Rogers (1969) identified the personal relationship between the facilitator and the learner as being critical to the facilitation of learning.

Positive outcome arising from the experience (14 occurrences). 'The aim of facilitation is the nurturing of self-directed, empowered adults' (Brookfield, 1986, p. 11).

Student-centred (18 occurrences). 'The term (facilitation) . . . implies a commitment to a client- or student-centred form of relationship' (Woolfe, 1992, p. 7).

Element of negotiation (8 occurrences). This would include '. . . a balance between confrontation and support in which students assume a major responsibility for their own learning and the tutor's role to debate, challenge, question, probe, encourage, guide, negotiate and mediate in an environment of mutual trust and cooperation' (MIHE, 1988, cited in McMillan & Dwyer, 1990, p. 190).

Element of feedback and reflection (8 occurrences). 'Facilitation aims to foster in adults a spirit of critical reflection' (Brookfield, 1986, p. 10).

Box 1 (cont)

Increased student independence (7 occurrences). 'The primary goal of nondirective teaching is to assist students in attaining greater personal integration, effectiveness, and a realistic self-appraisal' (Joyce & Weil, 1992, p. 264).

Motivation (4 occurrences). 'A good facilitator understands learners' goals (what they want to learn) and their motivation (why they want to learn), and finds the best ways of enabling them to achieve those goals' (Burnard, 1992, p. iii).

Social influences (4 occurrences). 'The stimulating effect in a person's behaviour of other people — even the mere presence of other people' (*Dictionary of Human Behaviour*, 1981, p. 117).

Process of communication (4 occurrences). Communication between the learner and the facilitator is important in establishing the learner's needs (Burnard, 1992a,b).

Climate of mutual trust, acceptance and respect (10 occurrences). 'The most effective basis for facilitating learning is an atmosphere of acceptance, understanding, and respect' (Rogers, 1951, p. 384).

The definition of facilitation as an active process and its use in physiology (lowered resistance, increased responsiveness, preferred route and increased ease of transmission) were combined. The justification for this is that the term related to an active, positive process in which change or the movement towards a desired outcome took place. Hence the category which emerged related facilitation to a *process of enabling change.*

Secondly, the *climate for learning* emerged as another category and incorporated mutual trust, acceptance and respect. The key factor related to the climate was the requirement that these characteristics would be reciprocal. The climate does not relate to the process but to the atmosphere created, which may well hinder or facilitate learning.

Thirdly, the *nature of the process.* This relates to the process or the activity of facilitation. The key characteristics are: student-centred learning, which encompasses negotiation; effective communication; and a collaborative, mutually beneficial relationship.

Finally, *student motivation and social influences* were viewed as related terms since they may influence learning positively or negatively. Motivation may be intrinsic or extrinsic. Generally, participation in adult learning is voluntary. It may be that the circumstances prompting this learning are external to the student (job loss, divorce, bereavement), *extrinsic* factors, but the decision to learn is the student's. Students are usually therefore highly motivated. Significant learning is more likely to take place when the subject matter is perceived by the student as having relevance for his or her own purposes (Rogers, 1969). This implies *intrinsic* motivation.

Following refinement, the 16 categories were reduced to 9. From these 9 categories, the defining attributes, antecedents and consequences were identified.

The defining attributes

The defining attributes which emerged from the literature are:

- Process of enabling change

- Climate for learning (mutual trust, acceptance and respect)

- Nature of the process (student-centred, negotiated and collaborative).

Concept analysis as outlined by Wilson (1969) cited Walker & Avent (1988) requires that the defining attributes are illustrated through their use in model, borderline, related, contrary, invented and illegitimate cases. Invented cases are constructed using ideas outside our own experience and in an illegitimate case the concept is used improperly (Walker & Avant, 1988). Examples of an invented and illegitimate use of the concept are not included in this paper.

Construct a model case

A model case is one that we are certain is an example of the concept and that all the defining attributes are present. Wilson (1969, p. 40) suggests that the model case is one in which the analyst can say 'well, if *that* isn't an example of it, then nothing is.'

A student on the enrolled nurse conversion course discusses learning opportunities and personal objectives at the start of the course. Ths student's prior knowledge and skills are valued by the teacher. The student suggests several goals which the teacher helps her to clarify and refine through discussion. The student negotiates a learning contract with the teacher and arranges a date to meet to discuss the progress towards the achievement of the learning goal.

In this case, the climate for learning is present because the teacher recognized the student's knowledge base and the student values the teacher's constructive comments and suggestions. The nature of the process is apparent through the use of negotiation and the student-centred focus. The process of change is evident through the development of a learning contract.

Construct a borderline, related and contrary case

The following case does not fulfil the criteria relating to the nature of the process and is therefore a borderline case.

The teacher accepted and respected the student's wish to focus on a particular area for her assignment; the teacher specified the written structure to be followed.

The climate for learning is apparent in that the teacher respected the student's wishes to focus on a particular area of interest. The completion of an assignment would indicate a process of change. However, the nature of the proccss is not apparent in that the structure of the assigment and assessment criteria were teacher-centred and not open to discussion.

Related cases involve the use of words and concepts similar to the concept of facilitation but do not contain all the critical attributes (Walker & Avant, 1988). Possible related cases would include words and concepts such as help, guide, enable, and catalyst.

Contrary cases are those that are clear examples of 'not the concept' (Walker & Avant, 1988, p. 41).

A tutor student on teaching practice is teaching a 'difficult' group for the first time. She proceeds to dictate notes to the class unrelated to the planned revision session without offering any explanation. The teacher seems unapproachable, the students leave the session totally bemused, not having covered the revision.

The climate for learning is not evident because the students did not feel comfortable in asking the teacher why the content of the session had been altered. The nature of the process was teacher-centred with no element of negotiation. The process of enabling change did not take place as the objectives were not expressed and the proposed revision did not take place.

The antecedents and consequences

Antecedents are the factors which must be present *prior* to facilitation taking place. The antecedents for facilitation identified in the literature are:

- Facilitator qualities (realness, caring and empathy)

- Access to a learning situation

- Motivation and social influences.

The facilitator qualities of realness, caring and empathy are antecedents because they are prerequisite to the process of facilitation. A facilitator possessing these qualities would be more likely to establish with the student a climate for learning, a defining attribute.

Access to a learning situation is an obvious prerequisite to learning and therefore must be considered as an antecedent.

The positive effects of motivation, and the social influence of another person affect the learning desire and performance. These factors normally occur as a precursor to the learning experience and make learning more likely and are classified as antecedents.

Consequences are those events or incidents that occur as a *result* of effective facilitation. The consequences of facilitation are:

- Reciprocal change (learning and understanding)

- Reciprocal feedback

- Increased independence.

Reciprocal change (usually measured through learning and understanding), and increased independence were considered the consequences of effective facilitation, in that the process needed to be initiated and implemented before the end result became apparent.

Empirical referents

'Empirical referents are classes or categories of actual phenomenon that by their existence or presence *demonstrate* the occurrence of the concept itself' (Walker & Avant, 1988, p. 43). The empirical referents for the concept facilitation the writer found difficult to identify and therefore these suggestions are made with caution.

Empirical referents may include the negotiation of individual learning contracts. Learning contracts help maintain a commitment to learner-centredness and should be individually planned (Henfield & Waldron, 1988). They act as a mechanism for facilitating learners in the achievement of specified outcomes (Jarvis, 1986).

The presence of facilitative behaviours such as: using open and closed questions; asking reflexive questions; summarizing and checking understanding (Burnard, 1992); and effective listening (Egan, 1990), could be observed and may indicate the presence of facilitative skills.

Limitations of the analysis

The limitations of the analysis arise from the depth and breadth of the literature which was accessed; it is impossible to determine if valuable sources were missed. Additionally, although the writer attempted to remain objective, it was the writer's interpretation of the literature which led to the identification, refinement and justification for the defining attributes, antecedents and consequenses. Although the use of the model provided a structure for the analysis, it may have been unnecessarily restrictive.

Conclusion

The concept of facilitation is used in a wide variety of contexts. However, through the analysis, the writer has been able to determine the defining attributes, the antecedents and the consequences of the concept facilitation. The antecedents are the facilitator qualities of realness, caring and empathy, access to a learning situation and the effects of motivation and social influences. The defining attributes are a process of enabling change, a climate for learning which includes mutual trust, acceptance and respect, and the nature of the process in which the interaction is student-centred, negotiated and collaborative. The consequenses of facilitation are reciprocal change as measured by learning and understanding, reciprocal feedback and increased independence.

This analysis has hopefully helped to clarify and refine the concept of facilitation. Effective facilitation requires that certain factors must be present (the antecedents) before the actual process of facilitation can take place (the defining attributes), which results in effective facilitation (the consequences). If the antecedents, the facilitator qualities, motivation and social influences, and access to a learning situation are not in place then the process of effective facilitation cannot begin.

The framework used for this analysis (Wilson, 1969, cited in Walker & Avant, 1983) provided a structure for the analysis, although the progression was not linear, but very much a process of revisiting earlier stages before being able to progress again. Discussion with others helped with the clarification of thought and highlighted areas for further consideration.

Acknowledgements

I would like to thank all members of the Department of Nursing Studies and the Education Department of the Institute of Advanced Nursing Education, London who are involved in the Master of Science and the Post-graduate Diploma in Education course, for their help in the preparation of this paper, especially Ann Garvey.

References

Bentley T (1994) *Facilitation providing learning opportunities for learning*. McGraw-Hill, London.

Brookfield S D (1986) *Understanding and facilitating adult learning: a comprehensive analysis of principles and effective practices*. Open University Press, Milton Keynes.

Brundage D H, Mackeracher D (1980) *Adult learning principles and their application to program planning*. Ministry of Education, Ontario.

Burnard P (1989) Teaching interpersonal skills: a handbook of experiential learning for health professionals. *Therapy in practice 10*. Chapman & Hall, London.

Burnard P (1992a) Professional development module: facilitating learning. Part (i): learning and communication. *Nursing Times* 88 (5): i–viii.

Burnard P (1992b) Professional development module: facilitating learning. Part (ii): the process of facilitating. *Nursing Times* 88 (6): i–viii.

Burns R (1982) *Self-concept development and education*. Holt, Rinehart & Winston, London.

Collins English Dictionary (1991) (3rd edn) HarperCollins.

Cross K P (1981) *Adults as learners: increasing participation and facilitating learning*. Jossey-Bass, San Francisco.

Dictionary of the English Language (1966, 1967) Unabridged edn. Random House, New York.

Dictionary of Human Behaviour (1981) Harper & Row, London.

Egan G (1990) *The skilled helper* (4th edn). Brookes/Cole, California.

Fontana Dictionary of Modern Thought (1988) (2nd edn) Brookes/Cole, California.

Henfield V J, Waldron R (1988) The use of competency statements to facilitate individualised learning. *Nurse Education Today* 8: 205–211.

Heron J (1977) Catharsis in human development. Human potential research project. University of Surrey, Guildford.

Heron J (1989) *The facilitators handbook*. Kogan Page, London.

Jarvis P (1986) Contract learning. *Journal of District Nursing*. November, 13–14.

Joyce B, Weil M (1992) (4th edn) *Models of teaching*. Allyn & Bacon, Massachusetts.

King E C (1984) *Affective education in nursing: a guide to teaching and assessment*. Aspen, Maryland.

Knowles M S (1975) *Self-directed learning: a guide for learners and teachers*. Cambridge Books, New York.

Knowles M (1984) *The adult learner: a neglected species*. Gulf, Houston.

Knowles M S *et al.* (1984) *Andragogy in action: applying modern principles of adult learning*. Jossey-Bass, San Francisco.

Macarther Institute of Higher Education (1988) In: M A McMillan, J Dwyer. Facilitating a match between teaching and learning styles. *Nurse Education Today* (1990) 10: 186–192.

Mak W M (1992) Experiential learning: the Confucian model. In: J Mulligan, C Griffin (eds) *Empowerment through experiential learning*. Kogan Page, London.

Maslow A H (1968) *Towards psychology of being*. Van Nostrand, Princetown, Massachusetts.

Oxford English Dictionary (1989) (2nd edn). Volume V. dvanda-follis. Clarendon Press, Oxford.

Penguin Dictionary of Biology (1980) (7th edn). Penguin Books, UK.

Quinn F M (1988) *The principles and practice of nurse education* (2nd edn). Chapman & Hall, London.

Rogers C R (1951) *Student-centred teaching. Client-centred therapy: its current practice, implications and theory*. Constable, London.

Rogers C (1969) *Freedom to learn*. Merril, Columbus.

Rogers C R (1983) *Freedom to learn for the 80's*. Merril, Columbus.

Spinks T. Clements P (1993) *A practical guide to facilitation skills — a real world approach*. Kogan Page, London.

Walker L O, Avant K C (1988) *Strategies for theory construction in nursing* (2nd edn). Appleton & Lange, Connecticut.

Wilson J (1969) *Thinking with concepts*. Cambridge University Press, New York.

Woolfe R (1992) Experiential learning in workshops. In: T Holls (ed) *Experiential training: practical guidelines*. Routledge, London.

19. 'Letting Go': Rationale and Strategies for Student-centred Approaches to Clinical Teaching

Elizabeth M. Rideout

To date the clinical practice portion of nursing education has tended to emphasise patient problems related to specific disease processes and the technical interventions needed to deal with those problems. Teacher-centred methods of education that place control of the process and content of learning with the teacher have seemed appropriate. However, the role and function of nursing is changing. Autonomy, independence and decision-making are more highly valued. In order that nurses develop these skills and abilities, a shift in focus in nursing education is required. This paper presents a rationale for more student-centred approaches to education. Strategies for clinical teaching will be described that emphasise collaboration between student and teacher. Suggestions designed to facilitate change in the roles of teachers and students will be offered.

Introduction

Clinical practice is an important component of any educational programme designed to prepare health professionals such as nurses, physicians and occupational therapists. The purposes of clinical experience in nursing education are similar to those for other professional groups and include enabling learners to integrate knowledge and skills associated with caring for patients and ensuring that students acquire the ability to provide nursing care (Woolley & Costello, 1988). The emphasis in clinical experience has been on the technical component of nursing practice with its focus on the performance of specific actions and skills. Traditional methods of nursing education have placed the control of the content and process of learning to nurse in the hands of the teacher. The purpose of this paper is to demonstrate that changing demands on the health care system, on the role of nursing and on approaches to teaching require that more control of the clinical practice component of nursing education be shared with students.

Rationale for change

Nursing has been described as consisting of three components: the technical with its focus on the performance of specific actions or skills; the rational which emphasises decision-making and critical thinking; and the emotive which encompasses the interpersonal or relational aspects of nursing (Bevis & Watson, 1989). Nursing education in general and the clinical practice portion in particular has tended to emphasise the technical component of nursing. The curriculum in most schools of

Elizabeth M. Rideout: '"Letting Go": Rationale and Strategies for Student-centred Approaches to Clinical Teaching' in *NURSE EDUCATION TODAY* (1994), 14(2), pp. 146–151. Reprinted by permission of the publisher Churchill Livingstone.

nursing has focused on basic disease processes and the technical interventions needed to deal with those diseases. However, the health care issues facing us are changing. The health problems associated with increasing numbers of elderly and those with chronic diseases require skills and abilities additional to the technical ones. The role of the nurse is also changing, from that of assistant to the physician where technical skills and abilities are most valued, to one of greater autonomy and independence, where the rational or decision-making component of nursing assumes greater importance (Bevis & Watson, 1989; Lindeman, 1989). Altogether the changing demands of nursing require the teaching of reflection, criticism, independence, creativity and inquiry. It is these qualities that are particularly needed for nursing in the future (Lindeman, 1989). Elements of discovery and innovation are important for nurses (and other health care professionals) to provide the care required (Schön, 1987). This dictates that the teaching–learning process be reconceptualised as a participatory process model, so students can develop the self-reliance to function in the rapidly changing situations that characterise the health care system of today and tomorrow (Lindeman, 1989). A move from traditional teacher-centred methods of nursing education to more student-centred approaches is required.

Definition of terms: student-centred and teacher-centred

To date nursing educators have relied on teacher-centred approaches to education that emphasise essential content and skills as defined by the teacher (Bevis & Watson, 1989). In this approach there is reliance on a subject or content orientation and the emphasis is on direct instructional techniques such as demonstrations and return demonstrations. The knowledge and skills to be acquired are identified by faculty and the evaluation is in relation to criteria specified by faculty (Miller & Seller, 1990; Stenhouse, 1975). A student-centred approach describes collaboration between students and faculty, where educational goals and the means to achieve the goals are determined through discussion and deliberation (Bevis & Watson, 1989). Although the faculty define the outcome objectives to be achieved, there is much opportunity for individual learning within the broad confines of the specified objectives.

Moving toward student-centred methods

Selecting clinical settings and patients

The traditional teacher-centred approaches to clinical teaching that emphasise the development of technical expertise (DeYoung, 1990; Woolley & Costello, 1988) would be familiar to most clinical nurse educators. These will be described and more learner centred strategies will be presented that should promote the development of nurses prepared to face the challenges of working in our changing health care system.

In the traditional approach to clinical teaching, students are assigned by the teacher to hospital and community practice settings and to patients within those settings. Patient assignments are made for students according to the student learning needs as identified by the teacher and based on course objectives. The choice of patients is often made in relation to the medical diagnosis of the patient and the resulting opportunity for skills practice. Information is provided by the teacher about the patient so nursing care can be planned for the 'typical' patient problems. Students then provide the care, modifying it as necessary as they learn more about individual patient needs. In the traditional teacher-centred method, placements for practice are also selected by teachers, based on the belief that students must be exposed to all clinical settings where nurses function. This is congruent with a content rather than process approach, where the focus is learning the specific knowledge and skills needed to function in diverse settings such as maternal–child, paediatrics, medicine, surgery and psychiatry.

A more student-centred strategy would promote student choice of placements for clinical practice and the selection of patients within those settings. Student input into choice of patients within settings would be encouraged in a student-centred approach. Students would select patients based on individual learning needs within the framework of course and programme objectives. In a system that allowed for student selection of clinical placements, some teacher control would be important to ensure that any statutory requirements for practice are met and a basic level of knowledge and skills is achieved while allowing individuals to pursue particular areas of interest. This approach would shift the focus from specific content to the process of nursing, from learning the nursing interventions for medical diagnoses to learning the process of care for common problems faced by patients and families, such as pain, grief and loss (Bevis & Watson, 1989).

Using clinical learning plans

Another student-centred strategy would be the use of clinical learning plans to facilitate the defining by students of individual learning objectives to be achieved in the clinical setting. Learning plans:

> 'replace a content plan with a process plan. Instead of specifying how a body of content will be transmitted (content plan), it specifies how a body of content will be acquired by the learner' (process plan). (Knowles, 1986, p. 39).

The roles of student and teacher must shift when learning plans are introduced. The teacher becomes the facilitator of self-directed learning and a content resource. The student assumes an active role in selecting objectives for learning from within the range of course and programme objectives. The outcomes for the student include expanded participation in planning learning experiences, enhanced ability for resource selection and acquisition, and increased skill in self-evaluation of current performance levels. Additional benefits are an increase in assertiveness and confidence that follows from the changed view of self and the modified relationships with teachers (Knowles, 1986).

Methods of clinical teaching

Record review

Record reviews are a useful strategy in clinical teaching (DeYoung, 1990). In the traditional, teacher-centred approach such reviews provide an opportunity to appraise the student's documentation of assessment and management of patients. The focus of the activity is the quality of the documentation; discussion of the interpretation of the data recorded is uncommon. The emphasis for the student is the meeting of teacher expectations for concise and accurate recording. In a more student-centred approach, record reviews could continue to provide a method for confirming precision of documentation while also providing an opportunity for discussion of the patient and the related care requirements (Edwards & Baptiste, 1987). In particular, the discussion could allow for a focus on the patient's particular response to illness rather than issues related to the completion of nursing care tasks. As such the record becomes a teaching tool and the educational strategy is a dialogue between teacher and student.

Pre- and post-conferences

Pre- and post-conferences are another part of the clinical practice experience of most nursing programmes. The pre-conference is held for 15–30 min prior to going to the clinical area. Traditionally it is used to question the students concerning their plans for the day; the primary purpose is to determine the degree of student preparedness to provide care for their assigned patient, and arranging times for teacher observation of skill performance. The pre-conference has been dubbed 'drill and grill' and it often resembles just that (Woolley & Costello, 1988).

The post-conference, which traditionally follows the clinical experience and lasts from 15–30 min, provides the opportunity for students to share their experiences and to learn from the approaches and interventions displayed by their classmates. The post-conference is sometimes referred to as 'facts and events' since it is used to describe within the group the events of the clinical session.

Changes in the format and use of pre- and post-conferences would provide another method of enhancing student-centred learning. For example, conferences could be student rather than teacher led. Rather than the 'drill and grill' routine, the conferences could provide the opportunity to meet individual learning objectives as outlined in student learning plans. Weekly rounds attended by students, nursing staff involved in the day to day provision of care as well as patients could replace the traditional conference. The content would shift from discussion of the day's events to mutual problem-solving around common issues of care as applied to particular patients. Opportunities for interdisciplinary conferences might also be provided, allowing for learning about the contribution of other health professionals to patient care.

The process of evaluation

Evaluation is an integral part of clinical teaching (Tower & Majewski, 1987). In the traditional approach, data for evaluation come from direct observation by the teacher of the quality of patient care provided by the student. The focus of evaluation is the extent to which the student meets the expectations of the teacher, as they reflect the course objectives (Bondy, 1984). This sets up what Bevis & Watson (1989) describe as an adversarial relationship between the student and the teacher/content:

> 'The students 'do battle' with the content, and the teacher tries to help the content to be learned' (p. 278).

In a student-centred approach to clinical teaching, evaluation would be shared with the student (Blomquist, 1985). This can be achieved in a number of ways. Any data supportive of achievement of learning objectives as specified in the student's learning plan can be incorporated into the evaluation. The use of student self-evaluation is also a student-centred strategy. To use self-evaluations effectively requires that students develop skill in self-evaluation and that teachers trust the judgements of students. Through the process of self-evaluation, students develop self-awareness, enhance self-esteem and increase their sense of professional development (Best *et al*. 1990).

Implications for faculty development

Changes in the roles of teachers and students are required if student-centred teaching strategies are to be effective. Students must be allowed and encouraged to move to self-directed learning while teachers must learn actions that facilitate independence on the part of students. Teachers need to 'let go', to see their role as assisting and facilitating the development within their students of the potential to be successful. The actions necessary for teachers are movement from roles of transmitter and authority figure to roles of model, guide and facilitator (Bevis & Watson, 1989; Grow, 1991). Faculty development is an essential feature of such a shift of focus. Strategies must be directed toward clarification and modification of the values and attitudes of the faculty as they adopt a new approach to education. They also need the knowledge and skills to assist learners to make the transition from teacher-centred to student-centred learners.

The establishment among the faculty of a philosophy of education that incorporates student-centred processes is essential if there is to be a successful transition from teacher-centred to student-centred teaching approaches. Specific faculty development activities could include reading and discussion of some of the recent literature such as that cited in this paper. In particular, reflection on personal values of education would be helpful (Miller & Seller, 1990; Schön, 1987). Workshops and training sessions on philosophy and practice of student-centred approaches should be presented (Rush *et al*. 1991).

Teachers must also learn about, and incorporate strategies that can help students become student-centred learners (see Grow, 1991; Pratt, 1988). Both Grow and Pratt identify that not all adult learners are self-directed and therefore willing and able to embrace student-centred strategies. Barrows (1984) offers a model for student development of the skills and confidence needed to increase control of their learning, and suggests that modelling is an effective first step, where the teacher models the desired behaviours. Coaching is a second activity, where students are actively engaged in dialogue about what they are observing, and how they are putting the data together. The process is more interactive with the teacher, and the learner is being coached in the processes of both patient care and interactive learning. The teacher becomes a facilitator and guide, as the student owns the ideas expressed. The teacher is also encouraging metacognition through this process: students are encouraged to think about thinking, to consider their questions and observations. The final stage suggested by Barrows is fading, where students begin to function on their own and the teacher is available to provide support and encouragement.

The support of administration is imperative (Rush *et al*. 1991). It is difficult if not impossible for teachers to make a shift from teacher-centred to student-centred approaches without the support of administration and other faculties. Changes in the administration's conception of teaching can be facilitated through discussion of teaching approaches. Often outside consultants are useful in such deliberations, since they bring a fresh perspective to a situation and may be seen as more knowledgeable (Rush *et al.* 1991).

Conclusion

This paper has presented the argument that more control of the clinical practice component of nursing education must be shared with students. Through more active participation in their learning, students would learn the skills and develop the qualities needed to function in a rapidly changing health care environment. Recent writings by experts in the field of curriculum development are encouraging such changes (Bevis & Watson, 1989; Lindeman, 1989), and schools of nursing are revising their curriculums to reflect these changing views (Programme Handbook, School of Nursing, McMaster University). Overall the need for such changes in nursing education are both feasible and essential as the expectations within nursing change, from an emphasis on the technically skilled individual whose role is to assist other members of the health care team, to that of a more independent practitioner skilled in the art as well as the science of nursing.

References

Barrows H (1984) A specific problem-based, self-directed method designed to teach problem-solving skills and enhance knowledge retention and recall. In: H G Schmidt, M L De Volder, (eds) *Tutorials in problem-based learning: New directions for training for the health professions.* Van Gorcum, Assen/Maastricht.

Best M, Carswell J B, Abbott S D (1990) Self-evaluation for nursing students. *Nursing Outlook* 38 (4): 172–177.

Bevis E O, Watson J (1989) *Toward a caring curriculum: A new pedagogy for nursing.* National League for Nursing, New York.

Blomquist K B (1985) Evaluation of students: Intuition is important. *Nurse Educator,* 10 (6): 8–11.

Bondy K N (1984) Clinical evaluation of student performance: The effects of criteria on accuracy and reliability. *Research in Nursing and Health* 22 (9): 376–382.

DeYoung S (1990) *Teaching nursing.* Addison-Wesley, Redwood City, Ca.

Edwards M, Baptiste S (1987) The occupational therapist as a clinical teacher. *Canadian Journal of Occupational Therapy* 54 (5): 249–255.

Grow G O (1991) Teaching learners to be self-directed. *Adult Education Quarterly* 41 (3): 125–149.

Knowles M (1986) *Using learning contracts.* Jossey-Bass, San Francisco.

Lindeman C A (1989) Clinical teaching: Paradoxes and paradigms. In: *Curriculum revolution. Reconceptualising nursing education.* National League for Nursing, New York.

Miller J, Seller W (1990) *Curriculum: Perspectives and practice.* Copp, Clark Pittman, Mississauga.

Pratt D D (1988) Androgogy as a relational construct. *Adult Education Quarterly,* 38 (3): 160–181.

Programme Handbook, BScN Programme. McMaster University, Hamilton, Ontario.

Rush K L, Ouellet L L, Wasson D (1991) Faculty development: The essence of curriculum development. *Nurse Education Today*, 11: 121–126.

Schön D A (1987) *Educating the reflective practitioner*. Jossey-Bass, San Francisco.

Stenhouse L (1975) *An introduction to curriculum research and development*. Heinemann, London.

Tower B, Majewski T (1987) Behaviorally based clinical evaluation. *Journal of Nursing Education*, 26 (3): 120–123.

Woolley A S, Costello S E (1988) Innovations in clinical teaching. In: *Curriculum revolution: Mandate for change*. National League for Nursing, New York.

20. Learning the Practice of Nursing: Views about Preceptorship

Vivien E. Coates and Ethna Gormley

The provision of clinically based education for nursing students is an essential part of their learning needs. In this article, the opportunity to enhance clinically based learning by means of preceptors is discussed and investigated. A case study was conducted of one college of nursing after the introduction of the Preregistration Diploma of Higher Education in Nursing (Project 2000) course. The study involved preceptors (62), nursing students (15), ward managers (4), senior nurse managers (2) and nurse teachers (8). The investigation involved quantitative and qualitative approaches, data being gathered through questionnaires and interviews. The results indicate that preceptors included functions such as being a role model and supervision of learners' skills but not assessment as part of their role. These views were supported by students, teachers and managers. Knowledge of the clinical area and experience were reported to be preceptors' greatest assets for the role but lack of time to work with students was cited as the greatest barrier. Extra resources required were reported to be protected time for the student and preceptor to work together and further in-service education. The implications of these results for clinically based learning opportunities in the future are discussed.

Introduction

Nursing is a practice-based profession and, thus, the quality of clinical nursing education for learners is fundamental to successful preparation for a nursing career. The importance of clinical education is widely acknowledged (English National Board, 1985; United Kingdom Central Council (UKCC), 1986; Bradshaw, 1989) but an urgent need for improvement in such education has been identified for many years (Fretwell, 1982; Davis, 1983; Paterson, 1994).

Project 2000 (UKCC, 1986) heralded a radically different form of nurse education leading to an award with academic as well as professional recognition. To improve learning opportunities, Project 2000 students are supernumerary when on placement in order to obtain educationally sound nursing experience. This change in the nature of clinical experience, removing emphasis from meeting service needs, is an important aspect of the new courses.

However, even within the Project 2000 programmes of nurse education at Diploma of Higher Education level, the provision of clinical education remains a challenge. Responsibility for clinical teaching is often ill-defined. It is acknowledged that neither ward managers (Orton, 1983; Chambers, 1994) nor nurse teachers (McHaffie, 1994; Paterson, 1994) fulfilled the teaching role satisfactorily.

Vivien E. Coates and Ethna Gormley: 'Learning the Practice of Nursing: Views about Preceptorship' in *NURSE EDUCATION TODAY* (1997), 17(2), pp. 91-98. Reprinted by permission of the publisher Churchill Livingstone.

Various ways of resolving the problem of clinical teaching of learners have been suggested and many believe that nursing skills should be taught in the clinical area by qualified nurses (Gott, 1983; Butterworth, 1994; Lathlean & Vaughan, 1994).

A system to help improve clinical teaching and learning is that of mentoring or preceptoring which was introduced to the UK from the USA (Morle, 1990). When Project 2000 was proposed, mentoring of students was regarded as vital for the success of the programmes but the meaning of the term was unclear (Collins, 1990; Donovan, 1990). However, attempts to clarify the terms mentoring and preceptorship have been made (Peutz, 1985; Morle, 1990; Ashton & Richardson, 1992; Morton-Cooper & Palmer, 1993).

In brief, 'Mentoring is concerned with making the most of human potential' (Morton-Cooper & Palmer 1993, p. 60). Although the precise meaning of such a broad definition is questionable, it could be applied to professional development needs at any stage in a nursing career. Preceptorship relates more closely to an educational relationship. According to Morton-Cooper & Palmer (1993, p. 99), preceptorship involves:

- access to an experienced and competent role model

- a means by which to build a supportive one-to-one teaching and learning relationship.

The English National Board has opted for the term 'mentor' for the nurse who facilitates clinical learning for Project 2000 students. However, in this paper the term preceptor is used as it appears to be the more appropriate word in the context of nurse learners (Morle, 1990) and is also the term used in the practice areas in which the study was conducted. Although it may be interpreted as described above by Morton-Cooper & Palmer (1993), in the literature and in practice the term remains ambiguous.

There is a lack of empirically based information on preceptorship in nursing (Marriott 1991; Earnshaw, 1995). Previous studies have considered supervision from single perspectives, such as from students (Earnshaw, 1995), teachers (Hardiman, 1993) or preceptors (Dibert & Goldenberg, 1995).

The purpose of this study was to investigate views about preceptorship after the introduction of the Preregistration Diploma of Higher Education in Nursing (Project 2000) course, using a case study approach. By seeking the views of preceptors, learners, teachers and managers, a more complete picture could be obtained and contrasting perspectives compared.

This was an exploratory study and it was envisaged that results would be used to develop future clinical teaching and learning opportunities.

Methods

This investigation takes the form of a case study of a college of nursing. Whilst the views concern staff in only one area health board, the issue has been considered from the perspective of key participants (Gilchrist, 1992). The college concerned was a reasonably typical example of a college of nursing following transition from a conventional system of nurse education to that of a Project 2000 course. The new course was validated by an institute of higher education and appropriate national board, but full integration between higher education and nurse education had not occurred.

The aims of the study were to:

- investigate preceptors' views about their clinical teaching role with nursing students on the Diploma of Nursing course

- obtain the views of nursing students, teachers and clinical managers regarding preceptorship.

The study was conducted in two parts. Firstly, the views of preceptors regarding preceptorship were sought using a survey approach and data were collected through questionnaires. Secondly, group interviews were held with separate samples of students and teachers, then individual interviews were held with ward sisters and senior nurse managers. By combining quantitative and qualitative approaches, greater depth of investigation is possible and it enables the validity of the data to be considered from contrasting perspectives.

Stage 1

The population for the study comprised staff nurses, grades D or E, with at least 1 year's postregistration experience, working in adult or children's nursing in the local area health board. All preceptors should have attended a 2-day preceptorship course. All the 150 nurses who met these criteria were included in the sample.

A questionnaire was used to gain data about preceptors' views. The questionnaire consisted of three sections and was designed to be brief in order to encourage participation. The first section concerned demographic data, for example clinical area and qualifications. The second focused on the role of preceptors in Project 2000 courses, such as perceived elements of the preceptor's role, influential and inhibiting factors. The third section concerned supernumerary status of students. This paper concentrates on the second section, which contained 10 questions. The choice of questions was influenced by personal experience of the authors and by literature on clinical supervision. Three questions were closed, requiring 'Yes', 'No', 'Don't Know', responses. Three questions required aspects of the preceptor's role to be rank-ordered. The four remaining questions were open-ended, needing brief answers. The content of the questionnaire was reviewed with three colleagues in nurse education. In this way, the content validity of the questionnaire was considered. Several drafts of the instrument were produced and gradually refined. Full psychometric testing of the instrument was not undertaken — this, upon reflection, is a limitation to the rigour of the study.

After gaining appropriate approval, the questionnaire was distributed via internal mail. An accompanying letter explained the purpose of the project, encouraged participation (which was purely voluntary) and assured confidentiality.

Stage 2

In stage 2 the following samples were drawn:

- Students were sampled according to which groups of students were in the college when stage 2 was conducted. From these student groups participants were requested, and a sample of 15 volunteers obtained.

- Teachers were also selected according to availability during the data collection phase; this involved eight individuals.

- Clinical managers were identified according to a list of wards on which students were placed. From this list, four managers at sisters level were randomly selected plus two senior managers with overall responsibility for areas in which students were placed.

The sample sizes used were small relative to the total populations. However, when using a case study approach the aim is to investigate an individual, group or other social unit thoroughly (Polit & Hungler, 1991), thus a large sample size may not be needed.

As convenience samples were used, bias may have occurred (Polit & Hungler, 1991). However, the results reflect a wide variety of experiences and appear to be credible, if not totally representative, of the target populations. In addition, the findings support themes identified through other studies which helps to endorse the validity of the data.

Data in stage 2 were gathered by semi-structured interviews. A similar range of topics was covered in each interview and with each cohort of participants. The interview themes were derived from the questionnaire. For example, staff nurses were asked, via the questionnaire, what factors helped them to be good preceptors. Subsequent interviews with students, teachers and managers also raised this issue. The interviews were audiotape recorded, with participants' permission, and transcribed.

Analysis

Descriptive statistics were used to summarize the data in the questionnaires about the views of respondents. The interviews were subjected to manifest content analysis (Berg, 1989) during which themes evident in the transcripts were identified and categorized. As this was a case study, it was intended that both sets of data would be considered together to gain an impression of the situation overall.

Results

Questionnaires were returned from 62 (41%) nurses. This is a poor response rate which indicated that the results may not be representative of the total population of preceptors. Those who respond may differ in some way from those who do not (Bryman & Cramer, 1990), and the extent or nature of any difference is unknown. The reason for the poor response in this study can only be surmised; perhaps conducting the study during a time of great change in health care causing uncertainty over future employment may have led to a disinclination to complete a questionnaire. Demographic data are summarized in Table 1.

Table 1   Demographic traits of the sample

Trait	Frequency
Clinical areas	
Medical	16
Surgical	19
Care of the elderly	10
Paediatrics	14
Specialities	5
Age	
21–30	43
31–40	12
41–50	6
51+	3
Years qualified	
1–5	16
6–10	20
11–20	8
21+	8
No response	10
Grade	
D	21
E	41
Other	2
Qualifications	
RGN/SRN	57
RGN+RMN	4
RSCN	2
RGN + degree	9
RFN	1

The majority of the respondents worked in medical or surgical areas, had a Registered General Nurse qualification and were aged less than 30 years.

The role of the preceptor nurse

The nurses participating in stage 1 were given a list of the duties of preceptors which had been identified in the course document from the affiliated college of nursing. The nurses were asked to rank the 10 duties according to perceived importance for the majority of student nurses. They were then asked to rank-order these duties according to which they believed they were best prepared to undertake. Their responses are listed in Table 2.

From the results shown in Table 2 it can be seen that acting as a role model was considered to be the most important aspect of the preceptor's role; teaching and learner supervision were ranked second and third, but assessing students was ranked joint eighth with the role of critic. The perceived adequacy of preparation for the various functions is also shown. Overall, the nurses reported that they were best prepared to be a role model but were not particularly well prepared to be a teacher of clinical nursing (ranked fifth) and felt inadequately prepared for the role of assessor (ranked eighth).

Table 2   Preceptors' views of their role and preparation

Proposed duties of preceptors	Rank order of aspects of preceptor's role	Perceived adequacy of preparation
Role model	1*	1†
Teacher of clinical nursing	2	5
Supervisor	3	2
Facilitator of learning	4	6
Friend	5	4
Motivator	5	3
Counsellor	5	7
Assessor	8	8
Critic	8	8
Protector	10	8

*1 = most important → 10 = least important
†1 = best prepared → 10 = least prepared

Through the interviews, similar information was sought from students, teachers and managers and Table 3 illustrates their perceptions of the main aspects of preceptors' work. The themes are ranked according to the priority expressed during the interviews.

Table 3   Main aspects of preceptor's role in order stated

	Student	Teacher	Manager
Educator/teacher	1	2	3
Supervisor	2	5	4
Counsellor/advisor	3	6	5
Facilitator of learning	4	4	1
Helpful/friendly	5	–	–
Role model	6	3	2
Assessor	7	7	6
Critic	8	8	7
Evaluating existing knowledge	–	1	–

(1 = most important → 8 = least important)

It is interesting to note that teachers, managers (and previously preceptors) thought that role modelling was a more important duty than the students. Students mentioned that any staff nurse could act as their role model, not just their appointed preceptor. All parties placed assessment rather low relative to other duties, which raises the question, if preceptors don't assess ability who should?

Benefits and hindrances to preceptorship

Preceptors were asked about factors which helped them to be good preceptors, and, conversely, those which hindered them. Their responses are illustrated in Table 4.

Table 4   Perceived benefits and hindrances to working as a preceptor

Benefits	Frequency of response
Knowledge	22
Experience	12
Being approachable	9
Communication skills	9
Backup support on ward	7

Other factors raised individually included: interest in the student, research orientated, knowledge of role, liaison with college staff, patience, confidence

Hindrances	
Lack of time	34
Workloads	22
Off duty	21
Staff shortages/skill-mix	16
Lack of knowledge/training	15
Being in charge of the ward	13

Other factors noted individually included: student preparation, short placements, student interest, personality clash, shortage of preceptors

Table 4 shows that the majority of respondents felt that knowledge and experience were their greatest assets to student learning; however, being approachable and having good communication skills were also important. The Table also shows that the main barrier to working as a preceptor is reported to be lack of time. Patient care has priority over teaching and little time is then left for teaching. Lack of time was reported to be a greater problem than lack of knowledge of their clinical area.

The results in Table 4 were supported by interview data. Ward sisters were well aware of the demands on preceptor's time:

> 'I feel they have a lot of pressures, and they are thinking about the patients, and I suppose when it comes to patient care, the student gets a secondary place.' [Ward Sister]

> '. . . trying to manage wards, manage groups of patients, be named nurses, be preceptors, and be all things to all men.' [Ward Sister]

> '. . . we have emergencies coming in and we have no bed for them . . . we are transferring patients continually . . . and the student is then left on her own.' [Ward Sister]

Students were also aware of the conflicting demands made upon preceptors:

> 'They have got their responsibilities in the ward as well — then along come all these students.' [Student]

'I think preceptors shouldn't be senior nurses, or left in charge of the ward. Because they don't have time.' [Student]

These problems are also recognized by managers, as is illustrated by the following quotation:

'I think it would work a lot better if our staffing ratios took into account the amount of time that was required for them to adequately fulfil their role as a preceptor — that right now is not done.' [Senior Manager]

Other factors to emerge from each sample of interviewees are summarized in Table 5.

Table 5   Summary of students', teachers' and managers' views of factors which influence the preceptor's role

Students' views	Teachers' views	Senior managers' views
Attitudes	Personal qualities/	Personality
Personality	personality	Adaptability
Student initiative	Fear	Interest
Knowledge	Lack of confidence	Length of time
Sister's attitude	(need positive support)	qualified
	Knowledge of student	Credibility
	Knowledge of curriculum	Knowledge
	Tutor education/support	Support from
	Open relationship with tutors	college staff

From Table 5 it would appear that personality is thought to play as important a part as professional criteria for successful preceptorship. Indeed, steps have been taken to address this issue:

'Some of them [preceptors] just plain don't have the personality for it . . . we asked people who are interested in undertaking the course and we try with the sister to look at their suitability for undertaking it . . . I think we are limiting the unsuitable people getting in there.' [Senior Manager]

This point illustrates that within the staff nurse role there is room for diversity. Whilst some nurses may have a particular aptitude for teaching, others may be better suited, for example, to management of care or quality assurance issues. It is important that the strengths of individual nurses should be maximized, but how objectively this is done will be considered in the discussion.

Additional resources required for the clinical area

The nurses were asked to indicate the nature of the additional resources (if any) which they envisaged would be necessary prior to working as preceptors to diploma students. Their responses are illustrated in Table 6.

Table 6 illustrates that the most frequently cited additional resource was the need for protected time to be allocated for preceptors and students to work together. This was mentioned by 38 nurses (61%).

Table 6   Additional resources needed by preceptors

Resources needed	Number of times cited by nurses
Time allocated for preceptor and student	38
More staff (including ward clerks)	30
In-service training	25
Clinical input from teachers	12

Although preceptors thought more staff were vital for the success of clinical teaching, a ward sister emphasized that the solution is not necessarily just more nurses:

'I think that a lot of the difficulties are linked with the turnover and the workload, as well as the number of staff. Too many nurses on the ward doesn't always make for better teaching. But I think the way the ward is organized could be more effective.' [Ward Sister]

This is an important point, as all possible ways in which work and time could be more efficiently managed must be considered.

The role of nurse teachers in clinically based teaching was reported to be a contentious issue in the literature and this was supported by the results of this investigation. By using a case study approach the views of several interested parties could be compared.

Only 12 preceptors thought it was important that teachers should be involved in the clinical area. However, the need for such involvement was emphasized during the interviews. Ward sisters mentioned that support from college teaching staff would help preceptors:

'I would have to say that the College here, the tutors are not over very regularly . . . we were told the role of the tutor was changing, and they would be over there in the wards for the students. That has not happened. The most of the support the students got was from clinical teachers.' [Ward Sister]

The teachers offered differing views on this subject. One teacher outlined that she felt her role was to support preceptors, for example concerning a ward which had not previously taken students on a management placement:

'and the preceptors were finding it difficult, and I spent time explaining what I expected the student should be doing, and to me, that is a big part of the tutor's role — is supporting that.' [Nurse Teacher]

Another teacher mentioned the conflict between being expected to be available to teach in the college and also to see students on placement:

'But you always have a class — you have to be in class.' [Nurse Teacher]

'But there isn't the time . . . if something else crops up, you can go on to something else and not get to the ward. Going to the ward isn't going to hold much water. You will be told to rearrange yourself.' [Nurse Teacher]

However, a colleague disagreed with this view:

> 'but where is the priority? . . . You could negotiate a class within your day. You can't negotiate the time with your preceptor . . . you can't just expect other people out there to suddenly apply something that they aren't even familiar with.' [Nurse Teacher]

It appears that there is conflict between the classroom and clinical roles of nurse teachers. Clarification of the teacher's role will help resolve this conflict.

The need for time for in-service training was cited as important by 38 preceptors (see Table 6). Although the standard provision was a 2-day preceptorship course, staff nurses suggested they needed more than 2 days and teachers supported this view:

> 'a 2-day preceptorship course doesn't give them the skills to teach . . . I think the preceptor should have a longer course.' [Nurse Teacher]

On a different theme, one of the senior managers expressed the view that investment in physical resources was needed:

> 'It would be nice if you had a resource room of some kind . . . an area where staff nurses could take them to elaborate on a point that has actually come up during their actual nursing practice that morning, and discuss it and talk it through. That is sadly lacking.' [Senior Manager]

Discussion

The majority of preceptors thought their knowledge and experience were their greatest assets to student learning, although being approachable and having good communication skills were also important. Students, teachers and managers stated that personality was as important as professional criteria for successful preceptorship. These findings would support those reported by others (Mogan & Knox, 1987; Bracken & Davis, 1989; Marriott, 1991). However, the attributes of an 'ideal' personality are not clear, although Darling (1984) has conducted some work in this area. From this study it would appear that 'ideal' personality characteristics are subjectively, rather than empirically, derived. Butterworth & Faugier (1992) discuss some of the attributes considered desirable in clinical supervision and note that it is a difficult but vital issue which requires further understanding if the role is to be successfully fulfilled.

Workloads, lack of time and of adequate training were reported to hinder preceptorship. Replacing the traditional student workforce since Project 2000 courses began contributes to the problem of staffing and skill-mix levels (Elkan et al. 1994). However, some problems may be mollified by, for example, reconsidering the organization of existing work. One of the sisters stated that it was the high turnover of patients causing constant moving of people and beds as much as the staffing levels which led to time constraints between preceptors and students. Marriott (1991) also notes that the organization of ward work influences clinical learning opportunities.

A senior manager noted that teaching must be allocated time in the same way that patient care is scheduled time. Protected time for preceptors and students to work together is needed. If preceptors are to be allocated more than one student then the amount of time must be increased accordingly. The provision of a place to work with students was seen as important as not all objectives can be achieved at a patient's bedside. Dibert & Goldenberg (1995) also acknowledge that preceptors take on this role in addition to other nursing duties and that they must have adequate support and resources to do so if the risk of 'burnout' is to be avoided.

Adequate preparation of preceptors is vital, but study days seem to be a scarce resource hindered by the cost of removing qualified staff from service. This situation has arisen despite initial reassurance that preregistration training, including practice placements, would be adequately funded (Working Paper 10, 1989). It was envisaged that such ' costs' would be offset against students' contribution to service needs during training.

In this study all parties supported preceptorship and thought it had the potential to make a positive contribution to nurse education. However, preceptors' learning needs must be facilitated (Dibert & Goldenberg, 1995). Clinical teaching and supervision is itself a skill (Mogan & Knox, 1987; Hinchliff, 1992; Titchen & Binnie, 1995) and it cannot be assumed that, by virtue of their knowledge and expertise, practitioners can automatically function as preceptors. In particular, it appears that preparation to undertake skills assessment is urgently needed, a point also noted by Westra & Graziano (1992).

Whilst several common themes emerged from the different cohorts, it appears that the role of preceptors has not been sufficiently identified to enable a standardized approach to the role to be established. A similar problem relating to both the name of clinical educators and their role was reported by Wilson-Barnett et al. (1995). Adequate preparation for preceptorship can hardly be provided whilst ambiguity over the role remains. There is an urgent need to clarify what is expected of preceptors to enable adequate development of the role to be undertaken.

Such issues must be addressed as it appears that the need for preceptors to meet students' clinical learning needs is increasing. Although it was anticipated that nurse teachers would be involved in the clinical teaching of Project 2000 students (UKCC, 1986) it appears that the nature of their clinical input has changed (Hardiman, 1993; Wilson-Barnett et al. 1995). Indeed, the commitment and opportunity for nurse teachers to contribute to a 'hands on' clinical teaching role is doubtful (Webster, 1990; Crotty, 1993; Clifford, 1995).

If teachers are to be involved in ward teaching, their work must be organized to facilitate this activity and be given as great a commitment as classroom teaching. If this is not done then other means of supporting preceptors must be arranged. Other approaches to nurse education, such as more lecturer/practitioner posts, whose responsibilities are unambiguously defined, should improve the situation (Lathlean & Vaughan, 1994).

Using a case study approach proved to be an interesting means of inquiry and has generated insights into practice-based education and learning in this specific area. The inclusion of perspectives from different groups of nurses and learners enhances the validity of the results and provides material for use in this locality to facilitate the development of the role of preceptors. The results indicate tangible factors which need to be addressed if clinical teaching and learning are to be improved. It is hoped that the results will be of interest to nurses elsewhere but the small sample size, the poor response to the questionnaire and lack of full psychometric testing of the research instrument must be regarded as limitations to the study. Although the extent to which these results can be generalized to other institutions and settings may be small, confidence can still be placed in these results as many findings help confirm trends reported from other studies.

Conclusion

To increase the future success of Project 2000 courses, student experience and staff morale, in-service training must take account of views and concerns expressed by practitioners and other relevant parties. The role of preceptors must be clarified to enable their functions to be clearly understood and supported. Sufficient resources to facilitate preceptor/learner's needs are required. The clinical responsibilities and role of nurse teachers must be clarified and then facilitated.

Clinical teaching of nurses of the future is too important an activity to be neglected. The potential for a first class system of nurse education exists and it is important that problems are addressed before the positive views of preceptorship diminish.

Acknowledgement

The authors wish to thank the N.I. National Board for Nursing, Midwifery and Health Visiting for funding this work. The contribution of the late Michael Hegarty (Senior Tutor) who was instrumental in the early stages of this project is also acknowledged.

References

Ashton P, Richardson G (1992) Preceptorship and PREPP. *British Journal of Nursing* 1 (3): 143–146.

Berg B L (1989) *Qualitative research methods for the social sciences*. Allyn and Bacon, Boston.

Bracken E, Davis J (1989) The implications of mentorship in nursing career development. *Senior Nurse* 9 (5): 15–16.

Bradshaw P L (ed) (1989) *Teaching and assessing in clinical nursing practice*. Prentice Hall, London.

Bryman A, Cramer D (1990) *Quantitative data analysis for social scientists*. Routledge, London.

Butterworth T (1994) Preparing to take on clinical supervision. *Nursing Standard* 21 (8): 32–34.

Butterworth T, Faugier J (eds) (1992) *Clinical supervision and mentorship in nursing*. Chapman and Hall, London.

Chambers M G A (1994) Learning psychiatric nursing skills: the contribution of the ward environment. Unpublished DPhil Thesis, University of Ulster.

Clifford C (1995) The role of the nurse teachers: concerns, conflicts and challenges. *Nurse Education Today* 15: 11–16.

Collins S (1990) The ENB pilot schemes: how plans have become reality. *Nursing Times Occasional Paper* 86 (31): 30–33.

Crotty M (1993) Clinical role activities of nurse teachers in Project 2000 programmes. *Journal of Advanced Nursing* 18: 460–464.

Darling L A (1994) What do nurses want in a mentor? *Journal of Nursing Administration* 14 (10): 42–44.

Davis B D (ed) (1983) *Research into nurse education*. Croom Helm, London.

Dibert C, Goldenberg D (1995) Preceptors' perceptions of benefits, rewards, supports and commitment to the preceptor role. *Journal of Advanced Nursing* 21: 1144–1151.

Donovan J (1990) The concept and role of mentor. *Nurse Education Today* 10: 294–298.

Earnshaw G J (1995) Mentorship: the students' views. *Nurse Education Today* 15: 274–279.

Elkan R, Hillman R, Robinson J (1994) Project 2000 and the replacement of the traditional student workforce. *International Journal of Nursing Studies* 31 (5): 413–420.

English National Board for Nursing, Midwifery and Health Visiting (1985) Professional education/training courses. Consultation Paper. ENB, London.

Fretwell J E (1982) *Ward teaching and learning*. Royal College of Nursing, London.

Gilchrist V J (1992) Key informant interviews. In: B F Crabtree, W L Miller (eds) *Doing qualitative research*, vol. 3, ch 4. Sage, London.

Gott M (1983) The preparation of the student for learning in the clinical setting. In: B D Davis (ed) *Research into nurse education*, ch. 6. Croom Helm, London.

Hardiman R H (1993) Teachers' experiences of their role following the implementation of Project 2000: a qualitative approach. *Journal of Advanced Nursing* 18: 1023–1032.

Hinchliff S (ed) (1992) *The practitioner as teacher*. Scutari Press, London.

Lathlean J, Vaughan B (1994) *Unifying nursing practice and theory*. Butterworth Heinemann, Oxford.

McHaffie H E (1994) Hands-on experience: do teachers need it? *Nursing Standard* 8 (48): 29–31.

Marriott A (1992) The support, supervision, and instruction of nurse learners in clinical areas: a literature review. *Nurse Education Today* 11: 261–269.

Mogan J, Knox J E (1987) Characteristics of 'best' and 'worst' clinical teachers as perceived by university nursing faculty and students. *Journal of Advanced Nursing* 12: 331–337.

Morle K M F (1990) Mentorship — is it a case of the emperor's new clothes or a rose by any other name? *Nurse Education Today* 10 (1): 66–69.

Morton-Cooper A, Palmer A (1993) *Mentoring and preceptorship: a guide to support roles in clinical practice*. London, Blackwell Scientific.

Orton H (1983) Ward learning climate and student response. In: B D Davis (ed) *Research into nurse education*, ch. 5. Croom Helm, London.

Paterson B (1994) The view from within: perspectives of clinical teaching. *International Journal of Nursing Studies* 31 (4): 349–360.

Peutz B E (1985) Learn the ropes from a mentor. *Nurse Education Today* 2 (6): 11–13.

Polit D F, Hungler B P (1991) *Nursing research principles and methods*. Lippincott, London.

Titchen A, Binnie A (1995) The art of clinical supervision. *Journal of Clinical Nursing* 4: 327–334.

United Kingdom Central Council (1986) *Project 2000: a new preparation for practice*. UKCC, London.

Webster R (1990) The role of the nurse teacher. *Senior Nurse* 10 (8): 16–17.

Westra R, Graziano M (1992) Preceptors: a comparison of their perceived needs before and after the preceptor experience. *Journal of Continuing Education in Nursing* 23: 212–215.

Wilson-Barnett J, Butterworth T, White E, Twinn S, Davies S, Riley L (1995) Clinical support and the Project 2000 nursing student: factors influencing this process. *Journal of Advanced Nursing* 21: 1152–1158.

Working Paper 10 (1989) *Working for Patients: education and training*. HMSO, London.

21. Continuing Professional Development
Ian McGill and Liz Beaty

In this chapter we explore the affinity between action learning and professional development and to show how action learning can support continuing professional development. The most well known use of action learning is in the management area but increasingly people are describing the enormous benefit action learning can have in other areas of professional development. We have designed programmes of action learning for professional groups, e.g. social services professionals, housing specialists, and health professionals. In higher education, action learning is being used in staff development programmes for managers, academic staff and administrators.

What are the generic features of professional development which make action learning such a useful process in these disparate areas?

What it is to be a professional

The term 'professional' is associated with work which is valued highly in society. The 'professions' — lawyers, doctors, social workers, accountants — are highly trained and often highly paid members of society. In this sense the term professional is a kitemark given to those who complete a rigorous and demanding training and then continue to develop their speciality within the profession through further formal training and experience. The professions are characterized by codes of conduct which they require of their members and also a degree of individual autonomy and responsibility for their working practice. Although professionals can belong to large organizations where their work is only one part of the whole, they tend to have a large amount of personal control and autonomy in their working practice. This brings with it a high level of responsibility and obligations for the maintenance of high standards and quality of work. The term professional is increasingly used to describe an attitude to work and not merely a type of work. We talk about a professional approach, meaning acting in a professional way: an approach to life and work which includes taking responsibility, being creative and not merely going through the motions and taking a questioning and critical look at our own individual practice. With this attitude individuals aim to use their knowledge and skill to develop working practice for themselves and for others. This professionalism can therefore be claimed by many more people than those in the traditional professions.

It is this second sense of professional which has a close affinity with action learning. Professionalism and action learning share the same values in taking individual responsibility for action and taking an active approach to development of the organization (where appropriate) and of oneself.

Ian McGill and Liz Beaty: 'Continuing Professional Development' from *ACTION LEARNING*, 2nd edn (Kogan Page Limited, 1995), pp. 198–208.

The nature of professional development

Professional development is the nurturing of an attitude to life and work which promotes a responsible, creative and proactive approach. The development of an individual with a professional approach goes beyond knowledge and skills to the core of personal growth and the ability to harness this growth into more effective action. It acknowledges that this development is never complete, there is always more one can learn about oneself and the complexity of the world in which we live.

Development of insight and wisdom

Whereas initial training can give us competence, professional practice requires the development of insight and wisdom in responding to the idiosyncrasies of the situations that face us. Professional development, therefore, crucially involves learning from experience. For a doctor, a lawyer, a teacher or a manager there is always a mixture of the expected and the novel in any situation. For a doctor, each patient has recognizable symptoms expressed through a unique individual context. In the classroom the teacher faces a blend of the known personalities and a unique interplay between them.

The challenge to the professional is to learn from experience in a way which does not cramp the fresh interest in each particular piece of work. Initial training can only provide the basic background for practice. Beyond this, a view of the unique circumstances must be involved in a judgement which becomes easier with experience and tacit knowledge built up over time. But as we build our experience, we may also become less attuned to the individual differences, become over-confident in our judgement and miss the signs of difference which are crucial to successful action.

Recognizing patterns in experience

We learn from experience through a process of observation, reflection and generalization and by recognizing patterns within the complexity of our experience. We also learn to tailor our actions by reference to our own internal store of experience which allows us to say, 'I have seen a situation similar to this before'. We learn to recognize emergent events so that they no longer take us by surprise. On the whole we do all of this naturally, without deliberate processes of record keeping.

We may also build up knowledge of our own individual habits, styles and tendencies. We learn to distinguish events that will challenge us from ones where we are comfortable and at ease. This store of self-knowledge is also fundamental to the development of professional practice.

Professional development and reflective practice

Although we all learn from experience, more and more experience does not guarantee more and more learning. Learning from experience tends to happen most effectively when the experiences are novel or where they are painful in some way. Our normal human reactions to events ensure that we think a great deal about things that have caused us pain: we search for a cause that will help us to act differently to the same stimuli in the future to avoid the pain. Over time, however, the same experience modified through the early learning will have less impact on us. For example, 20 years of teaching may not equate to 20 years of learning about teaching but only one year of learning repeated 20 times. Indeed, this repeated experience may have resulted in some inefficient or ineffective habits that may be very difficult to change.

Reflective practice, so important to professional development, is not an automatic result of experience. We need techniques and methods to encourage us to reflect and to enable us to learn from that reflection. Novel experience encourages reflection. Opportunity to experience novel situations may diminish with continued practice. We may need to seek the novel through deliberately exposing ourselves to new areas of work or different perspectives.

Painful experience can promote reflection. We think about what went wrong. Where the pain is great, however, this can lead to the opposite of reflection — a hiding from, or unconscious barrier to, thinking about it. In some circumstances then, we are likely to spend time reflecting whereas in others we may need help to face situations that we would rather not think about.

Most of our experience is neither particularly novel nor painful. There are, therefore, many times that our normal reactions to events are insufficient in themselves to encourage reflection. It is here that we need techniques and help from others.

The use of dialogue

There are things to be learnt from reflection with the aid of other people. For professionals the most immediate benefit can come from using various forms of feedback from customers and clients to encourage reflection. They are the other actors in the situation that we are reflecting about. Their perspectives, attitudes, responses and feelings provide rich data for our reflection on our professional practice. Moreover they focus our attention in a helpful way on the result of our work.

Peers can be very helpful in aiding our reflection. They are likely to be able to empathize, we may trust their professional ability to maintain confidentiality and so on. They aid our learning in that their own experience and knowledge adds insight into our reflections on our own practice. Unlike clients, they will notice our actions from the point of view of a professional. They will also be able to imagine clients' reactions to our suggested actions from this point of view.

A peer's view of the discipline can be an important focus for this reflection. On the other hand, a peer who is not in the same professional area could add a focus more on the process of professional action rather than on the content. The support of peers provides an opportunity for learning beyond that of private reflection by the individual.

While discussions do help us to reflect on our practice, rarely does a general discussion allow us to interrogate in a specific and deep way our own personal approach. It is easy to have a discussion about teaching and learning, for example, without feeling that there are any conclusions to be drawn about our own approach as a teacher. The concentrated and intentional process of deliberately reflecting with the aid of peers is altogether a more potent tool for professional development.

Developing appropriate links with others

A professional approach involves acknowledgement of our own limitations and a willingness to involve others or to take particular care with aspects of the work where we are less able. A newly trained professional will on the whole be more aware of the build-up of this experience than someone who is very experienced. After some time our ability to learn something new every day (or to believe that we can learn something new) tends to diminish. We may stop feeling like a learner and rely solely on our current skills and knowledge. It is at these times when the support and challenge of peers is crucial to our professional development.

Most of us experience a degree of isolation in our work. It is not so much that we work alone, more that we have few opportunities to reflect on our own practice. We can notice how other people work but we are unlikely to discuss differences unless they actively interfere with our own way of doing things. This can bring complacency and an increasing resistance to change. We may need to invest time in supporting our own development in a more formal way.

The need for emotional support

The professional's role is characterized by the responsibility that they have for their practice. This often means responsibility in relation to the welfare of other people, as most professional groups have clients who invest a degree of trust in their expertise. In doing these jobs there is an emotional content that is not so imperative in other work. We all have to relate to other people at work but the professional attitude requires the individual to take responsibility for the effects of their actions on other people. In some professional areas there are particular organizational strategies to cope with these pressures. Social workers, for example, have supervision on an individual basis, with a peer or more experienced member of the team, which provides a safe environment within which to discuss and to keep perspective on the emotional content of work. Most other professionals work without these formal processes.

The cycle of learning from action and reflection — how development occurs

We have shown above how reflection does not automatically follow from experience and how learning does not automatically follow from reflection. We need to make a further link between learning from reflection and consequent development of professional practice. For example, it is possible to identify some behaviour of mine that is interfering in the effective learning of students. My ability to change will depend on developing this understanding through reflecting on practice and in deciding what I could do to make a difference. In some cases I may conclude that I need to use different techniques of teaching, implying a knowledge base in educational practice. In other cases the necessary change may be to do with my personal style of interactions with students. Of course, to change habits or personal traits is more difficult than changing techniques of teaching. In either case I must not only decide what to change but also how to learn about or develop the skills involved in this change.

The cycle of action and reflection must therefore be enriched through knowledge-based or skill-based development. It is not enough to experience and to reflect: we must make a conscious effort to develop our knowledge and skill and this may require further development.

Continuing professional development

Professions are now recognizing the need for continuing professional development (CPD). The Institute of Personnel and Development (IPD) is a leading advocate of CPD and has set out guiding principles:

- Development should be *continuous* in the sense that the professional should always be actively seeking improved performance.

- Development should be *owned and managed* by the individual learner.

- Development should *begin from the learner's current learning state* and, while fitting appropriate organisation or client needs, would not be overinfluenced by someone else's ideals. CPD is a personal matter, and the *effective learner knows best what he/she needs to learn.*

- *Learning objectives should be clear, though they may be complex,* and wherever possible should serve organisational as well as individual goals.

- *Investment of time in learning should be regarded as being as important as investment in any other activity.*

(IPD, 1995, emphasis added)

The IPD has incorporated CPD into its professional standards because it ensures that professionals remain up to date, encourages their aspiration to improved performance, ensures commitment to learning as an integral part of work and helps to maintain the reputation of the profession. The IPD cites, as necessary, a minimum of five days or 35 hours CPD activity or the equivalent in learning outcomes per year.

The IPD professional draws up and implements a professional development plan (PDP) in order to structure their development. The PDP provides a focus and framework for identifying CPD needs, planning appropriate action, implementing learning activities, recording and reviewing progress. There is no uniform way to draw up a plan — each can be tailored to the individual. Support may also be sought from significant colleagues, mentors and managers. The PDP should take into account personal aspiration, professional development needs and an employer's requirements.

The IPD professional maintains a record of their CPD which lays emphasis on providing evidence of outcomes of the learning opportunities rather than just a list of inputs or activities. This requires analysing what was actually gained from having undertaken an activity. Reflection that enables a person to show what they have gained is essential to ensure that the process is really developmental.

Relevance of action learning

There are many means by which professionals can engage in their learning and development. The IPD cites professional work-based activities, courses, seminars and conferences, as well as self-directed and informal learning. The more formal elements include, for example, project management, secondment in and outside the

227

professionals' organization, professional, graduate and flexible learning programmes. The informal can include reading and writing for professional journals, voluntary work, and observation/reflection on events in the course of work.

However, engaging in the opportunities may not necessarily encourage the reflection which is so important for development to take place. As the IPD maintains:

> 'The most important aspect of CPD is the learning outcome, not the precise amount of input. Experience alone does not create learning: reflection is needed to gain real benefits' (IPD, 1995).

The IPD therefore encourages their membership to engage in reflection by inviting them to consider their approaches to learning as well as considering their learning styles. The personal record is designed to help the individual elicit responses to the questions: What did you learn from it? How have/will you use this?

The professional can make much headway with this individually. The IPD also suggest the use of their branches and groups with a named CPD coordinator to support members in the development and implementation of their plans. The coordinator may, *inter alia*, enable linking 'together members to encourage learning through peer group support, mentoring, appropriate events and access to learning resources' (IPD, op cit.).

We would like to make more explicit the use of action learning which can provide a coherent structure that encourages specific and explicit use of the whole learning cycle including the key element of reflection.

Our concern in this area is that the individual may be left very much to their own devices to engage in reflection in a potentially isolated, solitary way. Continuous professional development is rightly *owned and managed* by the individual. This principle highlights the responsibility and control for development and learning in the professional. This does not mean that the developmental process need be an isolated one.

Indeed we would assert that the process can be enriched by sharing. Action learning provides a structure for learning and a *social* context for reflection [see Chapter 10]. We believe this social aspect of learning is underrated. In a set each member is responsible for their own learning and responsible to other set members in supporting each other's learning. This is where dialogue, referred to earlier, is crucial. For set members to engage in a developmental dialogue, a balance of challenge and support behaviour is necessary. The skills to achieve such a balance are set out in [Chapters 8 and 9]. The process of dialogue creates the reflective conditions for learning. Focused development is provided by the professional's emergent plan for implementation.

We can now show how action learning meets the IPD's guiding principles, listed above.

Development should be *continuous* for the professional. That continuity can be maintained with the support of colleague professionals over time in a set described in [Chapters 2, 3 and 4]. We envisage that in the early years following acquisition of professional status, the support of a set would be particularly useful in order to attain an ease with the notion of reflection and learning how to learn.

In action learning the working assumption from which sets start is to *begin from the learner's current learning state*. As we state elsewhere, action learning works from where the set member is. No uniformity is imposed about where set members may be or ought to be. Linked to this principle is the clear recognition that *the effective learner knows best what he/she needs to learn*. The set member is encouraged to clarify what her learning needs are. An example of this approach in making CPD work for an individual is that drawn from self-managed learning (Cunningham, 1994). This is a rather more elaborate version of the approach of the IPD. The professional asks herself five key questions:

1. Where have I been?
   This is biographical in nature, drawing upon her background, previous experience, significant events in her learning about herself and the person she is.

2. Where am I now?
   This question invites her to articulate the skills and qualities that she possesses and what kind of person she is.

3. Where do I want to go to?
   This elicits important subsidiary questions: What do I want to do? What kind of person do I want to be? What skills and qualities do I need to gain to get/be there?

4. How do I get there?
   What learning programmes, opportunities and processes do I need?

5. How will I know that I have arrived?
   The questions that will provide evidence here include: How do I evaluate my learning? How will I assess myself so that I have the means to know that my learning goals are met? What measures do I need in order to assess myself?

Questions 1 and 2 enable our professional to clarify her learning needs. Question 3 is the basis for defining and setting her goals. Question 4, the *how* question, provides the means of attaining her goals. Question 5 provides the basis for her assessment of her learning achievements in the form of tangible evidence.

Returning to the IPD's principles, the approach, or variants of it, can help to ensure that our professional's *learning objectives should be clear, though they may be complex*.

Action learning reflects the last principle of CPD that *investment of time in learning should be regarded as being as important as investment in any other activity*. With, say, an annual cycle of CPD, the questions above could be spread over that period. Membership of an action learning set can provide the base for creating a personal contract that sets out what 'I' want to achieve with the agreement of significant others (such as colleagues in the set; line managers for project planning, implementation and review; joining a post-qualification programme). A contract and an agreement with others to go for it (even though it may be modified) helps to maintain momentum and tenacity. A planned intention to undertake something can remain at the planning stage for ever. With a challenging set the professional is encouraged to move from planning to implementation.

Having the continuing support and encouragement of an action learning set can provide the bridge over dips in motivation surrounding development. As we have shown earlier in the chapter, development can be painful and isolating as well as pleasurable and exhilarating.

Continuing professional development requires evidence for the person engaged in the process and, as in the example of the IPD, for the professional institute as well. The action learning set process creates the conditions and a framework for that evidence to be adduced. An action record of the set is itself evidence of the developmental process.

We endorse the approach being taken by the IPD and are aware of its application as a potential model for other professions. The formalization of continuing professional development in the IPD's approach has assisted us in conveying how action learning may be used by professionals to support and make effective their development.

Action learning and continuing professional development

As Pedler *et al.* (1991) put it:

> 'Action learning involves reconstructive learning, or reframing, as well as simple additive learning or error-correction. We can only learn when we are ready to do so, and what we have learned in the past, including the 'professional deformation' which comes from long practice, can take a long time to loosen and transform.'

Professional development demands a complex weave of reflective practice and opportunities for development of knowledge and skill. Reflection on practice is, however, the oil in the wheel of effective professional development. Action learning sets may ensure that development opportunities are better directed, i.e. act as a diagnosis of the need for more formal learning on courses etc., as well as a bridge between experience and learning.

Action learning can provide an environment within which the professional can describe their own feelings about the emotional content of the work. The set provides an opportunity to take a risk by exposing our normal professional practice to supportive yet challenging scrutiny by others.

Professionals on action learning programmes frequently comment on how difficult it would be to gain, at work, the quality of attention that they have available within the set. While many of us rely on our friends and partners for the support to cope with these emotions, action learning sets can add a more formal environment which provides empathy rather than sympathy; a focus on learning and future action rather than on merely coping with the moment.

The set provides a rich environment to consider alternative approaches. The presenter's attitudes may be challenged but they are challenged in order to foster learning. There are no hidden agendas and no loss of regard from showing vulnerability. This may be a refreshing change within a normally competitive working life. It is this action learning environment which can be so supportive of our continuing professional development.

References

Cunningham I (1994) *The Wisdom of Strategic Learning*. McGraw-Hill, Maidenhead.

Institute of Personnel and Development (IPD) (1995) *A Vehicle for Learning*. IPD, London.

Pedler M, Burgoyne J, Boydell T (1991) *The Learning Company*, McGraw-Hill, Maidenhead.

22. The Clinical Learning Environment
Robert Oliver and Colin Endersby

Introduction

Theories of teaching and learning go a long way to telling us how the individual may effectively learn, but they are by no means infallible in terms of their effectiveness in predicting learning outcomes. [Earlier chapters] have examined some of the factors that affect learning, such as memory, attention, perception and motivation. Even if we take these factors into account, learning may still be impaired by other factors which come under the collective term of "learning environment".

It is difficult to give an all-embracing definition of what is meant by a learning environment. Principally, as Quinn (1988) points out when describing the clinical learning environment, it is "a holistic notion involving every aspect of a clinical setting involving the students themselves". It is perhaps an impossible task, especially when considering the fact that much learning is interactive, to distinguish completely between outside factors such as the mentor, preceptor, systems used within the workplace, etc., and the individual's reactions to them.

If we accept that in some form the learning environment is a tangible concept, and that as such it can be measured, then we need to give some thought to the possibilities and implications of a relevant audit system. This will be discussed not in isolation, but rather with its natural partner, namely quality assurance, in order to give us some idea as to the standards that we must work towards.

The discussion will begin by examining briefly one of the most basic conditions required for learning to take place, namely motivation, and it will be seen that the learning environment itself is an interactive concept between the individual and outside factors.

Motivation and need theory

In identifying human needs, Maslow (1970) has postulated that some will remain relatively unimportant until certain other needs have been satisfied; hence the hierarchical nature of his model (Figure 1). The implications for the learning environment, and more specifically to individuals is briefly explored below.

Physiological needs

Although not normally associated with learning, this particular area does have an important role to play. Basic requirements such as having enough money to provide an adequate diet, living accommodation, and even the pressure of study causing sleep disturbances, are all important personal factors in determining how much learning will

Robert Oliver and Colin Endersby: 'The Clinical Learning Environment' from *TEACHING AND ASSESSING NURSES* (Baillière Tindall, 1996), pp. 91–101. Reprinted by permission of the publisher W B Saunders.

take place. Fatigue brought about through excessive travelling or even a hectic social life are well known to most of us and will eventually take their toll.

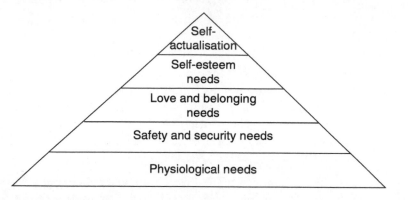

Figure 1   Hierarchy of human needs (Maslow, 1970)

Towards security

We are all aware of our need to feel secure and to have a sense of belonging in our personal lives and to the individual who is attempting to learn, these needs are just as important. The need for security is of particular concern in nursing where students move from area to area on a regular basis and frequently do not become a part of the ward team.

This, however, presents us with only half of the picture because, naturally, even whilst working in a ward area, particularly during long shifts, students often form affiliations with peers in preference to trained staff.

The need for security can be difficult to fulfil in the clinical environment for the learner, and yet Maslow emphasises its importance as second only to the basic physiological needs in his hierarchy. If we are to create an effective learning environment, we must therefore consider how best we can make the learner feel secure.

Perhaps the key to providing a secure environment lies in the sister/charge nurse being seen by the student as being responsible for controlling the clinical learning environment (Orton, 1981), although such a statement must not be made without analysing the possible reasons for it. Certainly in terms of learning, a climate conducive to integrating new information should be achieved, and it could be argued that this presents security in itself by ensuring continuity with the other facets of the student's world, i.e. ensuring that theory and practice are integrated.

The following strategies may be used in order to facilitate the student's perception of security:

1. Ensure that the teaching methods employed are in accordance with what the student perceives as the most effective learning method (Burnard and Morrison, 1991). It appears that students favour more structured teacher-centred

approaches, whilst those responsible for teaching nurses seem to favour students organising and carrying out their own learning sessions. Naturally the quality of student-centred learning method used is of paramount importance, although it should be said that threatening experiences, e.g. carrying out procedures when the student perceives their knowledge is inadequate, rarely help anyone to learn, and only increase the student's feelings of insecurity.

2. Reduce potential role conflict by ensuring that student nurses are not given instructions contrary to what they have been taught (Jones, 1978). This has been identified as a major source of stress, and close cooperation between nurse teachers and clinical staff is vital.

3. Ensure a comprehensive orientation programme as anxiety is often related to the initial part of the clinical experience (Sellek, 1978). It should be ensured that individual needs are identified at the beginning of the experience.

4. To reduce potential anxiety, it is important to ensure that students are well supported when caring for patients who are terminally ill (Birch, 1979).

5. Having an identified mentor/preceptor responsible for individual students will help to reduce initial anxiety [see Chapter 4], provided, of course that a degree of autonomy on the part of the student in choosing a mentor, is allowed.

6. Ensure, whenever possible, that the student has peer support.

It is often the case, as with student-centred learning, that the students themselves may feel under threat and that theories of teaching and learning which, in ideal conditions are effective, may, under certain circumstances have the opposite effect.

As a final word of caution to this short discussion on security, it is not helpful [making] direct comparisons between individuals, especially when one of those individuals is a mentor or preceptor and the other is a student. The only way to ascertain how an individual feels is, by gaining their trust, to allow them to express themselves. The individual who feels insecure will normally show reluctance to embark on a course of action where the outcome is not certain, and this of course is entirely normal. This can be largely overcome by a trusting relationship with a more senior member of staff, in which doubts, fears and deficiencies in knowledge can be freely expressed.

Towards a feeling of belonging

In terms of Maslow's theory, it is difficult to see, particularly in relation to short allocations to a clinical area, how a true sense of belonging can be fostered. Naturally, making the student feel valued and part of the team, if only in a relatively minor capacity, will go some way to achieving this.

As has already been mentioned, peer contact will often form the basis of feelings of security, particularly in the early part of the education process, and this may lead to a sense of belonging.

In the more general sense, however, the student member of a team should be made to feel that they have something useful to contribute, and whereas purely observational experiences are sometimes very useful and almost certainly unavoidable, they should be combined with a degree of involvement, even if this is only seeking and valuing their opinions and reflections.

Self-esteem

The people in the learning environment will be instrumental in making the student feel good about themselves and the contributions that they make. Generally speaking, high self-esteem will come about when the individual feels that they are valued by others and that they are an important part of the team. Personal experiences, opinions and even concerns, if dealt with properly can all serve to increase the student's self-esteem. Conversely, feeling as though they are "in the way", inexperienced and alone, quite apart from detracting from a sense of belonging and making them feel insecure, may also lead to a deterioration in self-esteem.

Self-actualisation

The pinnacle of human achievement is viewed by humanist psychologists as *self-actualisation*. It is characterised by a need for "goodness" with all that entails with our relationship with the world around us. The individual who self-actualises, for instance tolerates uncertainty, appreciates other people unconditionally and generally accepts their circumstances. Naturally, the individual will need to have the lower needs fulfilled before reaching this point, and Maslow is emphatic that few individuals ever reach this stage.

The clinical area as a learning environment

As with any profession, the workplace for which the individual is being educated to work in is of vital importance to the amount and quality of learning that takes place.

Clinical personnel

The role of mentors and preceptors has been discussed elsewhere in the text, although it is appropriate to revisit this topic briefly for the purposes of this discussion. In considering the learning environment as being partly the product of interactions between certain key individuals, it is perhaps relevant to examine the effects this may have.

In examining the learning environment, many authors have placed an emphasis on the ward sister as being perceived by students as being instrumental in creating and controlling the climate in which learning takes place (e.g. Fretwell, 1980; Orton, 1981). Where such a structure exists, it would indeed seem logical to deduce that such a key managerial and clinical position would have such an effect; however, Fretwell (1979) points out that, amongst other things, a hierarchical structure may actually be detrimental to learning, although this may be overcome by effective teamwork, negotiation and effective communication.

The nurse teacher attached to the unit should be able not only to add in some instances to the clinical expertise resource for the student, but also to act as a resource for staff involved in preceptorship and mentoring. The student will also have been allocated a personal tutor who will normally be outside of that particular clinical area. The role of the personal tutor may vary considerably from one college to another, and indeed the discussion on mentorship and preceptorship is as relevant to this role as it is to clinically based education. Suffice it to say that the personal tutor may assist with such matters as study skills, personal difficulties and individual academic tuition as well as acting as a valuable resource for the student.

Quite naturally, as health care is a multidisciplinary concept, other members of the health care team such as medical staff, physiotherapists and occupational therapists, will also be part of the learning environment.

Role-modelling

The organisational aspect of the learning environment should not be viewed as a separate entity. The organisation of learning experiences which are to be effective must be a multifaceted exercise in terms of interpersonal contacts, especially if it is accepted that a significant amount of learning occurs through "role-modelling".

Marson (1981) emphasises that effective teachers in the clinical situation are perceived by learners as having an attitude of care and concern for the welfare of others as well as having a commitment to the education of students in particular. Other authors (e.g. Ogier, 1989), have also emphasised the role-modelling component of learning. If we acknowledge that learning will take place as a result of role modelling, then we should examine some key areas that will determine its effectiveness.

Person-to-person conflict

Although a subject of much debate and diverse theories, it is worthwhile mentioning that there are times when people just do not get on with each other! The reasons can be many and varied; it may be differences of temperament, beliefs, attitudes — the list is almost endless. In [earlier chapters], the advisability of the student choosing their own mentor has been discussed, and this may overcome many potential difficulties.

As a general rule, it should be borne in mind that just as role-modelling may occur if the conditions are right for it to do so, so the student may miss learning opportunities or reject certain behaviours purely because they do not like the individual who exhibits them.

Clinical competence and expertise

It is a natural consequence of our discussion that the learning environment can only be effective if those personnel involved in it are well informed and clinically competent. It was mentioned earlier that both clinical and college staff should be teaching in a non-conflicting way. Updating personal knowledge should not merely be a "re-registering" exercise, but should be linked to practice, and should be an ongoing activity. The advent of the Framework and Higher Award gives nurses the opportunity to link learning directly with clinical practice.

Resources

The resources that any clinical area may have extend far beyond just journals and textbooks. The whole subject of audio-visual aids is covered elsewhere in the text, but for the purposes of our discussion here, a short list of possible resources is given. It will be noticed that a significant resource area can be developed for relatively little cost, and it is advisable to have a specific area set aside for such resources, and most certainly to have a named person responsible for it, perhaps on a rota basis.

1. *Journals*. Collected either from individuals who take particular journals on a regular basis, or by ward/unit subscriptions. Some discussion with ward/unit staff about the selection of these journals is essential in order to ensure their most effective use.

2. *Textbooks*. Find out whether there is a fund from which the finance for textbooks can be provided. Care needs to be taken to avoid hoarding (and hence probable use of) out-of-date/irrelevant texts.

3. *References*. There are several ways to build up a bank of relevant references. One possible way is for a member of staff to be delegated each month to scan the appropriate journals and to record a brief abstract of each one which could then form the basis of a reference section.

4. *Product information*. Manufacturers' information about their products which are being used in the clinical area is vital. Drugs, appliances and equipment will all have information relating to their use, as well as (in many cases) published research which justifies its use. All this information could be held centrally in a resource area.

5. *External agencies*. Information from self-help groups, national organisations and even relevant government agencies which may be applicable to the client group.

6. *Health education literature*. This is a superb resource which is readily available and usually free of charge.

7. *Projects and local research*. These may have been carried out by members of staff as part of a course, or by past students or medical staff.

8. *Department information*. Outlining the services offered by other departments in the hospital.

9. *Contact names*. Staff throughout the unit (or indeed outside) who are useful resources to the student (e.g. environmental health, dietician).

Education audit of the clinical learning environment

As already stated in the introduction, the clinical learning environment must be considered as a tangible entity, and as such, must be audited as a vital component of the overall education process. It comes as no surprise therefore that such an audit is a requirement of the course submission (ENB, 1990) in order that students are allowed to gain experience within that clinical area.

The approach that can be taken towards this subject can be geared towards participating either in an existing audit system or in developing a combined quality assurance/audit system as described below.

Although it has been said that the system combines quality assurance with an audit, this is in fact somewhat misleading, as the two concepts are inextricably linked. If a clinical area is being audited, then a measurable standard must be used in order to indicate whether aspects of that environment are satisfactory or unsatisfactory. It is for this reason that a brief explanation of the concept of quality is given below.

Quality assurance defined

The use of quality assurance tools in the clinical environment is now becoming a more familiar phenomenon although, due to the usage of generic systems such as "Monitor", and "QUALPACS", many nurses will not have had the experience of constructing a system of their own. The use of auditing systems in education, whether in the classroom or in the clinical environment, will follow the same basic principles.

Firstly, however, it is useful to define quality as a starting point, and the definition given below provides us with a sufficiently generic approach:

> 'The measurement of the actual level of the service provided plus the efforts to modify when necessary the provision of these services in the light of the results of these measurements.' (Williamson, 1982)

As with any area of any practice which attempts to evaluate the effectiveness of a particular system, the starting point is to devise a model (or adapt an existing one) so that we may have a basic framework with which to proceed. The model described below (Maxwell, 1984) has been seen as traditionally of use in the more familiar context of quality assessment in health. Bassett (1993), in examining Maxwell's model, has found that with adaptation it can be applied to nurse education.

Maxwell's model of quality

Maxwell (1984) identifies six dimensions in health care:

1. Access to services.

2. Relevance to need.

3. Effectiveness.

4. Equity.

5. Social acceptability.

6. Efficiency and economy.

In terms of the use for which this model was originally intended, the standards which will be applicable under each of the above dimensions will quite naturally be geared directly towards patient care, and will be dependent on how each one of the dimensions has been defined. Therefore, if we are to adapt the model effectively, then we need to redefine them. Bassett (1993), in looking at nurse education has redefined them as follows:

> *Access to services.* Flexibility of tutors working hours to allow access by students for a longer period each day.

> *Relevance to need.* Liaison with service managers/purchasing health authorities, e.g. ensuring that an adequate number of nurses are produced for each branch area.

239

Effectiveness. Identifying which teaching methods are most effective and in which situations.

Equity. Fair division of the budget between the various courses.

Social acceptability. Acceptability of the college by students, staff and purchasing authorities.

Efficiency and economy. Projected student costs must be accurate and competitive whilst maintaining high quality.

Naturally the above dimensions have been defined by Bassett in terms of the non-clinical learning environment (the college). What we have to do now is to examine these dimensions in terms of the clinical learning environment. In considering the example definitions below, the reader can extend them and make them more specific to their own area of practice.

Access to services. Availability of mentors, preceptors and resources to the student.

Relevance to need. Compatibility of clinical practice with student/curriculum learning outcomes.

Effectiveness. Effective learning facilitated through appropriate strategies by professionally credible preceptors.

Equity. Equality for all students, within the context of curricular and personal objectives, of experience and opportunity.

Social acceptability. Compatibility of clinical experience with student, college and national requirements.

Efficiency and economy. Uniform, economic and high quality integration of practice and education.

Standard setting

Having completed the above exercise, the next step in this process is to develop standards for each of the key words or phrases. Naturally, this is normally a function of a quality circle following extensive consultation with colleagues. It is relevant here though to pause briefly in order to examine the meaning of a standard statement and then to examine a method by which they can be classified.

Definitions (RCN, 1990)

Standard. Professionally agreed level of performance for a particular population which is achievable, observable, desirable and measurable.

Standard statement. A statement which describes the broad objectives of your standard.

Structure criteria. These relate to resources in the system which are necessary for the successful completion of the task/area under review.

Process criteria. These relate to actions undertaken by tutorial staff in conjunction with students, service managers, etc.

Outcome criteria. These relate to the desired effect of, e.g. education in terms of student behaviours, responses, level of knowledge and application of that knowledge.

The process described, by its very nature, does not permit short cuts to be taken but nevertheless some basic and fundamental errors do occur. Firstly, the standards are not validated within the area in question and hence are not appropriate. Secondly, consensus regarding the content of statements is minimal or absent, leading to conflicting practice. Thirdly, the process may be viewed from too narrow a perspective and may not take into account key personnel in an effective way. Naturally setting up an effective consultative process will overcome the first two difficulties.

One way of overcoming the third difficulty is to gather data from a variety of sources, e.g. the student, the mentor, the education staff and the clinical managers. Most common now is the practice of utilising student questionnaires about clinical placements. The practice of verbal discussions following clinical activity as a sole source of evaluation has been criticised (Beech, 1991) as being "negatively phrased and detached". It would seem logical therefore that, particularly within the context of being able to form direct comparisons based on some form of standard criteria, a questionnaire approach would be appropriate in most circumstances. The Delphi method has been used to evaluate clinical experiences with some success. This is a method which has been adapted from a system used to evaluate classroom sessions. The reader is referred to ENB (1987) where a full discussion of the method is provided.

The participation of students in the auditing process can actually be achieved by more than one route, firstly, as has been discussed, by the completion of questionnaires. These questionnaires may be fairly non-specific to the clinical area and may be directed primarily towards the quality of the learning environment; they may also include items such as systems for delivery of care. In rather rarer circumstances it may be geared towards more specific clinical aspects of the area. Secondly, there should be a student input into the audit system described above. Thirdly, there should be student participation in the curriculum planning process which should ideally be based on quantifiable information.

Summary

The need for security is of particular concern in nursing where students move from area to area on a regular basis and frequently do not become a part of the ward team.

Students often form affiliations with peers in preference to trained staff (Reid *et al.* 1991).

The following strategies may be used in order to facilitate the students perception of security:

1. Ensure that the teaching methods employed are in accordance with what the student perceives as the most effective learning method (Burnard and Morrison, 1991).

2. Reduce potential role conflict by ensuring that student nurses are not given instructions contrary to what they have been taught (Jones, 1978).

3. Ensure a comprehensive orientation programme as anxiety is often related to the initial part of the clinical experience (Sellek, 1978).

4. To reduce potential anxiety, it is important to ensure that students are well supported when caring for patients who are terminally ill (Birch, 1979).

5. Having an identified mentor/preceptor responsible for individual students will help to reduce initial anxiety.

6. Ensure, whenever possible, that the student has peer support.

The student member of a team should be made to feel that they have something useful to contribute.

Fretwell (1979) points out that, amongst other things, a hierarchical structure may actually be detrimental to learning, although this may be overcome by effective teamwork, negotiation and effective communication.

The nurse teacher attached to the unit should be able not only to add in some instances to the clinical expertise resource for the student, but also to act as a resource for staff involved in preceptorship and mentoring.

Marson (1981) emphasises that effective teachers in the clinical situation are perceived by learners as having an attitude of care and concern for the welfare of others as well as having a commitment to the education of students in particular.

The clinical learning environment must be considered as a tangible entity, and as such, must be audited as a vital component of the overall education process.

Maxwell identifies six dimensions in health care:

1. Access to services.

2. Relevance to need.

3. Effectiveness.

4. Equity.

5. Social acceptability.

6. Efficiency and economy.

A "standard" is a professionally agreed level of performance for a particular population which is achievable, observable, desirable and measurable.

A "standard statement" describes the broad objectives of your standard.

"Structure criteria" relate to resources in the system which are necessary for the successful completion of the task/area under review.

"Process criteria" relate to actions undertaken by tutorial staff in conjunction with students, service managers, etc.

"Outcome criteria" relate to the desired effect of, e.g. education in terms of student behaviours, responses, level of knowledge and application of that knowledge.

Related activities

Activity 1

Using the definitions given below, and, if required adding to them, write up to five key words or phrases that typify the dimensions e.g.: Access to Services: availability of staff, flexibility of service, resources, support.

Access to services.
Relevance to need.
Effectiveness.
Equity.
Social Acceptability.
Efficiency and economy.

Activity 2

Using one of the key words/phrases from Activity 1, write a standard using the four criteria below:

Standard statement.
Structure criteria.
Process criteria.
Outcome criteria.

References

Bassett C C (1993) Quality assurance in nurse education. *Nurse Education Today*, 13, 55–59.

Beech B F (1991) Changes: The Delphi technique adapted for classroom evaluation of clinical placements. *Nurse Education Today*, 11, 207–212.

Birch J (1979) The anxious learners. *Nursing Mirror*, 148(6), 17–22.

Burnard P, Morrison P (1991) Preferred teaching and learning strategies. *Nursing Times*, 87(38), 52.

ENB (1990) Regulations and guidelines for the approval of institutions and courses.

Fretwell J E (1979) Socialisation of nurses: teaching and learning in hospital wards. Thesis, Warwick University.

Fretwell J E (1980) An enquiry into the ward learning environment. *Nursing Times*, 76, 26. (Occasional Paper 69–75.).

Jones D (1978) The need for a comprehensive counselling service for nursing students. *Journal of Advanced Nursing*, 13(4), 359–368.

Marson S N (1981) Ward teaching skills — An investigation into the behavioural characteristics of effective ward teachers. Thesis, CNAA Sheffield City Polytechnic.

Maslow A (1970) *Motivation and Personality*, 2nd edn. Harper and Row, New York.

Maxwell R J (1984) Quality assessment in health. *British Medical Journal*. 12 May, 288.

Ogier M E (1989) *Working and Learning: The Learning Environment in Clinical Nursing.* Scutari, London.

Orton H D (1981) Ward learning climates and student nurse responses. *Nursing Times,* 77, 23 (Occasional Paper 65–68.)

Quinn F M (1988) *The Principles and Practice of Nurse Education,* 2nd edn. Chapman and Hall, London.

RCN (1990) *The Dynamic Standard Setting System: RCN Standards of Care Project.* Harrow, Scutari Projects, Middlesex.

Sellek T (1978) Satisfying and anxiety-creating incidents as identified by student nurses during the process of becoming an SRN. Thesis, Manchester University.

23. Communication and Control — The Essence of the Teaching Process (1)
Lesley B. Curzon

> 'You cannot speak of ocean to a well-frog — the creature of a narrower sphere; you cannot speak of ice to a summer insect.' (Chuang-Tze)

Consider the teaching activities outlined in [Chapter 1]. Each involves complex sets of relationships between teachers and learners, the most important being those resulting from *communication*. The relationships reflect, in part, the teachers' conscious manipulation of conditions, so that the students might achieve desired objectives. Manipulation of the teaching environment in relation to goals is, in effect, a type of *control*, a process which will be examined later. In this chapter we consider *communication*, i.e. the 'exchange of meanings' between teacher and students, without which there can be no effective teaching or learning, and *motivation*, i.e. the general desire of a student to enter into the learning process.

What is communication?

> *Communicate* [L. communicare (communis, common)], *v.t.* To impart, to give a share of, to transmit; to reveal; to give Holy Communion to. *v.i.* To share, to hold intercourse, to confer by speech or writing . . . communication, *n*. The art of communicating; that which is communicated . . . *(Cassell's New English Dictionary)*

The essence of communication is the transmitting and receiving of information through a common system of symbols, whether in the form of writing or other signs, expressive movements, or the spoken word. It takes place when the behaviour of one person acts as a stimulus for the behaviour of another; in the words of I. A. Richards, 'Communication takes place when one mind so acts upon its environment that another mind is influenced, and in that other mind an experience occurs which is like the experience in the first mind, and is caused in part by that experience.'

The following definitions of communication are of interest:

(a) 'the process by which people attempt to share meaning via the transmission of symbolic messages' (Stoner, 1982);

(b) 'an interactional process in which meaning is stimulated through the sending and receiving of verbal and non-verbal messages' (Tortoriello, 1978);

(c) 'the achievement of meaning and understanding between people through verbal and non-verbal means in order to affect behaviour and achieve desired end results' (Mondy, 1983).

Lesley B. Curzon: 'Communication and Control — The Essence of the Teaching Process (1)' from *TEACHING IN FURTHER EDUCATION: AN OUTLINE OF PRINCIPLES AND PRACTICE*, 3rd edn (Holt, Rinehart and Winston, 1985), pp. 69–81.

An important characteristic of man, which divides him from other creatures, is his capacity for the expressive vocalisation which we call *speech*. It may be that the early growth of civilisation depended in large part on man's ability to communicate with his neighbour by speaking, and the later stages of civilisation have reflected, in some measure, the invention of more complicated media of communication, such as the printing press and the radio. The development of formal teaching, in particular, is linked to the expansion of communication methods. From the spoken discourse to the printed textbook, the TV lesson and the computer, the teaching process has depended on the ability and technique of the teacher to convey to the learner in an appropriate form the fruits of human thought — that is, to communicate.

In the teaching situation, communication by the teacher is generally intended to influence the learner's behaviour. Its mode will be determined, therefore, by that situation which will reflect the lesson's objectives. To that end, communication in the classroom may be verbal or non-verbal, formal or informal, one-way or two-way, designed to elicit a verbal or non-verbal response, intended to state a fact or pose a problem. Its primary function in the teaching process is *the creation and maintenance of a community of thought and feeling which will lead to learning.*

Communication in relation to teaching

Class teaching requires the presentation of stimuli and the eliciting of learners' responses. Effective presentation of stimuli is, in itself, a form of communication. Whether pointing to a chart, tapping a ruler on a desk so as to attract attention or asking a subtle question which demands interpretation and insight for its solution, the teacher is engaged in the process of communicating. Consider, for example, the following situations in typical further education classes:

1. Day-release students are being taught the elements of vehicle maintenance. They and their tutor are examining a mechanism at which he is pointing. He states: 'Our next job is to lubricate the accelerator control linkage and cable and the pedal fulcrum. Here they are.' He then ensures that his statement has been understood.

2. Secretarial students are studying business documents. An overhead projector displays an illustration of a bill of exchange. The teacher says: 'This obviously isn't a cheque, which we looked at a few minutes ago! Why not?' Answers are elicited and considered by teacher and class.

3. BTEC students have been listening to one of their group reading his essay on 'Cures for Inflation'. He has reached his final sentence: 'Inflation can be cured, I submit, only by the abolition of the market price system.' The students turn their attention to the tutor, awaiting his reaction. He raises his eyebrows in mock, exaggerated surprise. The students observe, and understand, his reaction.

In these examples we can discern a variety of modes and media of communication. They include statements of fact, expressions of opinion, comment on opinion, questions, replies to questions, the posing of problems. The media and channels of communication include the voice, gestures (pointing, facial expressions — the so-called proto-linguistic signs, which are of great importance in the classroom), visual aids. In each of these varied examples of classroom communication will be found the following elements:

(a) an objective (e.g. to achieve an understanding of the functions of a bill of exchange);

(b) an awareness by the class teacher of the path to that objective;

(c) the creation of a link, or 'channel', between teacher and class, the effectiveness of which will be determined in large measure by the teacher's skill and the learner's initial motivation and continuing interest;

(d) the adoption by the teacher of appropriate modes of communicating his 'message', calculated to elicit responses and modify behaviour;

(e) the reception and comprehension of the message, of which the teacher becomes aware ('feedback').

Communication in the classroom is, therefore, not merely a matter of an instructor's addressing a class; it is the outcome of a number of interrelated activities. Where any one of these activities is omitted, the effectiveness of the communication may be vitiated or destroyed, so that the probability of successful learning is reduced accordingly.

Communication theory: a useful analogy

Attempts have been made in recent years to analyse the basis of information transmission so as to formulate a general theory of communication. The mathematical theory of communication, put forward by Shannon and Weaver, draws on information theory to present an explanation of communication systems which has important analogies with the teaching process. (The aim of information theory is the discovery of laws which can be couched in mathematical terms concerning systems designed to communicate or manipulate information. The term 'information' is used in a highly-technical sense as 'that which resolves uncertainty'; it can be measured in terms of changes in probability (Shannon and Weaver, 1949). In less formal terms, Paisley describes 'information' as denoting 'any stimulus that alters cognitive structure in the receiver . . . Something that the receiver already knows is not information' (Paisley, 1980).)

Consider a very simple system of communication, say, that existing where one person speaks to another. The system includes the following three elements:

(a) a *source* (or transmitter) — the speaker;

(b) a *channel* — the air which carries the speaker's voice;

(c) a *receiver* — the listener.

Such a system may be represented by the simple diagram in Figure 1.

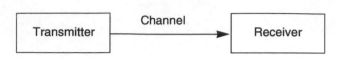

Figure 1

Shannon and Weaver utilised a relatively simple model of the communication process: a message flowed along a selected channel from source to receiver. Emitted signals were decoded by the receiver. In modelling information flow, the problems to be answered were: *'Who says what*, in *which channel*, to whom, and *with what result?'* The model was seen later to require modification since, in particular, it seemed to ignore the important role of feedback in the process of communication.

A later model emerged from the work of Berlo. He drew attention to the significance of feedback and stressed the significance of cultural influences and communication skills on the sender's message. Common experiences and shared meanings among participants were seen by Berlo as essential to effective communication (Berlo, 1960).

More recently, Barnlund has revealed the dynamic, transactional nature of communication. His model shows communication as a dynamic process ('continually responsive, continually changing') in which the interaction of all elements within the process must be studied. Each participant shares the processes of encoding and decoding; participants 'exchange roles' continuously during some types of communication. According to Barnlund, the process of communication should not be viewed as a unidirectional, linear activity, but more in the nature of a mutual, reciprocal, transactional phenomenon (Barnlund, 1980).

Certain general features have emerged from the above models. First, communication is viewed best as a process, that is, a series of sequential activities directed to some end. Secondly, communication involves an interpersonal relationship. Thirdly, communication involves 'traffic in symbols' which, by their very nature, are mere approximations to the concepts intended to be transmitted. Finally, communication, if it is to be effective, necessitates a community of meaning attached to its symbols.

Figure 2 is a diagram delineating the fundamental features in the communication process. (Note that 'noise' occurs throughout the system, and that the dotted line joining sender and receiver should be interpreted as suggesting an interchange of roles at many stages in the process.)

The system is made up of the following elements:

(a) an *information source* from which the message material originates;

(b) a *transmitter* which transforms (or 'encodes') the message into a form suitable for the channel;

(c) a *'noise source'* which interferes (not only in the auditory modality) with the flow of information between transmitter and receiver and reduces the probability of the message being received correctly to less than 1. (Indeed, as Shannon pointed out, the efficiency of a communication system as a whole is defined in part by the probability that noise will change the information content of the message. 'Noise' is used here in its communication engineering sense of unpredictable, random and unwanted signals that mask the information content of a communication channel.)

(d) a *receiver* which decodes the message encoded by the transmitter;

(e) a *destination* for the message;

(f) *feedback*.

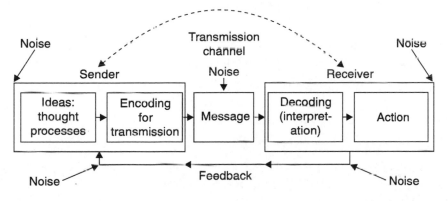

Figure 2

The analogy with the classroom situation in which a teacher is engaged in the processes of communication should be apparent. The importance when designing a lesson of allowing for the interference of 'noise' is clear.

The communication system of a typical lesson may be considered as consisting of the following elements:

(a) an *information source* — the brain of the teacher;

(b) a *transmitter* — the teacher's voice mechanism which produces a signal (words) which is transmitted through a channel (air);

(c) *'noise'* which distorts the signal and which may result from distractions in the classroom environment, for example, or an irrelevant meaning 'read into' the message on the basis of a previous experience;

(d) a *receiver* — the students' sensory organs;

(e) a *destination* — the students' brains;

(f) *feedback* — e.g. by question and answer.

Shannon and Weaver identify three levels of communication problems:

1. With what accuracy can the very symbols of a message be transmitted? — the problem of *technique*.

2. With what precision do the symbols convey the meaning of the message? — the problem of *semantics*.

3. With what effectiveness does the received and perceived meaning affect behaviour? — the problem of *effectiveness*.

These problems may emerge when a teacher analyses the lesson he has given, in the form of the following questions:

1. 'How accurately have I conveyed the meaning of the lesson, i.e. did I employ the appropriate mode of communication?'

2. 'How precisely, in practice, did the lesson content resemble that which I had in mind?'

3. 'How did perception of the lesson content modify the behaviour of the students as judged by their responses, and, in general, how effective was I?'

The analogy presented by the theoreticians' model emphasises for the teacher the complexities of communication and draws attention to some of the factors which are necessary for the attainment of teaching goals.

'Noise' as a barrier to effective communication

The best-planned lesson can fall on 'deaf ears' and there must be few tutors in further education who have not suffered the chagrin which arises from the confrontation of a teacher, anxious to present a carefully-prepared lesson, and a class, apparently indifferent and unwilling to participate. 'They didn't respond in any way!' 'I put everything I had into it — diagrams, models, notes — and it fell flat!' 'As soon as the lesson started, I could tell we weren't on the same wavelength!'

The effectiveness of communication in the classroom may be weakened by the deficiencies of the 'source' and 'transmitter', by 'noise' and competition from a variety of sources, and by inadequacies of the 'receiver'. Often, the very environment in which the class works acts as a 'noise source' which interferes with and distorts reception of the teacher's message. Physical conditions, e.g. lighting, temperature, seating, may be such as to distract from and therefore weaken reception of the message. A badly set-out room in which the teacher can be neither seen nor heard properly is a common source of interference with information flow. Where a classroom in a college is set out in formal 'school style', the recall of unhappy experiences or of failure associated with school may interfere with the reception of communication by adult students. Controlling the teaching environment, in the sense of ensuring that it does not function as a 'noise source', is an important task for the class tutor. This is not to be taken as implying that effective communication and teaching cannot take place save in a carefully-illuminated, thermostatically-controlled room! On the contrary, it is well known that extremely efficient instruction does take place in ill-ventilated Nissen huts or in badly-illuminated, noisy laboratories overlooking railway shunting yards. In analysing the reasons for poor communication, however, it is necessary to consider the effect on the class of *all* types of distracting stimuli including the physical environment.

The 'source' and 'transmitter' — the teacher himself — may be responsible for the erection of barriers to effective communication. His personality and mannerisms will obtrude on the communication process. An aggressive manner, a nervous disposition (which may reflect inadequate knowledge or poor lesson preparation), the proto-linguistic signs which are swiftly interpreted by students as evidence of hostility or lack of interest in the subject matter, may block the pathway to learning. Adolescents are often adept in the swift detection of insincerity, so that there is unlikely to be effective learning where the tutor reveals, by an inflexion of voice or a display of indifference in response to a question (so-called 'proto-linguistic symbols') that he is out of sympathy with the purpose of the lesson. An incorrect choice of the medium of communication — a long verbal explanation of the contents of a document, for example, rather than a discussion using its image projected on a screen — may weaken the effectiveness of message transmission. A lesson pitched at too high a level or out of sequence with previous lessons will usually ensure that the class is 'on a different wavelength', so that communication is impossible. A rate of delivery which is too swift for comprehension and assimilation of the message, or too slow to maintain interest, can prevent effective transmission. A badly-structured, disjointed lesson plan may produce signals so erratic that no part of the intended message reaches the class; the signals may also produce 'overtones' resulting in a distortion of meaning. (William James' reminder that 'the mind is, at every stage, a theatre of simultaneous possibilities', is of relevance here.)

The learner — the 'receiver' and 'destination of the message' — may function in a manner which weakens or renders meaningless the communication. He may be incapable of receiving or 'decoding' (i.e. comprehending) the content of a lesson because he is inadequately prepared. A strong desire to learn how to use a computer will not recompense for a total lack of knowledge of programming processes. A well-planned lesson designed to improve speeds of typing, utilising taped dictation, will have little value for those members of the class whose spelling is poor. Where effective interpretation of messages received by the senses is impossible because of lack of acquaintance with the technical vocabulary employed, comprehension of the message is impossible. Where there are variations in the learner's level of intensity of interest, his reception of information is influenced directly; there is no communication where the learner's mind is 'elsewhere'.

Effective barriers to communication may be set up where a teacher is unaware that the language he is using is, by reason of its structure, style and syntax, so far removed from that to which his class is accustomed that the disjunction of transmitter and receiver is almost total. The work of Bernstein in uncovering the different 'class codes' of communication is of great significance for the class teacher. Bernstein draws attention to the existence of two types of language-codes — 'working class language', a highly-predictable, 'public' language in which individual selection and permutation are severely restricted, and 'formal language' in which the speaker is able to make a highly-individual selection and permutation (Bernstein, 1971). (For a critique of Bernstein's views see the writings of Labov.)

Parry has enumerated the following factors as barriers to effective communication (teachers will recognise swiftly some of the causes of breakdown in lessons): limitation of the receiver's capacity (e.g. cognitive limitations, preventing recognition of exceptions to generalities — the 'reductive listening' which causes students to think that what is presented as new material is no more than old knowledge 'rehashed'); distractions (often from competing stimuli and environmental stress); the use of unstated assumptions (so that cognitive barriers arise between teacher and students, who are, effectively, at cross-purposes); incompatibility of 'schemes' of understanding (whereby differing reaction patterns and expectancies lead to misinterpretations); intrusion of unconscious or partly-conscious mechanisms (such as fear, leading to the rejection of disturbing and unwelcome information); confused presentation of information (which ignores the fact that as information becomes more complex, so, for many learners, comprehension difficulty is intensified) (Parry, 1966).

Probably the most effective barrier to communication in college classes is the learner's lack of motivation. In the absence of those conditions which arouse and sustain his interest in the learning process and its outcome, the chances of the teacher's eliciting the desired responses to a stimulus message are very slender. It is to the problem of motivation in the process of classroom communication that we now turn.

Motivation: its general nature

Motivation (*motes, movere* = to move) has been defined variously by psychologists as: 'the phenomena involved in a person's drives and goal-seeking behaviour'; 'the tendencies to activity which commence with a persistent stimulus (drive) and end with an appropriate adjustive response'; 'the arousal, regulation and sustaining of a pattern of behaviour'; 'the internal state or condition that results in behaviour directed towards a specific goal'. The term will be used here in a general sense to refer to a person's aroused desire for participation in a learning process. Dewey speaks of the teacher in his role of guide and director as steering a boat, '. . . but the energy that propels it must come from those who are learning'. The arousal, regulation and sustaining of the student's enthusiasm for learning, that is, the harnessing of his power of motivation in the service of the lesson, constitute an important task for the teacher.

The presence of motivation is considered by most teachers to be essential to effective communication and learning. Davies enumerates four effects of motivation that are of importance in instruction: motivation arouses, sustains and energises students; it assists in the direction of tasks; it is selective, in that it helps to determine students' priorities; it assists organising students' activities (Davies, 1971). Tutors in further education are aware of the relative ease of teaching highly-motivated students and of the frustrations and difficulties arising from lessons with students who, for example, see no link between their aspirations and the content of a curriculum. The former usually exhibit behaviour which is calculated to assist the process of communication; the latter may display a resistance which makes effective communication difficult or impossible.

Motivation: its psychological basis

Psychologists tend to speak of the concept of 'motive' in terms of that which accounts for a learner's energy, direction and persistence of behaviour; hence it becomes possible to *infer* a learner's motives from observation of his use of learned behaviour, from the direction of that behaviour and from its persistence in pursuing and attaining a goal. A learner's motives include those related to his physiological needs (hunger, sleep, etc.) and those related to self-esteem, ability to deal with his environment, etc. An individual's 'stored motives' depend on their strength and on the 'cues' in a situation which give him information as to the desirability of the goal and probabilities of attainment. Where motives are in conflict, the stronger motive generally prevails; where the motives are of equal strength, compromise or uncertainty will result.

Some psychologists speak of a 'motivational cycle' which is based on the following components: *need* (which arises when conditions felt to be necessary for optimal chances of survival veer from their optima); *drive* (some purposeful activity initiated by a need state of the organism); *goal* (the terminal point of the drive); *satiation* (resulting in the cessation of the drive activity).

Maslow (1908–70) saw motivation in terms of an individual's striving for growth; he sought to explain it by reference to a 'hierarchy of human needs'. He believed that at any given moment a person's behaviour is dominated by those of his needs which have the greatest potency. As his 'lower', physiological needs are adequately satisfied, motives at a 'higher' level in the hierarchy come into play. The hierarchy is made up as follows:

1. *Physiological needs*, e.g. hunger, thirst, leading to a desire for food and water.

2. *Safety needs*, e.g. security. (A highly-anxious student may be experiencing these needs.)

3. *Belonging needs*, e.g. friendship.

4. *Esteem needs*, e.g. success.

5. *Self-actualisation needs*, e.g. desire for self-fulfilment.

Motivation at levels 4 and 5 (often referred to as *intrinsic motivation*) is very important and should be taken into account in the planning of work which is related to the ultimate goal of the realisation of students' potential abilities.

Alderfer (b. 1926) has reformulated Maslow's hierarchy into three levels.

1. *Existence needs*, e.g. physiological and safety needs.

2. *Relatedness needs*, i.e. needs involving social and interpersonal relationships.

3. *Growth needs*, i.e. all those needs relating to the development of human potential.

In addition to Alderfer's hierarchy being based on a 'need satisfaction process', it incorporates a 'need frustration regression process'. Thus, where a student experiences repeated frustration in his efforts to satisfy some higher-order need, he will place greater importance on the preceding lower-level needs (Alderfer, 1972).

Herzberg (b. 1923) believes that persons are affected by 'motivators' and 'hygiene factors'. 'Motivators' are the factors directly associated with the *content* of an activity. He enumerates as examples recognition, responsibility and the feeling of accomplishment. To the degree that they are present, motivation will occur, having a positive effect on learning. 'Hygiene factors' are those primarily associated with the *context* of an activity. As applied to the classroom setting, examples of such factors are the style of instruction adopted by the teacher, security of the learner, interpersonal relationships in the classroom. When present, hygiene factors prevent dissatisfaction, but do not necessarily lead to satisfaction (Herzberg, 1959).

Motivation in the classroom

The teacher has the task of creating a learning environment which relates the learner's activity to his needs and aspirations, so that his competence is developed and strengthened and his sense of self-improvement heightened. This may necessitate a combination of teaching techniques which will deliberately keep alive, utilise and strengthen the learner's initial motivation. These techniques should take into account the following matters:

1. The individual learner's motivations and goals should be understood and the aims of the course should be clearly defined and explained to him.

2. 'Goals that are too hard or too easy to attain are neither motivating nor reinforcing when attained' (Hilgard and Bower, 1981).

3. Short-term goals should be seen to be related to long-term achievement.

4. Lessons should be planned by the teacher *and seen by the student* as part of a sequence eventually leading to the attainment of desirable ends.

5. Tasks set should be appropriate to the student's level of abilities. 'Nothing dampens motivation as much as an unrelieved diet of failure and frustration' (Ausubel, 1978).

6. Attainment of a required level of competence ought to be explained and accepted not as an end in itself, but as a key which opens the door to higher levels of understanding and achievement.

7. Lesson material and communication ought to be meaningful, ought to arouse intellectual curiosity and ought to involve students actively and personally. 'The intensity of our interest in an activity, as well as the amount of effort that we expend on it, depend on our feeling of personal involvement in that activity' (Kolesnik, 1978).

8. The level of communication during a lesson ought to be pitched carefully so that there is no 'comprehension gap' between teacher and student.

9. The fatigue which accompanies boredom and which destroys motivation ought to be avoided by a planned variety of teaching and learning activities. Cognitive drive should be maximised by arousing intellectual curiosity.

10. Assimilation of lesson material ought to be tested regularly.

11. Evaluation of test results ought to be conveyed to students as swiftly as possible and ought to be interpreted in the context of immediate and long-term aims.

12. Competence and mastery ought to be recognised and reinforced by praise.

13. Temporary failure ought to be considered by student and teacher as an occasion for a fresh attempt to overcome difficulties.

Does the absence of appropriate motivation preclude the success of a lesson? Ausubel suggests that the teacher should consider ignoring lack of motivation and concentrate on teaching the student as effectively as the situation allows. This, he claims will produce some degree of learning, and the motivation for further learning may result. Davies suggests that it is not always necessary to postpone learning until the appropriate motivation exists. The teacher should ignore initial motivational states and rely on lesson presentation which will capture and develop interest.

Effective *control* which, together with successful *communication*, helps to ensure the attainment of teaching objectives, [is considered next].

References

Alderfer C P (1972) *Existence, Relatedness and Growth*. Free Press.

Ausbel D P et al. (1978) *Educational Psychology — A Cognitive View*. Holt, Rinehart and Winston.

Barnlund D C (1968) *Interpersonal Communication*. Houghton Mifflin.

Berlo D (1960) *The Process of Communication*. Holt, Rinehart and Winston.

Bernstein B (1971) Social class and linguistic development in a theory of social learning. In: *Class, Codes and Control*. Routledge.

Davies I K (1971) *The Management of Learning*. McGraw-Hill.

Herzberg F (1959) *Motivation to Work*. Wiley.

Hilgard E R, Bower G H (1981) *Theories of Learning*. Prentice-Hall.

Kolesnik W B (1978) *Motivation*. Allyn & Bacon.

Labov W (1976) *Language in the Inner City*. University of Pennsylvania Press.

Maslow A H (1970) *Motivation and Personality*. Harper & Row.

Mondy R W et al. (1983) Motivation. In: *Management — concepts and practices*. Allyn & Bacon.

Paisley W (1980) Information and Work. In: *Progress in Communication Sciences*. Ablex.

Parry R (1966) *The Psychology of Human Communication*. ULP.

Shannon C, Weaver W (1949) *The Mathematical Theory of Communication*. University of Illinois Press.

Stoner J (1982) Communication. In: *Management*. Prentice-Hall.

Tortoriello T J (1978) *Communication in the Organisation*. McGraw-Hill.

24. Linking Theory and Practice in Teaching Basic Nursing Skills

Blenda E. Smith

In an attempt to integrate theory and practice in baccalaureate nursing education, students were taught nursing skills with two cognitive strategies (Vee heuristics and concept maps) that consciously identify and reinforce connections between scientific theory and practice. The research showed that students using Vee heuristics and concept maps, rather than traditional modes, were significantly better able to identify scientific principles to describe why specific steps of a nursing skill were done.

Introduction

Establishing links between theory and practice has been a challenge and a concern in nursing education for decades. Contemporary nursing leaders support the linkage as essential to professional nursing education and practice (Hawkins, 1981; Infante, 1985; Torres & Yura, 1974), yet the challenge of teaching integration of theory and practice continues.

When nursing is described as theory-driven, two perspectives emerge: nursing theory and scientific theory. Nursing theory gives a guiding framework for theorizing about concepts such as nursing, wellness, health care needs, and client systems. Scientific theory gives a fundamental basis to the practice of nursing, which is built on knowledge of the natural sciences (physics, anatomy, physiology, biology, and microbiology). Without precise identification of scientific concepts and principles, safe and comprehensive care is compromised.

This research focused on teaching strategies that develop links between scientific theory and basic nursing skills. A traditional approach to teaching basic nursing skills was compared with an innovative approach using two strategies that consciously link theory with practice. The strategies were *Vee heuristics*, which identify specific concepts, principles, and theories related to basic nursing skills, and *concept maps*, which teach students how to create schematic drawings of their mental understanding by organizing and linking relevant concepts.

Statement of the problem

When baccalaureate nursing students are taught in college laboratories with Vee heuristics and concept maps rather than with traditional modes, is there a difference in the ability to identify principles of scientific theory related to basic nursing skills? Is there a difference in performance of basic nursing skills in practice situations? Do students perceive learning as more meaningful?

Review of the literature

Teaching connections between theory and practice is not a new educational idea. Tyler (1949) urged that correlation of theory and practice was essential to professional education. The American Nurses Association (ANA) has called for professional nursing practice to be theory-oriented rather than technique-oriented (1965). The National League for Nursing (NLN) publication, *Characteristics of Baccalaureate Education in Nursing* (1987), supports theory-based thinking skills when it specifies that graduates "synthesize theoretical and empirical knowledge from nursing, scientific, and humanistic disciplines with practice" (p. 2).

In spite of the fundamental significance of natural science theory as the underpinning of nursing practice, Wilson (1975) sees curricula ill-defined and unstructured in terms of specific links between science theory and nursing practice. She finds the application of scientific theoretical knowledge in nursing education haphazard.

Akinsanya (1987) believes theoretical input from the life sciences must be clearly defined for nursing practice. He stresses the value of understanding concepts, principles, and theory from the life sciences in order to understand rationales for every nursing action. Akinsanya calls for (1) identification and categorization of nursing skills in relation to scientific underpinnings, (2) innovative curricular approaches to link theory and practice, and (3) the "progressive development of professional responsibility through a more conscious linking of theory with practice in nursing education" (p. 272).

Drew (1988) warns nursing not to devalue the theoretical knowledge base of the natural sciences, which helps to evaluate human responses and to direct nursing practice. She stresses that although technical skills can be performed without a clear theoretical understanding by technicians, professional nurses provide a higher level of care by giving comprehensive, theory-based care with knowledge from natural sciences.

Although theory-based care is essential, Fahy (1969) asserts that skill competence is the first responsibility of a practicing professional. According to Larson's (1984) findings, a nurse's technical competence is the attribute most valued by patients. Settlemyer (1978) believes that the small role of technical skills competency must be successfully accomplished for patient safety and the nurse's self-esteem before developing higher-level roles such as patient advocate, educator, counselor, researcher, and clinical expert. Infante (1985) defends the value of professional competence in skill performance for patients' needs. Nursing students reinforce the perception of practice as supreme. Mastery of skills is felt by nursing students as the "rite of passage" into nursing (Gendron, 1981). After many liberal arts courses, nursing students are finally introduced to "real nursing," the performance of nursing skills.

Yura *et al.* (1986, p. 226) support present nursing model curricula that develop "students who can discover, create, express meanings, and think, rather than merely accumulate facts." Curricula that integrate the practice of nursing with a well-defined theory base continue to be a major goal for professional nursing education.

A literature review of an educating theory by Novak and Gowin (1984) reveals the application of Vee heuristics and concept mapping in numerous classroom and science laboratory studies. Researchers find that using these strategies helps students organize and understand knowledge (Colling, 1984; Fuata'i, 1985; Gurley, 1982; Mollura, 1979). Learning to map is perceived by students as difficult although they claim to value consequential meaningful learning much more than rote mode learning (Colling, 1984; Fuata'i, 1985; Gurley, 1982). Presentation of content as a conceptual hierarchy with overt and repetitious reinforcement results in increased numbers of concepts and understanding of concepts in one's knowledge structure (Cullen, 1983; Mollura, 1979; Ring, 1969) Finally, Buchweitz (1981) finds that epistemological analysis of curricula with Vee heuristics and concept maps provides valuable assessment data.

Theoretical framework

The theories of Novak & Gowin (1984) and Ausubel (1978) form the major components of the theoretical framework for this research.

Meaningful learning

Novak views learning as occurring on a continuum, from rote mode (memorization) up to meaningful learning. Most school learning falls into the rote mode, i.e. learning is a verbatim incorporation of new knowledge into the cognitive structure and is not related to experience with events or objects. Meaningful learning is defined as a process of consciously integrating new knowledge with one's previous knowledge in ways that strongly link the two.

Since professional nursing's body of knowledge is based on knowledge (theory and facts) from the sciences and humanities, it is essential for students to recall, understand, and build on their prior knowledge from liberal arts courses. As students begin to learn basic nursing skills, prior knowledge from physics, anatomy, physiology, biology, microbiology, sociology, and psychology is fundamental to their understanding and practice. Nursing educators prefer "using the knowledge already at hand more effectively rather than continually increasing present amounts of knowledge. They seek to bring together and connect the concepts of different disciplines as a way of using present knowledge more effectively" (Yura *et al.* 1986, p. 225).

Structure of knowledge

The second component of the theoretical framework relates to the learner's structure of knowledge. Learners can construct mental pictures of their knowledge in schematic depictions called concept maps (Novak & Gowin, 1984). To draw concept maps, learners perceive concepts, recall prior knowledge, and connect new knowledge to prior knowledge in a conceptual hierarchy. Concepts are organized with the broadest concepts on top of the map and more specific concepts subsumed under larger ones. Linking words connect concepts to specify relationships between and among concepts. The more links that exist between various concepts, the more interconnected the concepts are in one's knowledge structure. Figure 1 is an example of a concept map for the basic nursing skill of dangling a patient.

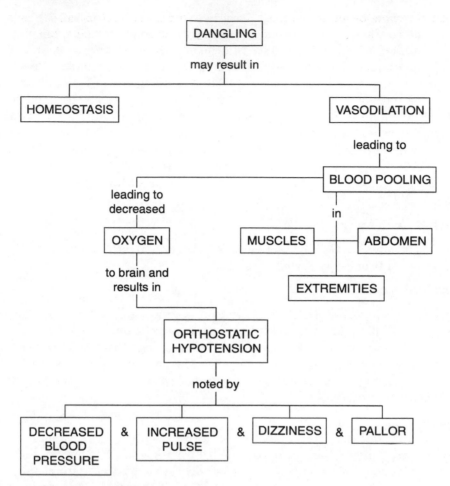

Figure 1   Concept map for dangling

Students identify new concepts and use prior knowledge from liberal arts courses in the process of learning basic nursing skills. Concept maps help the student and instructor to identify the student's knowledge structure about basic nursing skills. A bonus benefit of concept mapping is the ease with which misconceptions can be noted. When misconceptions can be identified and corrected before new learning occurs, learning can proceed more accurately. Mapping is, therefore, a powerful tool for clarifying misconceptions before new learning is built on prior misconceptions.

Linking theory and practice

The third component of the theoretical framework is the belief that learning should include both theory and practice perspectives. Clear linkages must be evident between practice and theory to conclude that practice is theory-driven rather than rote steps. It is the theory-driven nature of practice that gives intended meanings to procedural steps.

Learning the practice of nursing by understanding the theoretical basis of each practice step reflects optimal learning. To help conceptualize this theory/practice integration in learning, Gowin (1981) has developed the Vee heuristic, which asks a focus question about an educative event (i.e. learning a basic nursing skill) and answers with theoretical and practice perspectives. The particular "V" shape of the heuristic is not critical to its use but does represent the coming together of theory and practice in an educative event (Figure 2).

FOCUS QUESTION

How can a nurse begin mobilizing a patient safely?

THEORY	PRACTICE

PHILOSOPHY:

Humans value feeling healthy and secure.

THEORY:

Theory of gravity. Body system homestasis. Physiology of cardiovascular system.

PRINCIPLES:

1. Body constantly attempts to maintain homeostasis.
2. Baseline data is necessary to evaluate change accurately.
3. Rapid position change *may not* allow for body homeostatic mechanisms to avoid orthostatic hypotension [O.H.].
4. O.H. occurs when veins dilate and blood pools in muscles, extremities and abdominal spaces so that adequate blood supply cannot circulate to brain tissues.
5. Inadequate circulating blood volume results in pallor and decreased blood pressure.
6. Body response to decreased circulating blood volume is an increased heart rate for faster circulation of available blood.
7. Decreased oxygen supply to brain tissue results in dizziness and fainting.

CONCEPTS:

Homeostasis, Vasodilation, Dangle, Blood pooling, Orthostatic hypotension

VALUE CLAIMS:

Anticipating untoward patient responses:
a. avoids injury.
b. validates the quality of nursing judgments.

KNOWLEDGE CLAIMS:

1. Assess patient's color and pulse before "dangling".
2. Make position changes (lying to sitting to standing) *gradually*.
3. Assess patient's dizziness, pulse, skin color and moistness as soon as in sitting position.
4. If untoward effects noted, return patient to lying position and check for decreased blood pressure.
5. Wait to repeat "dangling" more gradually.

TRANSFORMATIONS:

Performance evaluation.

RECORDS OF EVENTS:

Observe nurse.

EVENT:

"Dangle" the immobilized patient.

Figure 2   Vee heuristic for dangling

Gowin sees "laying the Vee" on an event as a way of (1) analyzing previous knowledge (or identifying lack of previous knowledge), (2) understanding theory and practice of an event, and (3) constructing new knowledge.

The way to "read" a Vee is by first reading the focus question, which asks a fundamental question about what is to be learned in that specific Vee. Since the focus question is answered by the educative event (learning the basic nursing skill), the event is read next.

In order for an educative event to be theory-driven, the left side of the Vee is used to analyze the theoretical domain of the event. By listing all relevant concepts, one is forced to analyze what is being studied at a finite and definitional level. Next, principles are stated that reflect relationships among concepts to identify scientific knowledge. "Principles tell *how* events or objects appear or behave, whereas theories tell *why* they do so" (Novak & Gowin, 1984, p. 65). Theories are collections of principles organized into broad and inclusive systems of beliefs (e.g. the theory of gravity, learning theory). Even broader in interpretation is philosophy that expresses the overriding value of the entire theoretical domain. When the left side of the Vee is well developed, an educative event has a valuable theory base.

Once concepts, principles, theories, and philosophies are clarified, that understanding is used to underpin learning the practice side of the Vee. Moving up the right side of a Vee heuristic from the event, the practice domain is addressed by first making records of the event (e.g. observations of skill performance). These records are transformed into useful, "workable" data such as performance evaluations. Knowledge claims are the new pieces of information guided by theory and used in the practice of the event (e.g. specific steps of a basic nursing skill). Finally, value claims reflect the inherent worth and usefulness of the practice domains.

The right side of a Vee addresses practice aspects of an event within the framework of the theoretical left side. Interplay between left and right sides shows how (1) a basic nursing skill is theory-driven, and (2) prior knowledge (previously known scientific concepts, principles, and theory) guides the understanding of new knowledge (new practice skill). Although the "V" shape appears to suggest a split or separation of theory and practice, its purpose is to identify both so as to unite them in the event. Hence, a nursing skill is always grounded in theory.

Understanding the theory that guides nursing practice can be a nebulous, frustrating experience for students who are anxious to "do" nursing. Students perceive the laboratory as a place for practice rather than a place for analyzing theory as the driving force behind nursing practice. This concrete strategy is a powerful way to link theory and practice for nursing curricula.

Method

The study was quasi-experimental with a nonequivalent control group design. All students enrolled in a fall semester, junior-level, upper-division nursing course that taught basic nursing and assessment skills were invited to participate. Forty-two subjects comprised the convenience sample of students who volunteered (five chose not to participate). Students were divided in nonrandom fashion at registration into lab groups of no more than eight. Students had no knowledge of instructor assignment to lab sections at registration. There was no pattern of assignment, since the university registrar used a computerized registration system. Although much variability existed within each group, demographic data that were analyzed later established homogeneity between different lab sections for the following variables: age, sex, employment during the current semester, type and average number of employment hours per week, type or amount of prior work experience, type or amount of prior life experience, type or number of prior nursing-related courses, status as educationally disadvantaged, and cumulative GPA before beginning the semester with the research intervention.

Group design resulted from course structure and instructors' assignments to laboratory sections. Each laboratory section had one instructor for a three-hour weekly college laboratory practice time. Three instructors (the researcher and two other instructors) were scheduled to have two laboratory groups each per week. Instructors were introduced to the theoretical framework and taught how to use the two research strategies. Throughout the research, internal consistency between instructors and labs was assessed by periodic observers in labs. Each instructor taught both a traditional and a treatment mode each week to control for individual teaching differences. Each instructor's comparison and treatment groups could be compared with the others, since homogencity between groups was established.

Description of traditional and treatment modes

The traditional mode followed in the college lab required students to complete assigned weekly textbook readings, film viewing, and definitions of glossary terms before each lab. The students asked questions and discussed the week's basic nursing skills. Lab content was specifically itemized in the instructor's laboratory manual to assure that all instructors covered necessary course content. Next, the instructor demonstrated the skills. Finally, the students practiced the skills in the simulated setting and gave satisfactory return demonstrations to the instructor.

Lab structure for the treatment mode followed the traditional mode described, except as follows. In each treatment group's first lab, students were oriented to Vee heuristics and concept mapping. In subsequent labs, students used discussion time differently than comparison groups. Incorporated with student questions and discussion of basic nursing skills were one or two Vees each week that the researcher had made (in counsel with the other instructors) regarding the skills presently being learned. Vees were discussed for clarification of meaning. When appropriate, previous Vees were also referred to for building on prior knowledge. Vees were available as references to stimulate thinking of related principles while instructors demonstrated and students practiced skills.

Treatment students came to labs with one concept map of selected glossary terms each week. Their maps were discussed and a researcher-made map was reviewed on an overhead projector. Later, the researcher reviewed all maps (without grading) and returned them to students before the following week's lab so that comments could help with subsequent maps. Students received personal feedback from the researcher that clarified connections between concepts and the omission of important links. The researcher supported efforts of mappers as well as encouraged progress when evidenced. When misconceptions were identified on maps, the researcher made alterations in the map and explained a correct conceptualization to the student. Sometimes researcher-made maps were returned with the students maps for clarification when students seemed to need direction.

Measurement tools

Three measurement tools were used: short-answer questionnaires in which students identified scientific principles underlying 10 nursing skills; evaluations of skill performance in return demonstrations in the practice lab; and taped clinical interviews in which students discussed self-perceptions of meaningful learning, preferred learning modes, and components of practice labs.

Short-answer questionnaire

To answer the first research question, responses to 10 short-answer questionnaires were analyzed by identification of principles for nursing care based on theoretical knowledge from the natural sciences. Criteria were established for each question to distinguish the quality of principle identification. Examples of poor principle identification related to why the nurse checks the patient's pulse after dangling were "check for changes . . . to see how the circulatory system is handling the change . . . pulse may change . . ." An example of an excellent answer was "vasodilation causes blood pooling so circulating blood volume decreases and less oxygen goes to the brain; the heart responds with an increasing rate (pulse) to attempt to get more blood (oxygen) to the brain.' All principles expected for excellent answers were covered in course content through lectures, readings, videotapes, or lab discussions. Principles were also on Vee heuristics used as interventions with treatment groups. Answers were coded according to the clarity and inclusiveness of identified principles.

Analysis of variance (SAS General Linear Models Procedure) controlling for group and instructor was analyzed for each question and the mean of all short answers. Although no significant differences were noted when analyzed by instructors, results (Table 1) show that the single mean calculated for all short answers was significantly higher for the treatment groups ($F=8.98$, $p = .005$). Means for the treatment groups were higher for each question except the last question concerning isolation precautions. Statistical significance ($p<.05$) was found for five of the 10 questions, indicating that for those responses, students in the treatment groups were significantly better able to articulate scientific principles specifying why given actions were appropriate.

Table 1   Analysis of variance for short answers by group and instructor ($n=42$)

Short Answer Questions	Mean (Control Group)	Mean (Treatment Group)	F	p
1. Body mechanics	2.77	3.65	5.44	.03 *
2. Palpation of pulses	2.77	3.60	5.23	.03 *
3. Orthostatic hypotension	2.64	2.70	.02	.90
4. Clean/sterile gloves	3.28	3.40	.07	.79
5. Choice of stethoscope	2.55	3.60	5.97	.02 *
6. Pressure sores	2.59	3.40	3.10	.09
7. Skin inspection	2.41	2.90	4.30	.05 *
8. Blood pressure	3.09	3.75	2.63	.11
9. Percussion technique	2.09	3.35	7.17	.01 *
10. Isolation precautions	3.41	2.65	2.34	.14
Mean of short answers	2.76	3.30	8.98	.005 *

* $p<.05$

Return demonstrations of practiced skills

Return demonstrations of selected skills were required for all students to establish level of skill mastery in the college laboratory during the first week of the spring semester (approximately five weeks after the course with the research intervention was completed). Since all skills could not be checked due to time and faculty availability, only those skills were measured for which control and treatment groups differed significantly in their short-answer responses. To answer the second research question, the researcher investigated if those skills students described with qualitatively different principles were performed differently.

Results presented in Table 2 show that the treatment groups' means were higher for all return demonstrations. However, only body mechanics was performed significantly better when analysis of variance controlling for instructor and group was analyzed ($F=6.65, p = .01$). The mean for all return demonstrations was not significantly different.

Table 2   Analysis of variance for return demonstrations by group and instructor ($n=40$)

Demonstration	Mean (Control Group)	Mean (Treatment Group)	F	p
Body mechanics	1.7	2.3	6.65	.01 *
Percussion	1.2	1.3	2.41	.13
Choice of stethoscope	2.7	2.9	2.98	.10
Palpation of pulses	0.9	1.1	0.05	.82
Mean of all return demonstrations	1.6	1.9	2.96	.09

* $p<.05$

Taped clinical interviews

Audiotaped clinical interviews were conducted by lab instructors for their own students at the end of the course after final evaluation forms and conferences were completed in order to decrease threats to students' candor. Tapes were analyzed and coded. No significant differences were noted when analyzed by variations in instructors. Results showed one significant difference between control and treatment groups. Fifty percent of the treatment group and 15% of the control group felt that they answered the interview question about studying and learning differently after taking this course. Although reasons were not specified as related to interventions, a significantly greater number of treatment students did experience a change in learning and studying styles.

When asked why any given parts of the laboratory helped them to learn, the treatment and control groups responded differently. "Knowing what to expect" (content and action) was valued by the control groups while the treatment groups valued "putting it all together" and "being forced to think". The content analysis of clinical interviews indicated that "putting it all together" referred to connecting knowledge and skills.

Responses to treatment interventions

During clinical interviews, students in the treatment groups were asked to give candid responses about using concept maps and Vee heuristics for learning. Positive reactions to learning with Vee heuristics were identified by 81% of the treatment students. Representative positive comments included:

> 'At the time, they seemed stupid. Later I checked them and they helped me know why I was doing things. When you [instructor] said "remember the Vee principle . . ." I did check it and things made more sense. Vees were good to study with — clear and spelled out.'

> 'Vees were a great help. I used them to study and to understand rationales [for nursing actions] in my nursing care plans.'

> 'Vees pointed out exactly why . . . I need to know why I do things. Used them to review for the mid-term. Yes, they were okay.'

> 'Vees helped me see why we do it, and what's not so important.'

Feedback from instructors who taught with Vees identified the benefit of structured content in the Vees for incorporating information in laboratories. Instructors valued defining and clarifying the interrelatedness of theory and practice with Vees.

Sixty-nine percent of the students responded positively to concept mapping with such representative responses as:

> 'Maps were hard but with feedback they were incredibly helpful for pulling things together and for studying.'

> 'I didn't mind doing them. They gave me a chance to think of how things fit together. Maps encouraged me to refer to readings and notes where I might not have.'

'Hard to get the skill [mapping]. It forced me to keep trying and going to the books for reference in order to think it out. The feedback comments were very helpful.'

'. . . I would have liked to choose my own words [other than the researcher's list of relevant concepts]. At the end I began to see how a lot more words could be added and would fit.'

Instructors were less definitive in their opinion of concept mapping compared to Vee heuristics as applied in this research. Although instructors saw value in fostering conceptual organization of content and identifying misconceptions, map evaluation was seen as very difficult.

Conclusions

Students who were taught basic nursing skills with Vee heuristics and concept maps were better able to identify principles of scientific theory related to basic nursing skills. In the short-answer questionnaire, the overall mean and the mean for five of 10 questions indicated significantly better answers for treatment than control groups. Value in the treatment intervention is supported, since being able to articulate underlying scientific theory suggests that treatment students were better able than control students to link scientific theory to their practice, and to integrate prior learning with present learning of nursing practice. This integration of prior and present knowledge reflects meaningful learning as defined in this research.

There was a significant difference between treatment and control groups for mean scores of only one return demonstration, body mechanics. Research data did not support findings that the treatment groups' learning had improved overall skill performance in practice situations. Due to the issue of mastery learning of skills for passing the course, it may not have been realistic to expect differences in return demonstrations between control and treatment groups.

According to self-reports, students in control and treatment groups perceived their learning of course content to be meaningful. Both groups felt quite strongly that course content was meaningfully learned rather than memorized. However, short answer responses indicated that the treatment groups were significantly better able to state scientific theory originally learned in prerequisite courses and recalled in the present course. By definition, the integration of prior knowledge with present learning is meaningful learning.

Implications for nursing education

Nursing educators have long advocated the linking of theory and practice in teaching nursing. Most students had positive reactions to learning with Vee heuristics and mapping. They valued "putting it all together" in [the] lab. Vee heuristics helped students view nursing care as grounded in scientific theory such that nursing actions took on rational meanings. Concept maps helped students construct individual knowledge structures. Feedback to students from the researcher highlighted and corrected misconceptions that may have gone unchallenged. Those misconceptions would also have been the basis upon which new learning was added with resulting errors and confusion. The students exposed to Vees and maps were better able to identify underlying scientific principles of basic nursing skills, thus supporting the worth of these strategies that link theory and practice in teaching basic nursing skills.

Empowerment for creative thinking is an aim of professional nursing education (Yura *et al.* 1986). Rather than a sense of powerlessness that students often embrace (e.g. memorize this content for this lab), treatment students had some control over constructing an understanding that made sense to them based on their present knowledge structure. When strategies encourage students to take control of their own learning, their value is inestimable.

This researcher believes that prior knowledge is often ignored or undervalued in education, which results in fostering a lack of responsibility for cumulative learning, and in undermining the empowerment of students for self-educating as a lifelong process. The use of Vee heuristics highlighted the valuable interrelationship between prerequisite liberal arts courses and a present nursing course. If nursing educators hope to link scientific theory with the practice of basic nursing skills, content from prerequisite science courses needs to be consciously identified, built upon, organized by each learner, and incorporated into the processes of teaching and learning. Vee heuristics and concept maps can concretely integrate scientific theory and appropriate nursing practice.

References

Akinsanya J (1987) The life sciences in nursing development of a theoretical model. *Journal of Advanced Nursing*, 12: 267–274.

American Nurses Association (1965) American Nurses Association's first position on education for nursing. *American Journal of Nursing*, 65(12): 106–111.

Ausubel D (1978) *Educational psychology* (2nd edn). Holt, Rinehart & Winston, New York.

Buchweitz B (1981) An epistemological analysis of curriculum and an assessment of concept learning in physics laboratory. Unpublished doctoral dissertation, Cornell University, Ithaca, NY.

Colling K (1984) Educating for conceptual learning: A curriculum for educationally disadvantaged baccalaureate pre-nursing students. Unpublished doctoral dissertation, Cornell University, Ithaca, NY.

Cullen J F, Jr. (1983) Conceptual and problem solving: The use of the entropy concept in college chemistry. *Dissertation Abstracts International*, 44, 1747A.

Drew B J (1988) Devaluation of biological knowledge. *Image: Journal of Nursing Scholarship*, 20(1): 25–27.

Fahy E (1969, April) *Emerging trends in professional health practice affecting patient care.* Paper presented at the Fourth Annual Forum of the New England Council on Higher Education for Nursing, Boston, MA.

Fuata'i K A (1985) Use of Vee maps and concept maps in the learning of form five mathematics in Samoa College, Western Samoa. Unpublished master's thesis, Cornell University, Ithaca, NY.

Gendron D (1981) Symbolic acts and the development of a professional identity. *Nursing Outlook*, 29: 31–34.

Gowin D B (1981) *Educating*. Ithaca, Cornell University Press, NY.

Gurley L I (1982) Use of Gowin's Vee and concept mapping strategies to teach students responsibility for learning in high school biological sciences. *Dissertation Abstracts International*, 43, 1026A.

Hawkins J W (1981) *Clinical experiences in collegiate nursing education: Selection of clinical agencies*. Springer, New York.

Infante M S (1985) *The clinical laboratory in nursing education* (2nd edn). John Wiley & Sons, New York.

Larson P J (1984) Important nurse caring behaviors perceived by patients with cancer. *Oncology Nursing Forum*, 11(6): 46–50.

Mollura M F, Sr (1979) *A conceptually structured curriculum for teaching physiology*. Unpublished doctoral dissertation, Cornell University, Ithaca, NY.

National League for Nursing (1987) *Characteristics of baccalaureate education in nursing* (National League for Nursing Publication No. 15–1758). Author, New York.

Novak J D, Gawin D B (1984). *Learning how to learn*. Cambridge University Press, New York.

Ring D G (1969) An analysis of the cognitive influence of high school chemistry instruction on college chemistry achievement. Unpublished doctoral dissertation, Cornell University, Ithaca, NY.

Settlemeyer C (1978) Clinical evolution for clinical practice: Bridging the gap. *Pennsylvania Nurse*, 4–5.

Torres G, Yura H (1974) *Today's conceptual framework: Its relationship to the curriculum development process* (National League for Nursing Publication No. 15–1529). NLN, New York.

Tyler R W (1949) Trends in professional education. *American Journal of Nursing*, 49(1): 50–56.

Wilson J K (1975) *A study of the biological sciences in relation to nursing*. Churchill Livingstone, Edinburgh.

Yura H, Torres G, Chioni R, Frank E, Lynch E, McKay R, Stanton M, Carlsoa S, O'Leary H, Kelley J (1986) *Faculty-curriculum development*. (National League for Nursing Publication No. 15–2164). NLN, New York.

25. Clinical Audit: A Tool for Nursing Practice
Sue Kinn

Nurses are probably more aware of clinical audit now than at any time in history, but what do they actually know about it? Aware that for many, the words cause unnecessary fear and anxiety, the author has set out a simple guide to audit. The information in the article is based on a successful series of workshops on clinical audit she and her colleagues ran for nurses in the Greater Glasgow area.

Clinical audit is a buzz word in the NHS at the moment, although it is not always clear what is meant by it. The government white paper *Working for Patients*[1] defines audit as: 'The systematic critical analysis of the quality of care, including the procedures used for diagnosis and treatment, the use of resources and the resulting outcome and quality of life for the patient.'

Nurses have been looking at their work, or performing audit, for many years, but not calling it that. The current trend is for a more systematic and critical approach to the appraisal of health care[2]. For many, this is the first exposure to the techniques involved and can lead to apprehension about the process.

Audit is usually described as a cycle of setting standards, measuring current performance, comparing practice with standards and identifying the need for and implementing change[3] (Figure 1). This in itself is not audit, and a second tour around the cycle is required to see if the changes have made a difference. Audit is perhaps more accurately described as a spiral, because you do not start going round the cycle again from the same starting point.

In simple terms, audit is:

- Viewing what is happening now — the *real* situation

- Comparing this with what should be happening — the *ideal* situation

- Taking action to close the gap.

The ideal (or standard) set should be a realistic goal. If it is too high, it can lead to disillusion and the audit may fail. It is possible to set a 'gold standard' and move towards it through a set of intermediate stages. Nurses have had some exposure to standard setting exercises, the best known of which is the Dynamic Standard Setting System (DySSSy) developed at the Royal College of Nursing[4]. Standards for audit have to be set out in such a way that they are expressed as discrete items of practice which are measurable and observable. If this is not the case, there will be no means of determining whether the care given actually meets the standard.

Sue Kinn: 'Clinical Audit: A Tool for Nursing Practice' in *NURSING STANDARD* (1995), 9(15), pp. 35–36.

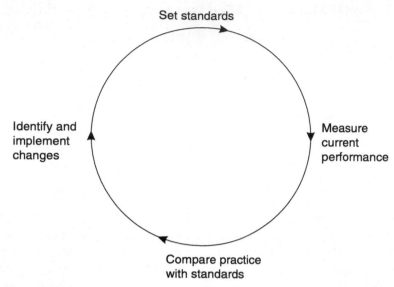

Figure 1   The audit cycle (3)

Measuring current performance, or collecting data, is often the most visible phase of the audit cycle. It is very easy to become involved in this stage and not move on to the more important phase of examining the data and comparing practice with the standards set. It is at this latter stage that deficiencies in care can be identified and necessary changes should become apparent.

Implementing change is a vital stage in audit. There is little point in setting standards and comparing real and ideal situations if no attempt is made to make changes when deficiencies are identified. The implementation of change is very difficult and will be successful only if everyone has been made aware of the audit taking place and felt involved, not threatened, by the process.

Audit can be carried out retrospectively, after care is complete, or concurrently, while care is still in progress. It is a method for continually reviewing the delivery of care and taking action to improve it when deficiencies are identified.

Why do audit?

For audit to be successfully integrated into the working day, there have to be benefits to the patients and professionals involved. Audit is about improving the standard of care given and benefits for the patient will include a better standard of care in a more effective service. For the professional, it can ensure skills are used in the most effective way, which can lead to enhanced job satisfaction.

Audit can also be an educational process. Very often the systematic and objective data collected can dispel perceptions people hold about their own work. The learning associated with this should increase knowledge and job satisfaction.

Nurses work in multidisciplinary teams whose members have different inputs to patient care. Audit is a useful tool in helping to promote communication between team members and co-ordinating team activities. Patient-centred projects can lead to better multidisciplinary working as the focus is the patient and the care he or she is receiving [is] from all professions, and not just one. An example of this might be a hospital-wide audit of pressure area care performed by the whole clinical team.

Different approaches to audit

Any aspect of care can be looked at. Traditionally, areas are broken down into:

• Structure (the facilities available)

• Process (the actions taken)

• Outcome (the result for the patient).

Looking at outcomes in nursing can be very difficult as there are not many areas where there is an obvious clear-cut outcome measurement.

Different approaches

Whatever aspect of care is looked at, there are a number of different approaches or methods that can be used[5]. Some nurses have had experience of the turndown approach to audit, using off-the-shelf packages such as Monitor or Qualpacs[6–8]. The process of these audits is set out for people to follow. The bottom-up (or project) approach requires more planning and research skills from the individuals concerned [4]. For those with little or no training in these areas, it can be quite daunting and difficult to get started.

At grass-roots level, it is important that nurses can use their own talents and expertise to set up audit projects without the need for large amounts of (often unavailable) extra resources. Projects should be designed to look at problems in areas where individuals, or teams, can put changes into place which will have a real effect on the immediate working environment. Advice from trained facilitators and constructive feedback on the results of ongoing projects can help overcome some of the fears described above.

The workloads of nurses are considerable and the main problem associated with breaking into the audit cycle is finding the time[9]. Once the first audits are performed the benefits can feed back, giving encouragement and stimulus for further audits to be undertaken.

Encouraging nurses to do audit

Many nurses lack confidence in their ability to perform audits, mainly due to their lack of research skills. There are some educational activities to encourage nurses to take part in audit, but they appear to be few and far between.

One initiative has been a series of workshops set up by the Area Nursing Audit Committee to try to improve knowledge levels about audit of nurses in the Greater Glasgow Health Board area. It became quite obvious to the organisers that these workshops were worthwhile and the quality of discussion and subsequent project work was very high. This suggests nurses have considerable talent which needs to be harnessed and channelled into constructive approaches to audit. The results of these workshops are discussed in more detail elsewhere[10].

As a result of the experiences obtained from the Glasgow workshops, the speakers pulled the material together into a booklet — *The Nursing Audit Handbook*. This consists of the transcripts of three lectures — 'An introduction to audit', 'The stages of audit' and 'Methods of audit' — accompanied by relevant handouts. It has been spiral bound in card to allow overhead slides to [be] copied and used by others wishing to provide workshops on audit.

The booklet is also suitable for those who wish to gain a basic understanding of audit. The text is illustrated with many examples of nursing audits and contains a list of some of the projects undertaken by attenders at the first series of workshops in Glasgow. There is a bibliography of useful books and journal articles relating to audit and quality issues in nursing[11].

Conclusion

Audit is a valuable tool which can help clinicians look at and find ways to improve areas of their current practice in a systematic and structured way. Some nurses may lack the confidence in their abilities to perform audits, often due to the lack of research skills, but when help and encouragement are given, worthwhile projects can be devised.

The local project design, or bottom-up approach, is more likely to be successful than a top-down approach, as it allows local design and standards and recent local data to be used. It also allows for a more rapid feedback of the results. With a little encouragement, even the most sceptical nurse can develop a worthwhile project, which can result in local changes having an effect on patient care.

For effective audit there should be:

- Local standards

- Local design

- Recent data

- A quality issue of interest

- Involvement for everyone (and keep them informed all the time)

- Brevity and simplicity ('keep it short and simple' — KISS).

By following these simple principles, it should be possible to perform small audit projects which do not take up too much time or use many resources, but have a positive impact on local clinical practice.

References

1. Department of Health (1989) *Working for Patients. Medical Audit. Working Paper 6.* HMSO, London.

2. NHS Management Executive (1991) *Framework of Audit for Nursing Services.* NHSME, London.

3. Fowkes F G R (1982) Medical audit cycle. *Medical Education* 16: 228–238.

4. Royal College of Nursing (1990) *The Dynamic Standard Setting System.* Scutari, London.

5. Redfern S J, Norman I J (1990) Measuring the quality of nursing care: a consideration of different approaches. *Journal of Advanced Nursing.* 15, 1260–1271.

6. Goldstone L A (ed). (1989) *Quality Counts in Nursing: The Monitor Experience.* Newcastle-upon-Tyne Polytechnic, Newcastle-upon-Tyne.

7. Kitson A. (1986) The methods of measuring quality. *Nursing Times.* 82, 3: 32–34.

8. Tomalin D A *et al.* (1992) Monitor and Senior Monitor: problems of administration and some proposed solutions. *Journal of Advanced Nursing.* 17: 72–82.

9. Malby R (1992) The process of change in nursing audit. *British Journal of Nursing.* 1, 205–207.

10. Kinn S *et al.* (1994) Practical audit workshops for nurses. *Journal of Advanced Nursing.* 20: 517–520.

11. Kinn S *et al.* (1994) *The Nursing Audit Handbook.* Glasgow University, Glasgow.

26.   Mentors or Preceptors? Narrowing the Theory-Practice Gap
Paul Armitage and Philip Burnard

The use of mentors in the clinical field has been debated in the recent nursing literature. The notion of the preceptor has also been considered. This paper compares the roles of the mentor and preceptor and offers some suggestions as to how those roles may help to narrow the theory/practice gap in nursing.

Ever since research reports appeared suggesting that a theory-practice gap existed in nursing (Alexander, 1983; Ogier, 1982; Orton, 1981) a search has been in progress for new roles for nurses in clinical practice and in nurse education which might ensure that what is taught in the theoretical component of nurse education corresponds, at least to some degree, with what happens in clinical practice. In this paper, two of these roles are reviewed and compared: the mentor role and that of the preceptor.

Mentors

The concept of mentorship had its genesis in the USA. A product of the feminist movement, the development of a new entrepreneurial spirit in the 1970s and of the business schools of the American universities, the idea of the mentor was taken up by some American nurse educators, notably, Lou Ann Darling (1984). It seems to have slipped into the folk-law of nurse education almost unnoticed and quickly became part of the educational language of the 1980s and 1990s (Burnard & Chapman, 1990).

Roles and functions

One of the problems surrounding the issue of mentorship is that there appears to be no common agreement as to the role and function of the mentor (Morle, 1990). Hagerty (1986) has referred to this as the 'definition quagmire'. If we do not have an agreed definition, we cannot assume that we are all talking about the same thing when we refer to mentorship. If this is the case, we cannot have an unified system of mentorship training nor can we develop general policies of organising mentorship.

At this point, some may want to argue for a variety of approaches to mentorship. Indeed, it seems likely that various forms of mentoring have been taking place in a variety of nursing situations over the years. On the other hand, it seems reasonable to call for *some* uniformity if the English National Board for Nursing, Midwifery and Health Visiting is to continue to recommend the development of mentors (ENB, 1987, 1988). Clearly, the ENB must have had some notion of mentoring in mind when they recommended it. If mentoring is to become a significant part of the education and training of nurses, then it would seem reasonable to call for some clarification of the concept.

Paul Armitage and Philip Burnard: 'Mentors or Preceptors? Narrowing the Theory-Practice Gap' in *NURSE EDUCATION TODAY* (1991), 11(3), pp. 225–229. Reprinted by permission of the publisher Churchill Livingstone.

The notion of the mentorship is sometimes tied to concepts such as 'wise, reliable counsellor' (ENB, 1987), or a close relationship in which 'attraction, action and emotion' meet (Darling, 1984). The suggestion is that the mentor will be an experienced practitioner who to a greater or lesser degree looks after and guides the neophyte nurse. An objection to this is that the notion of being looked after and guided in this way may not be compatible with the notions of adult education. Adult learning theory encompasses the needs of adults as autonomous learners who need to learn at their own pace and in their own way (Burnard, 1990; Jarvis, 1987; Knowles, 1978, 1984). It may be useful at this point to identify the stages in the disparity between adult learning theory and mentorship.

- Adults learn in a variety of ways and no single theory of adult learning seems likely to be developed, given the complexity of the issue.

- Given this apparent diversity, one should encourage their autonomy in the learning encounter.

- The mentorship relationship, given that the mentor is 'older and wiser' than the student, is less likely to encourage autonomy and more likely to foster dependence and conformity.

Preceptors or supervisors?

It may be argued, of course, that the mentorship relationship is a benign one in which the mentor stands back and allows the individual nursing student to develop in autonomous ways. In this relationship, the mentor is more of a facilitator than a surrogate parent. This seems more in keeping with the literature on adult learning but much is still dependent on how mentorship is to be defined. Morle (1990) has suggested that preceptorship is a more valuable concept in nursing than mentorship and quotes Lutz and Chickerella's definition of preceptorship:

> 'an individual teaching/learning method in which each student is assigned to a particular preceptor . . . so that she can experience day to day practice with a role model and resource person immediately available within the clinical setting'. (Lutz and Chickerella cited by Morle, 1990 p. 102)

The main and important difference between the mentorship and preceptorship is that the preceptor is more clinically active and more of a role-model than the mentor. The preceptor is more concerned with the teaching and learning aspects of the relationship, whilst the mentor, although also concerned with these things, seeks a closer and more personal relationship. The preceptor concept seems to encourage the 'sitting with Nellie' approach to learning, so that students learn 'on the job' by copying the skills of the clinical practitioners. This is only acceptable if 'Nellie' has the required skill levels. All the work that has been done on the 'theory-practice gap' suggests that this may not necessarily be the case.

Just to add a further dimension to the discussion, Rolfe (1990) suggests that *supervision* may be a more appropriate role for the qualified nurse who 'looks after' students in training and education. This concept of supervision has been developed in detail by Hawkins and Shohet (1989) who write convincingly of the need for those in training in the health professions to be offered the sort of supervision that has so far been available only to trainee counsellors and psychotherapists. Supervision does seem to be appropriate to those nurses working in the mental health field, given its focus on the interpersonal relationship and on the student's developing their therapeutic skills. Whether or not it is also a suitable framework for nurses in other fields remains more debatable.

In attempting to tease out the differences between mentorship and preceptorship, it may be useful to consider the preceptor role a little more closely.

Preceptors

Nursing theory and practice is changing rapidly. The increase of interest in the development of a discrete body of nursing theory, comprising nursing models (Meleis, 1985) and the take up of the idea of primary nursing (Manthei, 1980) has led to the need for change at the point of delivery of care. In order to facilitate a 'bottom up' approach to change in the clinical setting a change agent is needed at that level (Fairweather *et al.* 1974; Lewin, 1958; Wright, 1989). The skilled intervention of a nurse preceptor can be used in order to create the conditions for satisfactory implementation of the changes.

Fairweather *et al.* (1974) pointed out that there needs to be a change agent or 'outsider' who should have an active, personal and frequent involvement in the change. The outsider's role according to Fairweather is to act as a catalyst in activating the process of change.

Benner (1984) supported the use of a nurse preceptor in this way when she proposed that experienced nurses should sponsor less experienced nurses as they move toward competence in actual practical situations. Beckett and Wall (1985) considered that it was essential that 'clinical facilitators' should be employed at ward level to give

> 'direction by drawing upon their own experience to guide another individual along a pathway appropriate to the learner's needs . . . clinical facilitators are those who have a commitment to ongoing education; they derive their strength from their own expertise, self-worth and autonomy.'
> (Beckett & Wall, 1985 p. 68)

They also believed 'the process of communication, mutual support and acceptance' to be intrinsic in the idea of facilitation.

Kramer (1974) introduced the concept of the nurse preceptor role in an attempt to narrow what appeared to be the increasing differences between what is taught in schools of nursing and what occurs in nursing practice — the so-called theory-practice gap. The idea was that a clinical nurse teacher should become responsible for patient care, thereby giving learners the opportunity to observe her working as a practitioner. Goldenberg (1987) pointed out that 'preceptorship is a one-to-one relationship between an experienced nurse and a neophyte'.

However, nurse preceptor programmes have been used successfully to ease the transition from nursing student to staff nurse (Allanach & Jennings, 1990). The nurse preceptor is expected to demonstrate good nursing practice by role modelling

(Edmunds, 1983) and all staff who observe this practice in the care setting may improve their practice as a result.

Kramer (1974) defined the role of the nurse preceptor as follows:

> 'A nurse who has the ability to integrate education and work values so that realistic strategies for resolving conflict may be developed. Such a relationship allows for the trainee to work and identify with a competent role model. This involves not only observation by the trainee, but also planned two-way exchange of approaches and evaluation.' (Kramer, 1974 p. 32)

Raichura and Riley (1985) were not satisfied with the traditional clinical nurse teacher's role as they wanted a role for a clinical nurse who had 'responsibility for training and educating all nursing staff, for nursing care management style and practices'. Raichura and Riley found that the concept of nurse preceptorship suited their requirements when practised as nurse preceptors in a care of the elderly ward. They defined the responsibilities of the nurse preceptor as follows:

- Possess a strong clinical base and up-to-date knowledge of nursing practices and management

- Teach patient-centred care

- Be responsible for patient care

- Act as a role model for all staff

- Help all nursing staff to apply basic and advanced theoretical knowledge to practice

- Accept the role of member of the multidisciplinary team

- Discuss patient care with all nursing staff and other members of the multidisciplinary team

- Implement change in the clinical area

- Coordinate and utilise resources as and when necessary

- Involve ancillary, administrative, paramedical and medical staff in the training programme and gain their commitment

- Be involved in all ward duties.

However, Raichura and Riley do not include the personal characteristics of the 'ideal preceptor'. These were identified by Piemme *et al.* (1986) and included such virtues as: patience, enthusiasm, knowledge, organising ability, positive attitude, non-threatening/non-judgmental, flexible, open-minded, objective, sense of humour, maturity, mastery of clinical skills, assertive, advocate for learner, able to use resources, self-confident but knows own weaknesses, responsible, professional and respect for peers. It is difficult to see the practical utility of such lists except that they do give an indication of the nature and complexity of the role of the nurse preceptor.

This acknowledgement of complexity can help in developing the role of the preceptor from the point of view of training and education.

Clinical roles

Drawing on the definitions and discussion so far cited, the following roles could be identified for the preceptor in clinical practice.

Through example and discussion the preceptor may foster improvements in nursing care within the defined clinical area in order to develop high standards of patient care by peer group innovation and support.

As a result of the preceptor improving standards of nursing practice, changes could be created which would facilitate the implementation of primary nursing.

Once a system of primary nursing had been implemented, the preceptor would be in an ideal position to nurture it by giving continued support and encouragement to primary nurses who may experience difficulty adapting to the new roles. Clinical guidance and supervision — of the kind which may be offered by a preceptor — is very important when the traditional ward supervisory hierarchy is replaced by the decentralising effects of the primary nursing system (MacGuire, 1989).

In recent years, there have been many, sometimes confusing and often conflicting suggestions for reducing the theory-practice gap. However, recent evaluative research on the use of a preceptor assisting in the implementation of a primary nursing system (Armitage *et al.* 1990) has shown that the theory-practice gap can be narrowed in this way.

Conclusion

The roles of mentor and preceptor are different. The mentor role seems to be more about 'looking after' the learner nurse, whilst the preceptor role seems to be more concerned with enhancing clinical competence through direct role-modelling. Whilst the mentor clearly has a place in clinical nursing it can be argued that, given the clinical nursing emphasis, the preceptor role has more to commend it. This is particularly true given the increase of interest in primary nursing and in the development of nursing development units where clinical skills and competencies are paramount (Alderman, 1989; Wright, 1990).

When decisions have been made about whether or not to develop mentors or preceptors for helping to bridge the theory-practice gap, a new set of questions arise. First, how should the mentor or preceptor be chosen for his or her role? Should all trained nurses be considered for these tasks, should they be self-selecting or should educators and clinicians get together to identify criteria for selection? How should mentors or preceptors be trained and once trained how should they be supported and appraised? Such questions are beyond the remit of this paper but are ones that present themselves as soon as a college, school of clinical setting decides to modify the ways in which nurses seek to enhance the putting of theory into practice.

References

Alderman C (1989) Awaiting developments. *Nursing Standard* 4, 8: 20–23.

Alexander M F (1983) *Learning to nurse: integrating theory and practice*. Churchill Livingstone, Edinburgh.

Allanach B C, Jennings B M (1990) Evaluating the effects of a nurse preceptorship programme. *Journal of Advanced Nursing* 15: 22–28.

Armitage P, Champney-Smith J, Owen K (1990) Primary nursing in long-term psychiatric care. *Senior Nurse* 10, 3: 4–6.

Beckett C, Wall M (1985) Role of the clinical facilitator. *Nurse Education Today* 5: 259–262.

Benner P (1984) *From novice to expert*. Addison Wesley, Menlo Park.

Burnard P (1990) *Learning human skills: an experiential guide for nurses* (2nd ed). Heinemann, Oxford.

Burnard P, Chapman C M (1990) *Nurse education: the way forward*. Scutari, London.

Campbell C (1984) Bring in the specials. *Nursing Mirror* 159, 12: 22–26.

Chickerella B G, Lutz W J (1981) Professional nuturance: preceptorship for undergraduate nursing. *American Journal of Nursing* 81, 1: 107–109.

Darling L A W (1984) What do nurses want in a mentor? *The Journal of Nursing Administration* 14, 10: 42–44.

Edmunds M (1983) The nurse preceptor role. *Nurse Practitioner* 8, 6: 52–53.

ENB Circular (1987/28/MAT) Institutional and course approval reapproval process. Information required: criteria and guidelines. HMSO, London.

ENB Circular (1988/39/APS) Institutional and course approval/reapproval process. Information required: criteria and guidelines. HMSO, London.

Fairweather G W, Saunders D, Tornatsky R, Harris R (1974) *Creating change in mental health organisations*. Pergamon, Oxford.

Hagerty B (1986) A second look at mentors. *Nursing Outlook* 34, 1: 16–24.

Hawkins P, Shohet R (1989) *Supervision in the helping professions: an individual, group and organisational approach*. Open University Press, Milton Keynes.

Jarvis P (1987) *Adult learning in the social context*. Croom Helm, London.

Knowles M S (1978) *The adult learner: a neglected species* (2nd ed). Gulf, Texas.

Knowles M S et al. (1984) *Andragogy in action: applying modern principles of adult learning*. Jossey Bass, San Francisco.

Kramer M (1974) *Reality shock*. Mosby, St Louis.

Lewin K (1958) The group decision and social change. In: E Maccoby (ed) *Readings in social psychology*. Holt, Rinehart and Winston, London.

MacGuire J M (1989a) Primary nursing: a better way to care. *Nursing Times* 85, 46: 50–53.

MacGuire J M (1989b) An approach to evaluating the introduction of primary nursing in an acute medical unit for the elderly — II: principles and practice. *International Journal of Nursing Studies* 26, 3: 243–251.

Manthei M (1980) *The practice of primary nursing*. Blackwell, Boston.

Meleis A I (1985) *Theoretical nursing*. Lippincott, Philadelphia.

Morle K M F (1990) Mentorship — is it a case of the emperor's new clothes or a rose by any other name? *Nurse Education Today* 10, 1: 66–69.

Ogier M E (1982) *An ideal sister?* Royal College of Nursing, London.

Orton H (1981) *Ward learning climate*. Royal College of Nursing, London.

Piemme J A, Kramer W, Tack B B, Evans J (1986) Developing the nurse preceptor. *Journal of Continuing Education in Nursing* 17, 6: 186–189.

Raichura E, Riley M (1985) Introducing nurse preceptors. *Nursing Times* 81, 46: 40–42.

Rolfe G (1990) The role of clinical nurse supervision in the education of student psychiatric nurses: a theoretical approach. *Nurse Education Today* 10, 3: 193–197.

Tiffany R (1984) The Marsden Experience. *Nursing Mirror* 159, 21: 28–30.

Wilson-Barnett J (1985) Learning from the specialists. *Nursing Mirror* 160, 2: 33–34.

Wright S C (1989) *Changing nursing practice*. Arnold, London.

Wright S G (1990) *My patient — my nurse*. Scutari, London.

Reflective Practice

In essence reflective practice is a retrospective process concerned with thinking about action (Boud *et al*. 1985). This process is in three stages:

1. Reframe the experience through discussion with others.

2. Work through the experience using positive feelings and dealing with negative feelings.

3. Re-evaluate the experience and integrate new skills and knowledge.

Schön (1990) supports the idea that the emphasis in reflective practice is on students being able to see the consequences of their actions for themselves and determining the relationships between input and output. He sees the role of the facilitator in this process as that of 'guide' and the student as 'explorer', indicating that there is a really important role for the facilitator to play.

Reflective practice in nursing and midwifery has been practised by some for many years but has only relatively recently been formalised with the emergence of a theoretical foundation and a range of supporting literature. Reflection is now recognised by the professions as a required competency for nursing and midwifery practitioners (ENB, 1989), and as such, frameworks to encourage reflection are now a requirement of any nursing/midwifery curriculum.

The overall goal of facilitating reflection is to foster both an intellectual and action-oriented approach to nursing and midwifery education, encouraging analytical reflection as a precursor to action and change (Glen *et al*. 1995). In order to promote reflective practice in others it is first essential to ensure that you yourself fully understand the concept and have the appropriate skills to reflect effectively on your own practice. Learning to reflect and learning from those reflections is a very individual process. Some people are more naturally reflective than others but reflection is a skill that can be learned, practised and refined by anyone.

One of the main strategies within the professions to promote reflective practice is the introduction of the personal profile in the form of an individual portfolio. Basically, a profile is the vehicle used to record reflections on practice and experiences and is increasingly being recognised as an important learning tool. Professional work is exceedingly complex and often very fast moving. Reflection provides the opportunity to stand back for a short period of time from what you are involved in, think about it for a while and learn from that process. The opportunity then emerges to use that learning to change practice or behaviour in some way; sometimes the change may be simple and straightforward, sometimes it might be more complex and personal and have a significant impact on personal development and practice.

There has now been a great deal written about reflection and the extracts which follow are merely a cross-section of views and ideas about the topic for you to read, explore and gain greater insight into the concept and its application to your role as teacher and assessor.

References

Boud D *et al.* (1985) *Reflection: Turning experience into learning.* Kogan Page, London.

Glen S *et al.* (1995) Reflecting on reflection: a personal encounter. *Nurse Education Today* 15(1): 61–68.

Schön D (1990) *Educating the reflective practitioner.* Jossey-Bass, San Francisco.

27. The Clinical Learning Spiral: A Model to Develop Reflective Practitioners

Lynette Stockhausen

Reflective practice in clinical nursing is an exciting concept. Much of the literature on reflection has been derived from education. Recently the Australasian Nurse Registering Authority Committee (ANRAC) endorsed reflective practice as a registering prerequisite competency for beginning nurse practitioners. This paper examines the concept and development of an action research clinical learning spiral to foster reflective practice of both undergraduate students and their clinical teacher in the practice setting. The innovation of a mutual group, that is, teacher and students interacting through reflection to create a co-operative learning environment is explored. In designing the spiral a number of models were consulted and incorporated.

The action research clinical learning spiral adds structure and focus to the process of reflection-on-action and provides an avenue for students and the clinical teacher to set mutual goals of action to trial for future experiences. This process of reflection allows the clinical facilitator to be an integral component of success to the students learning in the clinical context.

Reflective practice

Reflective practice in nursing is an exciting concept. Although practised by nurses for many years, only recently has available literature regarding reflective practice in nursing emerged (Garrett, 1991; Jarvis, 1992). However, the concept of reflection is not new. Philosophers, educationalists and practitioners have been developing views of reflection since Aristotle first introduced practical judgement and moral action (McKeon, 1974). Since then much has been written and researched regarding reflection. Some of the significant contributors to this school of thought include Dewey (1933), Kolb and Fry (1975), Kemmis (1985), Boud, Keogh and Walker (1985), Zeichner (1983), Schon (1983) and Benner (1984).

The process of reflection is an integral factor in the organisation of our daily activities. From the first time we look in the mirror, to when we retire at night, we replay on our minds the days events, often analysing them and re-examining what has occurred in our lives. Boud *et al.* (1985) note that 'reflection comprises of those intellectual and affective activities in which individuals engage to explore their experiences in order to lead to new understandings and appreciation'. Their definition implies that reflection is goal orientated and that feelings and cognitive abilities are interwoven. The underlying assumptions being that individuals are in control of the activity, that reflection can take place in isolation or in association with others, such as peers or the

Lynette Stockhausen: 'The Clinical Learning Spiral: A Model to Develop Reflective Practitioners' in *NURSE EDUCATION TODAY* (1994), 14(5), pp. 363–371. Reprinted by permission of the publisher Churchill Livingstone.

clinical teacher, and finally that reflection is not an end in itself, but, preparation for new experiences.

Learning through practice and reflective processes have been expounded by Kolb (1984) within the terms of his experiential learning theory. The theory suggests that learning, change and growth are facilitated by cyclic processes. Such experiences involve direct experiences, reflection on the experience, and abstract concept formation from which behaviour may be modified to aid new experiences. Similarly, reflection has been viewed as the link between theory and practice (Schön, 1987).

Reflection as perceived in this context suggests that learning is facilitated by early active engagement in practice. Without reflection, experiences would remain unexamined, with the full potential for learning by the participants not fully realised. Within the education literature on reflective practice there is a dimension of an 'elusiveness' to learning that is personal, developmental and embedded in the experience of the learner (Boud, 1988). In order to actualise these learning episodes the role of the clinical teacher becomes an integral part of the reflective process. As such, the clinical teacher, rather than being external to the process of learning, is an essential and strategic component to that learning. The clinical teacher has the opportunity to become captured in the developmental and cyclic nature of the total experience, facilitating, not controlling, the clinical experience.

A framework for reflective practice

Reflection has been identified as a prerequisite competency for beginning nurse practitioners in Australia (ANRAC, 1990). In order to facilitate students' achievement of this competency, a framework to encourage reflection within nursing curricula was required. As such, the Clinical Learning Spiral (Stockhausen, 1991) was developed for the purpose of incorporating and developing reflective processes in undergraduate nursing clinical practice. The spiral has been trialed successfully with a cohort of second year students and their clinical teachers in a Bachelor of Nursing programme.

The framework of the spiral incorporates the theoretical elements of clinical education and structures the management of the clinical experience. Inherent within this framework are those elements necessary to successfully prepare, induct, implement and evaluate reflective clinical practice experiences.

The Clinical Learning Spiral was developed utilising other models of experiential learning with particular reference to the Action Research Cycle (Carr & Kemmis, 1986), the Reflective Process Model (Boud, 1985) and the Critical Experiential Learning Model (Chuaprapaisilp, 1989). Each of these models when integrated provides a framework that incorporates all aspects of undergraduate clinical experiences. It was felt that no one model alone consolidated features of clinical experiences that captures the balance, transference and significance of theory and practice and is uniquely nursing orientated.

An overview of the development of the Clinical Learning Spiral with reference to the previous models are contained in the following discussion.

The Action Research Model (Carr & Kemmis, 1986) has four cyclic phases of planning, acting, observing and reflecting. These four phases are linked into a cycle that recreates itself into a self reflective spiral (Figures 1 and 2). In this sense no component of the model can be conducted independently of the other. The Carr and Kemmis model premises that a group and its members, collectively and collaboratively undertake the four phases of the cycle. Practice is viewed within a political, economic, historical and social context. From this perspective, examination and reflection of practice leads to a new social consciousness and change. Bartlett (1990) suggests 'that actions are intentional and are to be understood in the social context of their occurrence'. As such, deliberation and analysis of ideas about 'nursing' as a form of action, based on our changed understanding, is highlighted.

The process of reflective learning as postulated by Boud *et al.* (1985) involves three stages that are interrelated and cyclic in nature. Following an initial experience the first stage of the reflective process is 'returning to the experience'. Here students recollect the events that have occurred and re-examine their reactions to those events. The chronological sequence of events is recalled in a descriptive rather than judgmental manner. The second stage is 'attending to feelings', which allows for emotions to be identified, examined and challenged. The focus on feelings heightens the learners' self awareness and enables them to enhance and retain positive emotions and discard negative feelings. The final phase is that of 'processing', where the events that occurred during the experiential phase are reconstructed by the learner in order to make sense of them. This phase requires indepth reflection and introspection.

As the learners process their experiences, Boud *et al.* (1985) suggest that a re-evaluation occurs. During this activity students link new data to what is already known (association), seek relationships amongst this data (integration), determine the authenticity of ideas and feelings (validation) and create a personal understanding or knowledge about the event (appropriation). Through the use of the Reflective Process Model students are able to actively construct and arrange their knowledge of the world thus developing their own interpretational schema.

The Critical Experiential Learning Model (Chuaprapaisilp, 1989) uses elements of the Carr and Kemmis model. It was developed specifically as a framework for learning from clinical experiences in nursing. Chuaprapaisilp's model has three phases: preparation for practice, managing the experiential learning process and reflecting on the experience.

During the first phase, students undertake several preparatory activities. This may include orientation to the clinical environment and the delineation of structures and procedures (development of personal learning objectives and undertaking client assessments) at the commencement of the experience.

The second phase involves the facilitation of the learning experience. There are five strategies in this phase which provide a plan to the total process. These are: structuring, organising, controlling, facilitating and emancipating. In the structuring phase of the clinical experience, the clinical teacher assesses the clinical environment and then facilitates activities within a set time frame. The second strategy of organising involves prioritising activities in order that students receive adequate supervision in meeting their objectives. The clinical teacher and students also decide at this stage the format of debriefing sessions.

During the subsequent facilitating stage the clinical teacher provides ongoing individual consultation and explores avenues to provide successful clinical experiences for the student. The facilitation of student learning requires clinical teachers to control their own teaching within a set time frame. In this sense the clinical teacher does not provide all the answers for the students. Instead teaching strategies which foster self-directed learning and critical analysis of issues is encouraged, such as student learning contracts. The final strategy is emancipation which encourages students to challenge approaches to nursing care and make decisions for change.

The final phase of reflection, as outlined by Chuaprapaisilp, is similar to the Boud *et al.* (1985) model but with the inclusion and introduction of a critical theory approach to experiential learning. In this phase the clinical teacher attempts to create a democratic atmosphere where, together, students and clinical teacher, clarify objectives, structures, processes, roles and assumptions during debriefing sessions.

The clinical learning spiral

The Clinical Learning Spiral (Figure 1), developed by the author (1991), draws on the previously discussed models and personal reflective experience as a clinical teacher. The model was developed to emphasis the importance of reflective practice to the professional growth of a beginning nurse practitioner. The integration of Carr and Kemmis, Chuaprapaisilp and Boud *et al*'s key concepts provides a model that is clinically and goal orientated. This acknowledges practice by the self and others as a central tenet of professional education for nurses.

The Clinical Learning Cycle detail (Figure 2) is represented by the preparative, constructive, reflective and reconstructive phases.

The Preparative Phase begins as the individual considers the demands of the experience ahead, the resources required, the environment (sight, sounds, smells), the people (roles, relations, reactions and conflicts), the climate (social, political) and their role as learners in the clinical setting (reflector, participant, observer, facilitator) (Emden, 1991).

There are two components to the preparative phase. The first is related to on campus classroom teaching and university laboratory sessions. This incorporates the development and exploration of nursing skills within a controlled learning environment. The second component is the briefing session which is conducted before the commencement of a clinical experience or day. This first phase assists the teacher of the clinical experience and the students to establish the parameters of the experience. During the briefing students are given the opportunity to identify personal and professional objectives to achieve during the clinical experience. At this time the clinical teacher fosters a climate for the students to achieve their objectives and may explore possibilities for creating new learning opportunities.

The Preparative Phase allows the students to identify other resources (such as specific client needs or specialist departments) within the clinical environment that would create learning opportunities. The benefits of student initiated personal objectives highlights the students own learning needs and creates motivation to learn. The Preparative Phase can also be conducted on a one-to-one basis between students and the clinical teacher. Students have identified that this process of individual negotiation has been beneficial in providing them with the opportunity to set personal goals for their experience and plan the care for their clients (Stockhausen, 1991).

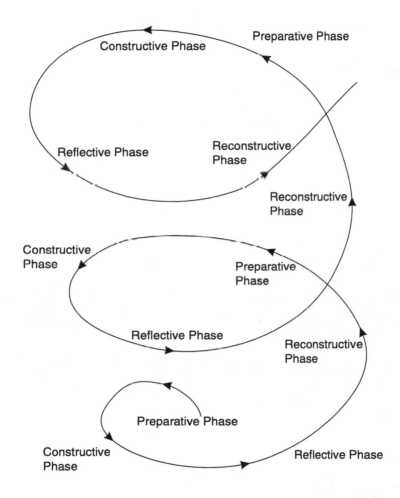

Figure 1   The clinical learning spiral

Each phase throughout the spiral is facilitated by journal writing which has been identified as the most widely used expression of reflection (Zeichner, 1986). Students and clinical teachers are encouraged to write about events of significance which occur whilst undertaking clinical experiences.

The Constructive Phase allows students to undertake actual nursing skill development. This second phase incorporates the experience or actual practice of

291

nursing which takes place during the practicum. The clinical experience is viewed from a perspective of 'completeness' (beginning, middle and end). Observation of the students during this phase is crucial as reflections between the observer and the observed can heighten the experience and reveal different perspectives of the same experience.

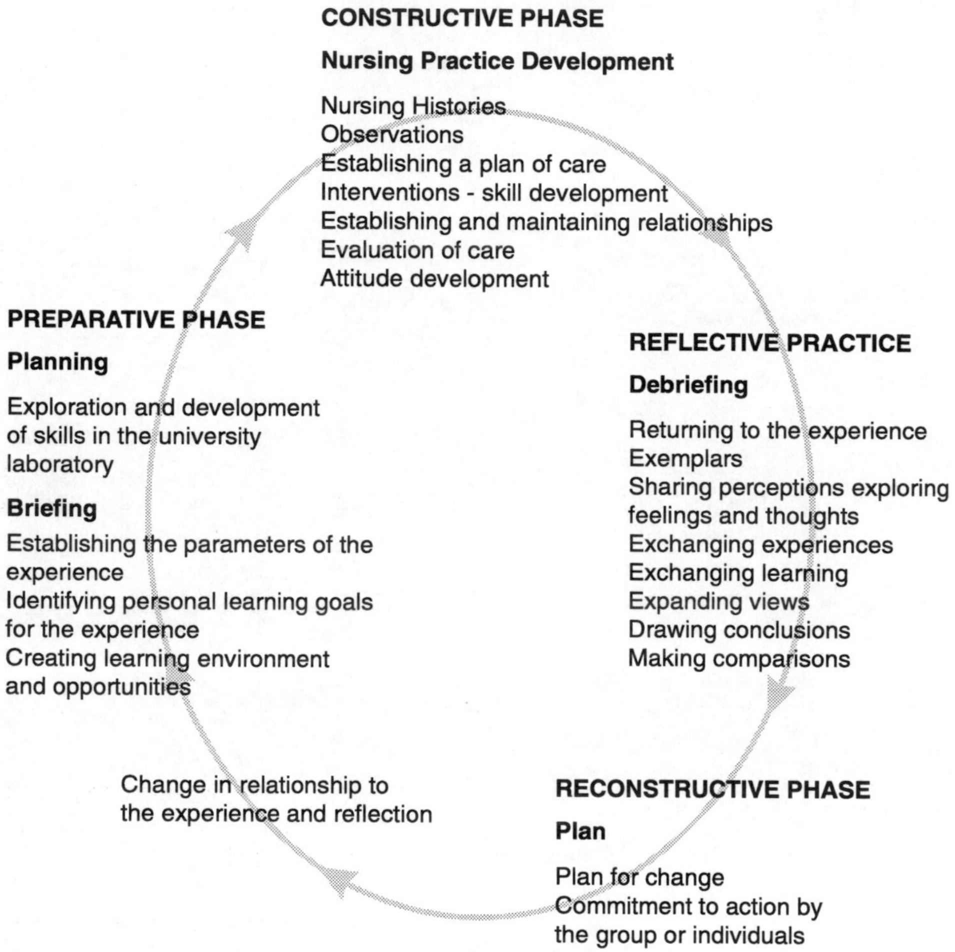

CONSTRUCTIVE PHASE

Nursing Practice Development

Nursing Histories
Observations
Establishing a plan of care
Interventions - skill development
Establishing and maintaining relationships
Evaluation of care
Attitude development

PREPARATIVE PHASE

Planning

Exploration and development
of skills in the university
laboratory

Briefing

Establishing the parameters of the
experience
Identifying personal learning goals
for the experience
Creating learning environment
and opportunities

REFLECTIVE PRACTICE

Debriefing

Returning to the experience
Exemplars
Sharing perceptions exploring
feelings and thoughts
Exchanging experiences
Exchanging learning
Expanding views
Drawing conclusions
Making comparisons

Change in relationship to
the experience and reflection

RECONSTRUCTIVE PHASE

Plan

Plan for change
Commitment to action by
the group or individuals

Figure 2   The clinical learning cycle

The Constructive Phase is the actual experience the students and the teacher share in the clinical environment. This phase takes into consideration the dimensions of practice such as care planning, psychomotor skills, attitude and interpersonal communication development and evaluation of care. The establishment and maintenance of relationships, especially with the client and staff of the agency, is also highlighted within this phase.

The third phase of the clinical spiral is the Reflective Phase. Time is allocated for purposeful inquiry so students can deliberate on aspects of their development as a nurse. Consideration is given to others involved in the student's practice such as the patient, peers, registered nurses, the clinical teacher and other health care professionals.

The reflective phase is facilitated by a debriefing process. This allows the students the opportunity to 'return to the experiences' of the Constructive Phase and highlight significant exemplars and events from the day. Debriefing may occur at intervals throughout the day, but always at the end of a clinical day or experience.

The reflective phase can be initiated at anytime on a one-to-one basis between a student and clinical teacher, peer or registered nurse. It is particularly important to provide a reflective phase for constructive feedback to students following some aspect of their nursing practice development. This may be, for example, a psychomotor skill, interpersonal interaction or professional enquiry. Later, during the group reflective phase, students have the opportunity to share personal reflections from their previous one-to-one reflection or share extracts from their journals. During the group reflective phase the rest of the group share their experiences. The students sense of excitement, anxiety and relief, or how the patient felt or responded is explored. Horsfall (1990) notes that as students 'share each others' challenges, achievements and experience' it is possible that vicarious learning takes place. This phase also sets the scene to examine complexities, differences and subtleties not found in text books but learnt, or made explicit, as a direct result of being submerged in the experience.

The learning processes espoused by Boud *et al.* (1985) identify the importance of allocating time during which students can share feelings, thoughts and perceptions of their experiences. In this forum, students have the opportunity to exchange ideas, consider other points of view, draw conclusions and make comparisons from their clinical experiences. As a consequence of this planned reflection students arrive at a deeper and more meaningful understanding of the practice of nursing.

The final stage of the Clinical Learning Spiral involves the reconstruction of the learning experience. The Reconstructive Phase provides the students and the clinical teacher the opportunity to plan for change. The change may be in the form of alternate nursing strategies/interventions in patient care, or changes in behaviour that foster interpersonal relationships or personal and professional development. There is a commitment to action as a result of the constructive and reflective phases. This is akin to the Action Research Cycle (Carr & Kemmis, 1986). Re-evaluation of the experience helps expand views and develop strategies for future action (Boud, 1988).

The Reconstructive Phase ideally develops into a set of negotiated, mutual goals set by the group as a consequence of reflections on experiences, journal entries and discussions during debriefings. Hedin (1989) notes that at the heart of clinical practice is 'the development of meaning to the learner and the avoidance of imposing an other meaning on the learner'. It is the participants of the clinical experience who decide if reflections develop into action. Not every day will produce a new action as some reflections will not lead to any new consequences. Mutual goals are reconstructed from the constructive and reflective phases of the clinical learning spiral, as a direct result of practice. The intention is to make modifications to, or develop goals that can be acted upon. It is imperative that a commitment to action as a consequence of reflection is realised. For action to occur without reflection leads to uninformed, unintentional behaviour. Reflection prior to and subsequent to action can ensure mutual goals are carried forward to the next situation or spiral.

The clinical learning spiral in action

Using the Clinical Learning Spiral has provided structure to promote and develop reflective practitioners, enabling the ANRAC competencies within the reflective practice domain to be achieved. With active participation in all phases of the spiral students have begun to develop the art of reflection. Through self-expression using journal writing and involvement in debriefing sessions students have had the opportunity to examine their practice, feelings and beliefs, and the consequences of these for patient care. This has been achieved through active participation in all aspects of the spiral. Students and the clinical teacher reflect on what is important to them and then contribute towards the maintenance of a supportive group as they pursue mutual goals of clinical practice.

The phases of the spiral and the processes involved are highlighted by using an example from previous research, by the author, for which the spiral was developed.

Spiral 1

Preparative phase

During the briefing students identify their anxieties at being accepted by the staff of the organisation. Some students have used their journals to write about their impending experience. Students also explore strategies to overcome their fears. To help establish the parameters of the experience and rapport with the organisation and ward staff, as clinical teacher, I undertook the hospital's orientation programme and introduced myself to the ward staff prior to the students' first day.

Constructive phase

A number of registered nurses are asked either by the charge nurses or myself (the clinical teacher) to assist students with their learning goals. Students, registered nurses and clinical teacher interact throughout the day.

Reflective phase

Students record in their journals learning incidents related to interactions and establishing interpersonal relationships with the registered nurses. Some of these reflections are shared with the group at debriefing, 'I found the staff extremely friendly'. As the students' clinical teacher I also wrote and shared my experiences with the students as I had received positive feedback from the staff regarding the students' courtesy and attentive patient care. During debriefing the students were aware that their fears regarding the staff had been unfounded.

Reconstructive phase

The students and clinical teacher decide to set a goal to: 'Maintain and foster the collegial relationships established on the first day'.

Spiral 2

Preparative phase

The students discuss the implications of the previous set goal to their nursing practice development. Students write and discuss their expected interactions with registered nurse. Objectives for the day are identified that incorporate these ideas.

Construction phases

Students and registered nurses interact throughout the day providing patient care and fostering student skill development.

Reflective phase

'I found "my RN" willing to help me, show me procedures', 'The Registered Nurse was receptive and open to my questions' and 'The RN took the time to explain the procedure to me'. These were some of the journal or spoken comments of the reflective phase. Students discussed the significant impact the Registered Nurse, as a role model, made to a perceived positive or negative clinical experience.

Reconstructive phase

Students and clinical teacher examine the implications of their debriefing and aim to: 'Respect the Registered Nurses knowledge and input into the clinical experience'. Action from this goal was recorded as: provide feedback to the Registered Nurses for their invaluable input into student learning.

Whilst the process did not finish after the second spiral it is evident from the example provided that the Spiral is a worthwhile framework to be utilised in the clinical education. It provides the students with evidence of the significance of their lived experience. If students had only been informed about the contribution the Registered Nurse can make to clinical practice this may not have meant as much to the students as actually being immersed in the context. Students experienced first hand that the Registered Nurse can make a positive contribution to their learning.

Conclusion

In an environment of trust, students and the clinical teacher expose their actions, thoughts and feelings; hold them up for examination, reconstruct them and then transform them. In so doing, students are likely to question and challenge their preconceived assumptions about nursing practice. The clinical practice experience is facilitated by the clinical learning spiral and a supportive clinical teacher. The clinical experience becomes a time to collect and analyse judgements, reactions and impressions about what is actually going on in a particular setting. Greater exploration of the social, political, historical and economic dimensions to practice are encouraged.

Schön (1983) asserts that through reflective practice students develop a critical understanding of 'the repetitive experiences of a specialised practice', and can make new sense of the situations of uncertainty or uniqueness which they experience. These experiences lie within a lived context which is connected to the learners' reality within that context.

The phases contained within the Clinical Learning Spiral provide a framework for the clinical teacher to use students' experiences as the catalyst for their next learning experience. The spiral is dynamic and flexible. It is not meant to be static or followed strictly from one step to the next. There is no limit to the number of spirals that can occur. Reflection and reconstruction may occur between a student and clinical teacher throughout the experience and may only take a matter of minutes.

Developing reflective practitioners becomes an avenue to generate explanations of practice situations and build upon practice knowledge. Aligning and complementing student and clinical teachers' reflections on clinical experiences has the potential to provide more meaningful learning for students and rewarding teaching experiences in the practicum.

References

ANRAC. Nursing Competencies Assessment Project, (1990) Report to Australasian Nurse Registering Authorities Conference. Nurses Board of South Australia, Adelaide.

Bartlett L (1990) Teacher development through reflective practice. In: J Richards, D Nunan (eds) *Second language teacher education*, p. 203. Cambridge University Press, London.

Benner P (1984) *From novice to expert: excellence and power in clinical nursing*. Addison-Wesley, Menlo Park.

Boud D, Keogh R, Walker D (1985) *Reflection: turning experience into learning*, p. 19; p. 30. Kogan Page, London.

Boud D (1988) How to help students learn from experience. *The Medical Teacher*, 2nd edn. Churchill Livingstone, London.

Carr W, Kemmis S (1986) *Becoming critical: knowing through action research*. Deakin University Press, Melbourne.

Chuaprapaisilp A (1989) Improving learning from experience through the conduct of pre and post clinic conferences: Action research in nursing education in Thailand. Unpublished PhD thesis, University of NSW, Sydney.

Dewey J (1933) *How we think*. D C Heath, Boston.

Emden C (1991) Becoming a reflective practitioner. In: G Gray, R Pratt (eds) *Towards a discipline of nursing*. Churchill Livingstone, Melbourne.

Garrett S (1992) Reflective practice as a learning strategy. In: G Gray, R Pratt (eds) *Issues in Australian Nursing* 3. Churchill Livingstone, Melbourne.

Hedin B (1989) Expert clinical teaching. In: *Curriculum revolution: reconceptualising nursing education*, p. 82. National League for Nursing, New York.

Horsfall J (1990) Clinical placement: prebriefing and debriefing as teaching strategies. *The Journal of Advanced Nursing* 8(1) (Sept–Nov): 5.

Jarvis P (1992) Reflective practice and nursing. *Nurse Education Today* 12: 174–181.

Kemmis S (1985) Action research and the politics of reflection. In: D Boud, R Keogh, D Walker (eds) *Reflection: turning experience into learning*. Kogan Page, London.

Kolb D (1984) *Experiential learning: experience in the source of learning and development*. Prentice Hall, New Jersey.

Kolb D, Fry F (1975) Towards an applied theory of experiential learning. In: C Cooper (ed) *Theories of group processes*. John Wiley, London.

McKeon R (1974) *Introduction to Aristotle*. Random House, London.

Schön D (1983) *The reflective practitioner*. Temple Smith, London.

Schön D (1987) *Educating the reflective practitioner*. Jossey-Bass, London.

Stockhausen L (1991) Reflective practice: the mutual group. Reflection in undergraduate nursing practice. Unpublished masters dissertation. University of Queensland, Brisbane.

Zeichner K (1983) Alternate paradigms in teacher education. *Journal of Teacher Education* 334(3): 3–8.

Zeichner K (1986) Preparing reflective teachers: an overview of instructional strategies which have been employed in preservice teacher education. *International Journal of Educational Research* 11(5): 565–575.

28. Reflecting on Reflection: A Personal Encounter

Sally Glen, Alison Clark and Maggie Nicol

This paper reports a retrospective study of a Senior Lecturer in Nursing Studies experience of supervising a student teacher who, as part of her teaching placement experience, utilised 'Critically Reflective Analysis of an Educational Event' as a means to assess her teaching in the practice setting. The Senior Lecturer and student nurse teacher used an external 'advisor' to facilitate their meta-reflection on the theoretical perspectives that informed the process in which they were engaged. The paper raises the following questions for consideration — What is the link between ability to reflect and quality of practice? Is it possible to utilise reflective tutorials as a means of assessing professional competence whilst at the same time encouraging personal and professional development? Is the ability to reflect on practice dependent on the context? Should we assume that all practitioners have the necessary skills to supervise students in practice and what preparation and support is needed? The paper demonstrates that by introducing 'Critically Reflective Analysis of an Education Event' into the student teachers' curriculum the role of both supervisor and student teacher was challenged and changed. The paper also demonstrates that reflective tutorials are not wholly a retrospective business. They are creative, or recreative of a teaching experience, as well as to some extent representing it. Finally, even if one cannot speak in Kuhnian parlance, of a conceptual revolution, it would seem legitimate to say, in Schön's terms, that the contextual frame in which professional problems are addressed has undergone significant change.

> 'We need to develop reflective practitioner teachers . . . This requires a system of tutorial mentor support which serves as a powerful role model.'
>
> (Gallego & Walters, 1991)

Introduction

Reflection has become part of the language of professional education (Gore, 1987). Professional bodies advocate the development of reflective practitioners (English National Board, 1989) and educators make claims for education for reflective practice (for example, French & Cross, 1992; Meerabeau, 1992; McCaugherty, 1991). However, the discourse amongst nurse educators has become increasingly muddled in the past few years as terms such as 'reflection', 'empowerment', and 'critical' have been bandied about, often with little explicit indication of the perspectives and commitment underlying them (Barnett, 1987). Thus the notion of 'reflection' is so popular that it is in danger of becoming totally devoid of meaning (Kotthamp, 1990).

While there is an abundance of educational literature encouraging practitioners to be more critical and reflective (Schön, 1983, 1987, Fish *et al.* 1989; Powell, 1989; Gallego

Sally Glen, Alison Clark and Maggie Nicol: 'Reflecting on Reflection: A Personal Encounter' in *NURSE EDUCATION TODAY* (1995), 15(1), pp. 61–68. Reprinted by permission of the publisher Churchill Livingstone.

& Walters, 1991) there is a dearth of practical advice on how this may be achieved. This paper reports a retrospective study of a senior lecturer's experience of supervising a student teacher who utilised 'Critically Reflective Analysis of an Educational Event' as a means to assess her teaching in the practice setting.

Literature review

One might argue that conceptual clarity does not matter. The phenomenon of reflection can be discussed whatever it happens to be. However, in documenting the process of facilitating reflective practice with a student teacher, the potential to become entrapped in rhetoric was very real. Conceptual clarity does matter if one is to resist degenerating into polemic.

The literature, however, shows no unanimity with regard to definitions of reflection (Goodman, 1989; Weiss & Loudan, 1989). Shulman (1987) describes reflection as:

> 'What the teacher does when he or she looks back at the teaching and learning that has occurred and reconstructs, re-enacts and/or recaptures the events/emotions and the accomplishments of a given experience.'

Reflection is a process through which a professional learns from experience. A number of writers have been engaged in the exploration of professional or action-related understanding. The work of Polanyi (1967) allows legitimacy to 'tacit knowledge' in any human pursuit, and implies its proper predominance in practically oriented knowledge domains. From a different starting-point, Ryle (1949) [makes] a cognate distinction between 'knowing how' and 'knowing that', according to the former a far from subsidiary role. Schön (1983, 1987) in his account of professional knowledge indicates how transferable systems of thought can derive from as well as being able to inform intelligent practice, through a process which he terms 'reflection-in-action'.

For Schön (1983) the notion of reframing lies at the heart of reflection. Reframing alters the way in which data from reality is seen (Munby, 1989). Effective facilitation of adult learning involves challenging students to examine their previously held values, beliefs and behaviours, and confronting them with perspectives of the world which diverge from those they already hold (Shulman, 1984).

Adult education is not a matter of acquiring a set of fixed competencies but, through a praxis of continual reflection in action, is a process of lifelong learning (Brookfield, 1986). Mezerow (1981) addresses the dilemma of adult development, growth and change when he writes of perspective transformation.

Janson & Van der Vegt (1991) also underline the importance of critical self reflection. They describe a critical dimension as: 'reflexive self-regulation' as where individuals can attempt to initiate change through recognising the traditionally accepted ideologies of practice. Reflection on experience enables the student teacher to view her experience within broader contexts: social, political, economic and educational. It is the ongoing dialogue of the reflection and feedback that helps to transform, in this instance, a student teacher's personal understanding, into educational knowledge. Dialogue has clear merits in educational terms in constantly reminding students that learning is a two-way process. At best, the dialogue should be a 'critical dialogue', a collaborative process, in which the supervisor constitutes a resource to assist the student teacher to reflect critically on her experience and possibilities for future development. Dialogue has as its focus the expansion of an individual's understanding of her own achievements and aspirations and by extension the setting of her goals (Glen & Hight, 1992). It is from the dialectic that develops through the interaction of the differing perspectives (supervisor's and student teacher's), practical with theoretical, experienced with naive, that mental structures and thus meaning and knowledge are reconstructed. The synthesis of personal perceptions strengthens the accuracy of the interpretations.

The goal of reflection

Stones (1984) points to the importance of supervisors having a clear overall goal. Part of the role of the supervisor is to cultivate reflective self-consciousness about the student's symbolic representation, forcing a theoretical wedge between herself and her own representation. The overall goal of facilitating reflection is to foster both an intellectual and action oriented approach to nursing and midwifery education, encouraging analytic reflection as a precursor to action and change.

The study

The following study offers insight into the way in which 'reflective tutorials' were utilised for monitoring the progress of a student teacher during her teaching practice. This study itself is an example of 'reflection-on-action' (Schön, 1983) that is, it illustrates the nature of the learning potential for both supervisor and student teacher. The implications of introducing such strategies are highlighted as issues requiring further study.

Methodology

The senior lecturer utilised Kolb's (1975) learning cycle and Schön's (1983) ladder of reflection (Figure 1) as a framework to review the nature of the reflective tutorials. A student teacher consented to the recording of her tutorials. These were subsequently transcribed and analysed. In addition, the student's reflective diary was explored to give greater insight into her experience.

The student's diary was central to the process described. MacIntyre (1984) has argued that narrative history is 'the basic and essential genre for the characterisation of human actions' (p. 80).

The force of this is, in part, to deny that one can make sense of separate, disconnected bits of behaviour, 'basic actions', and construct our understanding of other people and what they are doing out of these building blocks. On the contrary, to understand what someone is doing is to place it both in casual and temporal order in the agent's history and in the history of the social and other settings that give meaning to the action, that is, to locate it within a story or narrative of events. Unless we set actions in context in this way, MacIntyre argues, they are simply unintelligible.

In order to develop a comprehensive understanding of the concept of reflection Goodman (1991) suggests that three factors require examination: the focus of reflection; the process of reflection; and the attitudes necessary to be a reflective teacher.

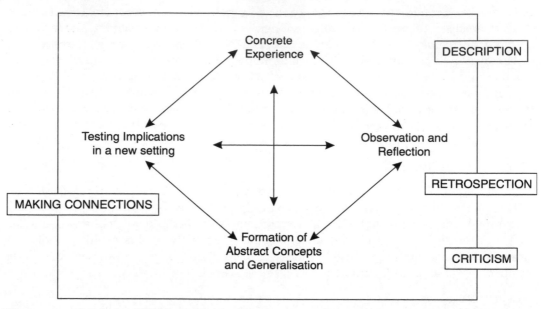

Figure 1   Schön's (1983) ladder of reflection superimposed on Kolb's cycle of experiential learning

However, in order to analyse the data in such precise terms, the senior lecturer had to reflect on the total process of supervision sifting out and isolating the factors that had both direct and indirect influence on the nature of the tutorials. In doing so it was recognised that the context was important and factors such as the students and senior lecturers past experience and expectations had an overall influencing affect, in addition to the philosophy of the student's course, the working ethic of the college of nursing and midwifery, and finally the relationship between the two colleagues (student and lecturer). In setting these aside to focus on the nature of the tutorials themselves it was important not to eliminate them totally from the discussion.

The data presented in this paper explore the focus of reflection, the process of reflection and the nature of the relationship between supervisor and student nurse teacher.

The focus of reflection

Goodman (1991) suggests that the focus of reflection is the teaching event. However, it became apparent in this instance that the event was more the vehicle for reflection, rather than the focus itself. It was not so much what the student *did* that was important, but what was *learnt* (Benner, 1984). The focus of reflection for this student concerned three interrelated issues. First, what had been learnt from the event. Second, how that learning built on previous learning, and third, how future learning needs, and opportunities to fulfil them, were identified and translated into action. The learning which occurred was both personal and professional. In professional terms this encompassed the fundamental methods and skills of teaching, the difficulties encountered in teaching, and how actual practice related to educational theory.

Discussion also included management of the changing role from practitioner to teacher of nursing. In personal terms, the learning was about developing self-awareness. Dimensions involved how the student felt about the event, the emotions it evoked, and how she interpreted the event in the light of past experience and its anticipated influence on future performance. Initially judgements about the event were made in very personal terms, how 'good' or 'bad' it felt. Discussion of the event had to focus therefore on the concrete facts about what occurred — plus sometimes painful deliberation on why it felt 'good' or 'bad' — to a broadening of perspective from the student teacher's performance to other factors which may have influenced intention and/or behaviour within the context in which she was operating; for instance, the student's mood, motivation, expectations, the expectations of nurse teachers within the college, the setting and even the time of day. Thus the parameters for analysis of the event were broadened. A decision about 'effectiveness' being made in the light of personal as well as contextual information available. The following extracts illustrate some of these points (i.e. method, skill development and self-acceptance):

> 'I thought it would be useful to see whether I'm facilitating or whether I am just taking over . . . I don't know whether I've achieved that? I've tried very hard not to go in and say 'this is how you should do it' . . . I find myself as the leader, the focus of it . . . I tried to keep us on the subject . . . I did feel quite positive, certainly my voice does say 'yes . . . mmm . . . right'. I did try and probe them . . . valued what people were saying, yes, I think I achieved what I set out to do . . .'

> 'It made me aware that careful planning pays dividends, thinking things through, even things like how to put feedback on the board . . .'

> 'What I must do is learn to accept something as being 'just OK' or even 'not very good'. My constant striving for perfection will make me unhappy otherwise . . .'

Thus both personally and professionally the student teacher developed a double way of regarding herself, one prospective and essentially practical, the other retrospective and essentially contemplative.

Van Manen (1977) refers to these components of learning as 'levels'of learning, with social, moral and political issues at level three. There is an implicit hierarchy in the way those are described. The authors have some concern with this model as both breadth and depth of learning needs to be kept within focus. The focus of learning may differ for each student depending on their point of entry and past experience. For some students a concentrated focus may need to be given to teaching methods and skills, with only superficial explorations of other issues, for others, who came to the course with sound clinical teaching experience, exploration of theory to practice or vice versa, or 'higher' issues may be more appropriate. Each component however needs to have equal value, the emphasis being determined by the learning needs of the student teacher. What is not explored in that educational literature is the notion of the developing person as a teacher developing personal awareness, and a recognition that there must be a boundary between the role of supervisor in educational counselling and the nature of reflection in personal therapeutic terms.

Process of reflection

In theory the process of reflection requires the supervisor and student to shift from a purely descriptive exercise, through retrospection and criticism of an event, to search for and develop clearer and deeper conceptual frameworks, towards a state of informed and theoretically improved practice (Schön, 1983, 1987; Fish, 1989). In order to facilitate this process, a framework for reflection was negotiated between student teacher and supervisor (Fish, 1989; Bodley, 1992).

This framework had three key components:

- Identification of events for reflection

- Definition of a structure for reflection

- Establishment of an effective working relationship between supervisor and student teacher.

Identification of events for reflection

Rather than limit the reflective tutorials to analysis of the more traditional teaching sessions, such as lectures or working alongside a student in the clinical area, the student teacher was encouraged to explore a wider range of experiences, for instance, the result of a meeting with ward staff on care planning, one-off chats with students over coffee, supporting a trained nurse after a stressful event, or giving career advice. This framework challenged the traditional definition of the role of the teacher in the clinical area, i.e. working alongside student nurses at a patient's bedside. The role of the teacher, in this instance, was seen as having a wider frame of reference: educational support and advice, counsellor, facilitator of change as well as clinical practitioner, if appropriate. This was very much dependent on the setting the student teacher chose to work in, and the expectations of the practitioners she was working alongside.

The effectiveness of most professionals is largely dependent on the knowledge and know-how they bring to each individual case, problem or brief (Eraut, 1985). Much of this knowledge comes from experience with previous cases. Therefore its use involves a process of generalisation of some idea, procedure or action that was used in a previous situation which is considered to be applicable to the new one. Eraut (1985) argues that one way to develop the knowledge base of a profession would be to study this generalisation process to make it more explicit so that it can be criticised and refined, and to give close attention to specifying the condition under which any given practical principle or generalisation was held to apply.

The problem with such an open framework was in determining which events were 'worthy' of the time needed for reflection, when neither supervisor or student were sure of its value. The reality was a process of discovery as the following dialogue illustrates:

> S.T. 'I'm not sure, I think you suggested this (ward report) . . . somebody said you could use this. I have difficulty seeing this as teaching thing, but it obviously is input as a teacher.'
>
> 'I don't know, if you know, what that point is . . . in advance . . .'

S.L. 'No I don't think I do know . . 'cause it's like . . . I may run out of questions to ask . . . different perspectives to look at something . . .'

Each situation therefore has its own potential for learning, with each partner learning from what the other had to offer. The main point here is that 'practice' is far from being all of a piece (Barnett, 1987). It follows that 'being critical about professional practice' needs to be unpacked, analysed and properly developed.

Definition of a structure for reflection

The structure had to meet the course objectives, as well as the student's and supervisor's goals. It also involved devising strategies which would enable reflection to occur (see Figure 2). The course required the student teacher to undertake reflective tutorials and keep a reflective diary. Within the tutorial, however, other skills were required. One strategy that was found useful in facilitating reflection was the use of metaphor (Kotthamp, 1990).

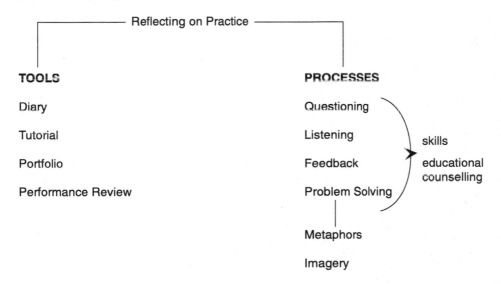

Figure 2   An example of some of the strategies enabling reflection

An area of conflict that was encountered concerned the fact that the reflective tutorials were part of the summative course assessment strategy thus requiring judgements to be made about the quality of the experience. This proved difficult and appeared to be in tension with the notion of reflection as a developmental tool. One issue we debated was whether a student teacher could perform badly, and therefore be said to have failed in the traditional sense, but reflect well on what they had learnt from the experience, and thus be deemed to have achieved the purpose of reflection.

The role of the supervisor here, the authors felt, was to clearly communicate the expected standard of performance, in helping the student teacher reflect on the behaviour which may be below the level required. It was important not to personalise judgements, i.e. not condemn the person just point out the unacceptable behaviour. In this instance such a situation did not arise. However the notion of using reflection as a means of summative assessment needs further exploration in terms of both its reliability and validity.

Establishment of an effective working relationship

The model of supervision was based on a strong relief that both supervisor and student each had a role to play in its success (Schön, 1987; Fish, 1989). For the student teacher, the process was one of self-exposure, positive appraisal of her strengths and weaknesses, and dynamic action planning. For the supervisor the process of leading the student along the 'ladder of reflection' (Fish *et al.* 1989) was a synthesis of strategic planning, problem solving, educational counselling, appraisal and performance review. On analysis, the key skills identified for the supervisor were active listening; ability to give constructive criticism; and facilitation combined with a willingness to reflect on one's own performance and knowledge. In addition the senior lecturer found that an appreciation of attribution theory and personal construct psychology proved particularly helpful in understanding the way people construe situations and make judgements about the event, and helped in offering the student a different perspective from which to look at her practice.

The importance of the dialogue between the student and supervisor has been stressed in the literature (Schön, 1987; Glen & Hight, 1992). The extract shown in Table 1 illustrates some of the important components.

Table 1   Student-supervisor dialogue: important components

Dialogue	Components
S.T. '. . . I could have spent the whole time on just working out drops or the whole time on the other . . . whether in retrospect I should have done that I don't know . . .'	The problem-area of concern
S.L. '. . . look at it in terms of what was possible at that actual time of day . . . in terms of greatest need . . .'	Refraining
S.T. '. . . that's practical . . . in real life we are not always going to be able to do things at the best time . . . I was concerned there was too much information . . .'	
S.T. '. . . and they should understand the relationship between the two . . . you have related the two quite well'	Positive feedback 'looking for the gains and losses'
S.T. '. . . obviously there was a gap in their learning . . . there was me that could teach them, probably in the ideal world I'd have gone in the afternoon, there would have been no interruptions, we'd have enough time to cover both . . . more time for practice . . . it's not ideal . . . OK in the given circumstances . . . I think I overcame most of the negative factors . . .'	Self questioning Learning to give own 'pat on the back'
S.L. '. . . What about practice issues, do we have a responsibility to take that further?'	
S.T. '. . . I suppose I'm not sure whether that matters . . . I don't know . . . I have to assume, no I don't . . . if it was my ward . . . I'm in a funny position, only visiting as it were . . . it's quite frustrating . . .'	Wider issues opening up the debate

It illustrates the way in which the supervisor facilitated the process of 're-framing' the event (Mezerow, 1981; Schön, 1983, 1987; Munby, 1989), giving positive feedback through clarifying the situation, and confronting the student with issues to be explored (Mosey, 1981). The use of non-judgmental language, essential to the development of an effective relationship (Schön, 1987; Kotthamp, 1990), is also evident.

The student teacher is describing a clinical teaching session (on the use of drip regulators). To her consternation the students could not remember the formula for regulation of intravenous fluids, and recapping on this had taken up valuable time leaving the student feeling that she had skimped on both issues.

Discussion and implications for practice

The purpose of the reflective tutorials seemed to be to convert a work experience with some learning into a learning experience about work. Experiential knowledge therefore becomes propositional, yet as Jarvis (1992) states, the experiential is always ahead of the theoretical (propositional). One question was dominant throughout data analysis, to what extent does the use of reflective tutorials differ from the more traditional method of observation and assessment? The reflective diary, written by the student following her tutorials, illustrates that for her it was a different experience, and reveals a developing understanding of the process of reflection:

> '. . . I learnt that I hadn't really reflected, I had described what happened and how I felt, but I hadn't worked out what I had learned . . .'

> '. . . I think I am closer to seeing what reflection is, its probing each situation to pick out the learning that has occurred . . . not a natural skill, it has to be developed . . .'

> '. . . the reflection sessions with (supervisor) was really interesting although exhausting. A lot of really deep thought, probing at a deep level. I feel I understand the process better now, she (supervisor) keeps probing until she gets a comment or reaction from me.'

> 'It was clear that I took something on board, thought it through, and then there was almost a eureka. That seems to be the point where I reflected and learnt from the experience. I don't know if I could do that on my own, it's the level of debate that appears to be the key . . .'

It is clear from the data analysed that practice was the vehicle for reflection, the focus being what could be learnt from everyday practice (Figure 3). The level of debate was dependent not only on the skills of the supervisor, but also on the motivation of the student. The role of reflection was to convert a black and white, two dimensional picture of the event or experience into a technicoloured, multi-dimensional perspective.

Finally, where professional education increasingly attaches a high priority to monitoring, grading, assessing and profiling, its customers must concern themselves more and more with the self they present to the world.

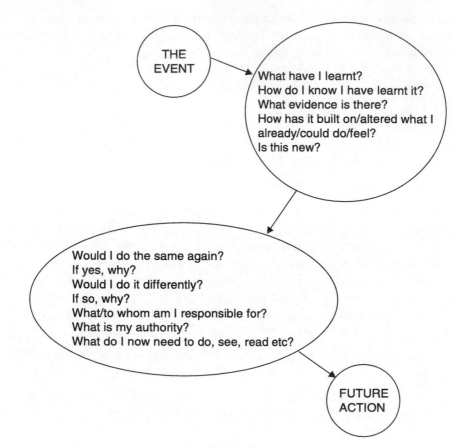

Figure 3   A process of learning about practice

The process is captured in Bradbury's (1984) novel *Rates of Exchange*, where the magical novelist, Katya Princip, explains what it is like to live in a totalitarian state, constantly aware of the secret police:

> 'It is a state of mind, you know, to be watched. We like, don't we, to see our lives from the inside. But if you are watched you see them from the eyes of those others. You can't remember anymore if you really have an inside, or if the inside is already the outside. You become like an actor.'

Through reflection, one finds the possibility of living life more richly 'from the inside': of acknowledging and starting to make sense of those experiences, motives and feelings one really has instead of continuing to present the image which those around us find acceptable. Our conception of 'the good' must, to borrow a phrase from Bernard Williams (1985): 'grow from inside human life'.

The inclusion within student teachers' curricula of strategies to encourage reflection on practice has many implications. Before students and their supervisors can be expected to implement them, consideration of the following questions is essential.

- What is the link between ability to reflect and quality of practice? This is alluded to in the literature but concrete evidence is lacking. There is perhaps a case for some direct assessment of student teacher's performance in the clinical placements, provided a 'shared culture' for assessment can be negotiated between the College of Nursing and Midwifery and the Institute of Higher Education (Chatterton, Roberts & Huston, 1989).

- Is it possible to utilise reflective tutorials as a means of assessing professional competence; whilst at the same time encouraging personal and professional development? The notion of educational counselling needs further exploration within the debate relating to the use of reflective practice within nursing and midwifery education.

- Is the ability to reflect on practice dependent on the context, that is, to what extent does the learning environment foster the attitudes and skills necessary for reflection? Is there a danger of perpetuating the 'theory–practice gap', expecting students to achieve what they do not observe in practice?

- Should we assume that all practitioners have the necessary skills to facilitate students in practice, and what preparation and support is needed? It is tempting to suppose that understanding life and living it are different processes and that one may interfere with the other: life is lived forwards but understood backwards (Wollheim, 1984). This paper has demonstrated that reflective tutorials are not wholly a retrospective business. They are creative, or recreative of a teaching experience as well as to some degree representing it. But this is: 'the only alternative to a more baneful relation to the past to which we are otherwise condemned' (Wollheim, 1984).

The unexamined personal and professional life is incomplete without that self-examination which requires sensitivity to the particulars of life's experience and to its pattern.

Conclusion

This study has attempted to illustrate how reflective tutorials were successfully established as part of the assessment strategy for teaching practice. By introducing the concept of 'Critically Reflective Analysis of an Educational Event' (Gallego & Walters, 1991) into the curriculum, the role of both supervisor and student was challenged and changed. The process of monitoring and supervising student teachers is traditionally hierarchical in nature, expert to novice. In this instance the relationship was one of partnership, success depending on equal commitment and motivation, and an openness on the part of both to learn from and through the experience.

Reflection on the experience of implementing this strategy into one College of Nursing and Midwifery highlighted many benefits. However, it is a costly exercise as it requires a closer and more intensive teacher–student relationship.

Finally, as Barnett et al. (1987) document from an empirical base, practice has begun to manifest a shift comparable with that of precept. Even if one cannot speak in Kuhnian parlance, of a conceptual revolution, it would seem legitimate to say, in

Schön's terms that the contextual frame in which professional problems are addressed has undergone significant change.

References

Barnett R (1987) Beyond the reflective practitioner? Notes on the development of critical abilities in professional education. Anglo-Swedish Seminar No 4. Professional training in the context of Higher Education, parallels in the training of nurses, teachers and others. Stockholm, Sweden 6–11 October 1987.

Benner P (1984) *From novice to expert: excellence and power in clinical nursing practice*. Addison Wesley, California.

Bodley D (1992) Clinical supervision in psychiatric nursing: using the process record. *Nursing Education Today* 12: 148–155.

Boud D, Keogh R, Walker DR (1985) *Reflection: turning experience into learning*. Kogan Page, London.

Bradbury M (1984) *Rates of exchange*. Arena, London.

Brookfield SD (1986) *Understanding and facilitating adult learning*. Open University Press, Milton Keynes.

Carr W, Kemmis S (1986) *Becoming critical*. Falmer Press, Lewes.

Chatterton D, Roberts ?, Huston F (1989) The assessment of work experience. CNAA Development Services Briefing Paper 18, May 1989.

English National Board for Nursing, Midwifery & Health Visiting (1989) *Preparation of teachers, mentors and supervisors to the context of Project 2000*. ENB, July 1989, London.

Eraut M (1985) Knowledge creation and knowledge use in professional contexts. *Studies in Higher Education* 10 (2): 117–133.

Fish D (1989) *Learning through practice in initial teacher training: a challenge for the partners*. Kogan Page, London.

Fish D, Twinn S, Purr B (1989) How to enable learning through professional practice. West London Press, London.

French P, Cross DC (1992) An interpersonal-epistemological curriculum model for nurse education. *Journal of Advanced Nursing* 17: 83–89.

Gallego A, Walters P (1991) Preparation of health care teachers for the future. *Nurse Education Today* 11: 94–99.

Glen S, Hight N (1992) Portfolios and 'an effective' assessment strategy. *Nurse Education Today* 12 (6): 416–423.

Goodman J (1991) Using a methods course to promote reflection and inquiry amongst pre-service teachers. In: R Tabachnick, K Zeichner (eds) *Issues and practices in inquiry orientated teacher education*. Falmer Press, Lewes.

Gore JM (1989) Reflecting on reflective teaching. *Journal of Teacher Education* 15 (3): 9–26.

Jansen T, Van de Vegt (1991) On lasting innovation in schools beyond institutionalisation. *Education Policy* 6 (1): 33–46.

Kemmis S (1981) *The professional development of teachers through involvement in action research project*. University Press, Geelong, Victoria, Australia.

Kolb DA (1975) *Experiential learning*. Prentice Hall, New Jersey.

Korthagen FAJ (1985) Reflective teaching and pre-service teacher education in the Netherlands. *Journal of Teacher Education* 36 (5): 11–15.

Kotthamp, R (1990) Means for facilitating reflection. *Education & Urban Society* 22 (2): February, 182–203.

Macintyre A (1982) *After virtue*. Duckworth, London, UK; (2nd edn) 1984 University of Notre Dame, Notre Dame, Indiana.

Marton F *et al.* (eds) (1984) *The experience of learning*. Scottish Academic Press, Edinburgh.

McCaugherty D (1991) The use of a teaching model to promote reflection and the experiential integration of theory and practice in 1st year student nurses: an action research study. *Journal of Advanced Nursing* 16 (5): May, 534–543.

Meerabeau L (1992) Tacit nursing knowledge: an untapped resource or a methodological headache? *Journal of Advanced Nursing* 17: 108–112.

Mezerow J (1981) A critical theory of adult learning. *Studies in Adult Learning* 32: 3–24.

Munby H (1989) Reflection-in-action and reflection-on-action. Paper presented at the Annual Meeting of the American Educational San Francisco, Research Association.

Perry W G (1970) *Forms of intellectual and ethical development in the college years: a scheme*. Holt, Rinehart and Winston, New York.

Polanyi M (1967) *The tacit dimension*. Doubleday, New York.

Powell J (1989) The reflective practitioner in nursing. *Journal of Advanced Nursing* 14: 824–832.

Reason P (1988) Experience, action, metaphor and dimensions of post-positivist inquiry. In: R Woodman, W Passmore (eds) *Research in organisational change and development*. JAI Press, Greenwich.

Ryle G, (1949) *The concept of mind*. Hutchinson, London.

Schön DA (1983) *The reflective practitioner: how professionals think in action*. Basic Books, New York.

Schön DA (1987) *Educating the reflective practitioner*. Jossey Bass, San Francisco.

Shulman LS (1984) The practical and the eclectic: a deliberation on teaching and educational research. *Curriculum Inquiry* 14: 183–200.

Shulman LS (1987) Knowledge and teaching: foundations of the new reform. *Marvans Educational Review* 57 (1): 1–22.

Stones E (1984) *Supervision in teacher education: a counselling approach*. Methuen, London.

Van Manen M (1977) Linking ways of knowing with ways of being practical. *Curriculum Inquiry* 6 (3): 205–228

Weiss J, Loudan W R (1989) Clarifying the notion of reflection. Paper presented at the Annual Meeting of the American Educational Chicago, Illinois, Research Association.

Williams B I (1985) *Ethics and the limits of philosophy*. Harvard University Press, Cambridge, Massachusetts.

Wollheim R (1984) *The thread of life*. Cambridge University Press. Cambridge.

29. Reflective Practice and Nursing

Peter Jarvis

Reflective practice is a frequently used but infrequently defined concept in nursing at the present time. Part of the reason for the lack of definition lies in the fact that there is no theory of practice. This paper lays the foundations for a theory of practice and paves the way for one useful way in which the relationship between theory and practice can be understood. It is suggested that thoughtful practice is often mistaken for reflective practice, but that the latter can only exist where practice is not taken for granted and so the outcome of practice is more learning from experience. The paper also maintains that for reflective practice to be practised within the profession it is necessary both to have the structures within which it can be encouraged and the theoretical foundation whereby efficient practice need not only be judged in terms of 'value for money'.

Ever since the popularisation of Schön's (1983) seminal book, reflective practice has been a constant theme among some groups of professionals, which is not surprising since they had lost some confidence in themselves as a result of the attacks on the professions in the 1970s by such writers as Illich (1977). Yet reflection was no new idea when Schön wrote his book; Dewey (Wirth, 1979) had emphasised it and Freire (1972), Habermas (1972) and Mezirow (1981), for example, had all been writing about it before this work was published. Freire, for instance, discussed the relationship between reflection and action and argued that congruence between the two was a form of praxis and there are certain similarities here to Argyris' and Schön's (1974) espoused theory and theory in use: Habermas had explored reflection in a variety of forms in his *'Knowledge and Human Interests'* in which he argued that self-reflection is a form of science, and here he combined critical sociology with Freudian analyses: Mezirow was influenced by Habermas and he produced a typology of reflection with seven different levels. Yet it was Schön's book, focusing as it does on the professions and professional practice, which attracted a tremendous amount of attention — an important study which has raised so many ideas about reflection as a result.

It might even be claimed that the idea of *reflective practice* is a bandwagon, upon which many professionals have jumped because it provides a rationale for their practice. At the same time it has not really helped to solve the problem of the relationship between theory and practice, even though some had hoped that it would. For others, the ideas provide justification for their practice, as if it is something unique. Cervero (1988), for instance, claims that:

> '. . . to *reflect-in-action*, is the core of professional artistry. Professionals reflect in the midst of action without interruption; their thinking shapes what they are doing whilst they are doing it. The goal of reflection-in-action is to change indeterminate situations into determinate ones, and

Peter Jarvis: 'Reflective Practice and Nursing' in *NURSE EDUCATION TODAY* (1992), 12(3), pp. 174–181. Reprinted by permission of the publisher Churchill Livingstone.

the key to successfully completing this problem-setting activity is to bring past experience to bear on current action' (p. 44).

But consider this statement:

'Repetitive thinking and praxis can be seen as disengagement in that our capabilities are thus liberated so that they can be applied to the solution of tasks which can only be tackled via inventive praxis (or thinking).' (Heller, 1984, p. 129f).

In very different language, Heller seems to be communicating a very similar set of sentiments to those of Cervero — the idea is to reflect in action in order to problem solve. Cervero may be a little easier to understand — and he is writing about the professions; Heller is certainly more difficult, more technical — only she is writing about everyday life!

The point is that both of them are writing about action or performance, and they are doing so from very different perspectives. That they are writing about the same phenomenon — action — is significant in itself. It does point to the fact that, while there is not yet a theory of professional practice, there has been considerable research into action which might form the basis of such a theory. Before one is formulated, however, it is impossible to discuss in a meaningful manner the relationship between theory and practice, since neither term is clearly defined.

The purpose of this paper, therefore, is 3-fold: first of all to discuss a theory of practice, then to ask what is reflective practice and, finally, to ask whether reflective practice can exist in a profession.

Towards a theory of practice

Perhaps the most significant thing about the two quotations from Cervero and Heller is that they were both writing about action. Professional practice is about action in a specific type of location, and everyday life is also about action which can occur in any location. Therefore, in order to understand professional practice it is necessary to understand action — it is necessary to have a theory of action in order to have a theory of professional practice. Indeed, Schutz (1972) uses the idea of meaningful social action and this might be considered to be an adequate description of professional practice. Many writers have expounded theories of action (Berger & Luckmann, 1959; Maddens, 1979 *inter alia*; Goffman, 1959; Merton, 1968; Parsons, 1951; Schutz, 1970, 1972) and it would be impossible to explore them all here. However, some of the ideas are taken here in order to formulate a theory of practice. Once it is accepted that it is essential to have a theory of action, it must also be recognised that it is also necessary to understand why actions do not occur in professional practice, and so it is necessary also to have a theory of non-action. Unfortunately, fewer scholars have explored non-action, but it is also a social phenomenon which is as worthy of study as is the study of action.

Understanding action does not only refer to the type of action or non-action which is occuring; a number of other factors enter the equation including — the relationship between thought and action, the level of consciousness of the actor, the social context within which the action is performed, and also such phenomena as the intended outcome of the action, and so on. Thus it may be seen that to devise a theory of practice is a complicated process and that it is not possible within this paper to work it out fully. Suffice to note that the theoretical basis of this has been developed more thoroughly in 'Paradoxes of Learning' (Jarvis, in press) which starts from the theoretical perspective of '*Adult Learning in the Social Context*' (Jarvis, 1987) and develops this aspect much more fully. However, in the following paragraphs this position is outlined.

Berger and Luckmann (1967) claim that all 'human action is subject to habitualisation', that is that when actions are repeated they become more taken for granted. There is an almost predetermined order through which the actors move as the following sequence suggests:

1. creative/experimental actions (which are new and being worked out in practice),

2. repetitive acts (which are acts that are thoughtfully repeated during the normal process of living),

3. presumption (where actors presume upon the situation and act almost unthinkingly),

4. ritualism (where actors merely go through the motions mindlessly) and,

5. alienation (where the mindless repetition of actions becomes self-destructive).

Berger and Luckmann claim that all actors habitualise their activity and in professional practice there is a sense in which professionals do repeat many of their performances and so they may feel compelled to habitualise many of their actions, so that these five forms of action may become the first stage of a theory. In addition, there are at least three forms of non-action:

1. anomic, when actors do not know how to respond,

2. prohibited, when they are prevented from responding by other people or circumstances,

3. non-response, when actors just do not respond for whatever reason.

Schutz (1970) seeks to relate action to the thought processes. In the first instances many actions are planned so that actors have a picture in their mind's eye about what they want to do (Schutz, 1970) and these, Heller (1984) suggests, are based upon probability, that is 'acting with sufficient ground'. Now this is significant in professional practice because it still occurs even though the practitioner has considerable knowledge and experience. Indeed, there is always a probability factor in planning but its level is diminished as a result of that knowledge and experience. Herein lies a relationship between theory and practice — it is a pragmatic relationship rather than a deterministic one — that is, that theory may be learned in a classroom situation and then it constitutes part of the biography that an actor brings to the planning stage of thoughtful action. Here it is used by the actor in planning professional performance, which takes into consideration the situation within which the action is performed, the known theory and other contingencies, and the probability that the action will achieve the desired results. Theory is valid, then, if it can be operationalised reasonably successfully, but there should never be precise congruence because action is always based on levels of probability. Even if actors feel certain that their actions will produce specific outcomes, there is always a possibility that this will not occur. During action itself there is also a form of 'reflexive monitoring of action' (Giddens, 1979), that is that the actors are consciously aware of what they are performing and of what is happening, and at the end of an act there is a form of retrospection (Schutz, 1970) which is a review of what has gone before.

However, the level of attention, or consciousness, given to an action can vary from almost zero to a very high level of concentration. All of these factors enter into any discussion about a theory of action and Table 1 outlines some of the possibilities that there are for understanding different forms of action.

It may be seen from Table 1 that any theory of action is extremely complicated and that this is but one stage towards constructing it. However, it is important to see that thus far in the theory the idea of reflection has not yet entered into the discussion. Professional practice is about meaningful conscious action in a specific field and seeking to learn from practice and so improve it constantly, and so become experts. Experts are those who have acted frequently within a specified field of practice and know that the level of probability in their practice is recognised but restricted because of their own knowledge and expertise. Even so, the dangers of habitualisation for experts may be greater than for many novices in the field, for the latter are still performing experimental and repetitive actions; they are still learning to become professional practitioners but, by contrast, the experts have done it all many times before.

Table 1   A theoretical analysis of conscious action

Category of action	Level of consciousness		
	Planning	Monitoring	Retrospecting
Non-action			
Anomic	None	None	High
Prohibited	Low–High	None	None–High
Non-response	None–High	None	None–High
Action			
Experimental	High	High	High
Repetitive	High–None	High–Low	High–None
Presumptive	None–Low	None–Low	None
Ritualistic	None	None–Low	None–High
Alienating	None	None–Low	None–High

Towards an understanding of reflective practice

Professional practice — note the term *practice* — does mean just that it is an occupational field in which actions are repeatedly practised! Expertise is gained through successful practice. However, all actions are subject to habitualisation and run the danger of degenerating into presumption, ritualism and, eventually, alienation.

This is certainly true when actions are performed in isolation or even upon things — but it should not occur when there is interaction between people because people are unique and interpersonal relationships should mean that people interact in a unique and humanistic manner, so that all actions should be carefully planned and monitored — even though they have been performed many times previously. The danger, however, is when people become cases they become almost dehumanised in the minds of the practitioner, and this occured most easily when professionals were taught, as they used to be, to be detached from their clients (patients) in order to protect themselves psychologically and emotionally, and to treat their clients as cases. When people become objects then the danger of actions moving from the carefully planned to the taken-for-granted is enhanced but, by contrast, when professionals treat their patients as unique human beings then the danger of the practice becoming mindless decreases and the level of consciousness required by practice remains high.

The idea of reflection has not yet entered into this discussion and, perhaps, what many people mean when they discuss the idea of reflective practice has already been covered in this discussion: that is, actions are carefully planned in relation to the theory known to the professional and consciously monitored, so that the outcomes of the action will be beneficial to the patient. But the question must be asked whether this is sufficient? What happens when the actions which are being monitored seem to be going wrong, or when retrospection indicates that the action has not produced the anticipated outcome? Perhaps, then, the theory described above is no more than the basis upon which thoughtful practice can be performed. Schutz (1970) suggests that:

> 'Men [sic] stop and think only when the sequence of doing is interrupted, and the disjunction in the form of a problem forces them to stop and rehearse alternative ways — over, around or through — which their past experience in collision with this problem suggest.' (p. 134)

Reflection then, occurs when the monitoring or the retrospecting indicates that the probability factor had been greater than was anticipated. The anticipated outcome has not materialised. The practitioners are forced to inquire why this is so and a new potential learning situation has arisen from which they can learn new knowledge and new skills. Additionally, reflection can occur as a result of practitioners analysing the expected outcomes of action to see whether they could have been achieved more efficiently, although this is probably less likely to occur because it always seems harder to ask why actions have been successful than to investigate why they have failed to achieve their anticipated ends.

Now it has been argued elsewhere (Jarvis, 1987) that all learning begins from the disjuncture that occurs between people's biography and experience, so that the potential new learning situations are created wherever this disjuncture occurs. All learning in practice starts from this point: paradoxically, reflective practice may begin at the point where the taken for granted is questioned so that a potential learning situation is generated. However, that problem need not only be induced by the experience, by the fact that the anticipated outcome has not occurred, it can be self-induced or other-induced. In other words, a colleague or a good manager can pose a question that leads a taken for granted situation to be transformed into a problem and

317

into another potential learning situation. Good managers, then, do not need to supervise in an oppressive manner, but they do need to be able to recognise when professional performance is in danger of becoming presumptive or ritualistic and then they need the ability to create a situation where reflection can occur — but this calls for specific professional knowledge and skills from management! In addition, the good reflective practitioners can also ask questions of themselves and about the taken-for-granted in their practice which can lead to new learning. This, then, is where reflective practice begins — where practitioners are problematising their practice and learning afresh about both the knowledge and the skills and attitudes that their practice demands.

In contrast, it may be seen that the bad manager seeks conformity of practice, expects presumptive or even ritualistic actions and the procedures of practice may result in action being prevented. It is, therefore, necessary to examine a theory of learning in practice at this point. Naturally, this must be experiential — an approach to learning that has become popular in recent years. However, Jarvis's (1987) research into learning demonstrated how reflective skills and reflective knowledge stem from disjuncture, that is — from questioning why the outcome has occurred. Table 2 shows the different types of learning that may occur.

Table 2   A typology of learning

Category of learning	Type of learning
Non-learning	Presumption
	Non consideration
	Rejection
Non-reflective learning	Pre-conscious
	Skills
	Memorisation
Reflective learning	Contemplation
	Reflective skills
	Experimental knowledge

Each of the reflective forms of learning can have two possible outcomes — conformity or change

Reflective knowledge is the process of learning new knowledge from the experience, which is adding to the body of theory, while reflective skills is creative/experimental action. New skills, new ways of doing things are tried out as a result of reflecting upon why a performance has achieved the outcome it has. This means that the professional performances will consistently be experimental and creative but this does not necessarily mean that they will be innovative, because reflective learning can demonstrate the validity of the procedure and the knowledge as easily as it can show that there are new and better ways of doing things.

Reflective practice then is more than just thoughtful practice, it is the process of turning thoughtful practice into a potential learning situation and, significantly enough, it is the utilisation of good theory in practice in what must always be a situation of probability — but the professional reflective practitioner is always trying to ensure that the outcome of any action is close to what is anticipated by the theory and the previous experience combined.

Reflective practice in the profession

The question might be posed as to whether a profession, like nursing, can have reflective practice. Jarvis (1983) distinguished between the structures of the professions and the professionals who practise within them. No profession can be said to have reflective practice, whatever claims the profession may wish to make to the contrary — that would be merely a form of public relations — something to be believed only after considerable research! Professionals, by contrast, can practise reflectively. This does not mean that they all will, only that the possibility exists that they all might! By contrast, it might be said of a profession that it has the structures within which it is possible to practise reflectively, or even thoughtfully, or that there are procedures laid down that encourage reflective or thoughtful practice. This is rather different from claiming that nursing is a form of reflective practice — good nursing might well be — but not all nurses are necessarily good nurses, nor are all managers good managers, and so on.

What then is needed to have reflective practice? In the first instance, it could be claimed that the ability to reflect is essential. In a major piece of research in America, Carnevale and colleagues discovered that learning to learn was identified as the first new basic skill required in the workplace (Cheren, 1990). Now, everybody has the natural ability to learn but what they might not have is the opportunity or the encouragement to learn. Cheren suggests that, while traditional educational jargon might be discounted, the significant factors include helping practitioners to read more purposefully and also helping them manage their own learning. This is something that managers, if they are aware, could do and it is also something that nurse educators should also be doing (Jarvis, 1991). Indeed, if practitioners do not learn in the situation of professional practice, those non-learning situations might also lead to mere ritualism in the professional performance, and this might actually move into situations of non-action, because the practitioners do not know what to do in specific situations.

Naturally, to have thoughtful and reflective practice takes time. Heidegger (1968) has a wonderful example in his book on *thinking* from which this discussion might commence:

> 'A cabinetmaker's apprentice, someone who is learning to build cabinets and the like, will serve as an example. His learning is not mere practice, to gain facility in the use of tools. Nor does he merely gather knowledge about the customary forms of the things he is to build. If he is to be a true cabinetmaker, he makes himself answer and respond above all to the different kinds of wood and to the shapes slumbering within wood — to wood as it enters into man's dwelling with all the hidden riches of its nature. In fact, the relatedness to wood is what maintains the whole craft. Without that relatedness, the craft will never be anything but empty busywork, any occupation with it will be determined exclusively by business concerns. Every handicraft, all human dealings are constantly in that danger . . .

> Whether or not a cabinetmaker's apprentice. while he is learning, will come to respond to wood and wooden things, depends obviously on the presence of some teacher who can make the apprentice comprehend.'
> (pp. 14–15).

He goes on to explain why teaching is more difficult than learning since it requires the teacher to create a situation in which the learner learns, so that it might be argued that, the management of practice is a highly skilled occupation. Two other things in this passage seem most important about reflective practice: the first is that there must be time to perform the craft and see the possibilities that lie within the wood or else it will be merely 'busywork' and the second is that, if there is not time, it will be an occupation determined exclusively by business concerns. Here then are elements about the structure of the occupation, not only does it need people trained to help others learn in practice but it requires the time to allow practitioners to do so or else it will merely be like some other business.

Reflective practice takes time, but today's practice often appears to be conducted in an ethos which encourages both the performance of 'correct' procedures and efficiency. Efficiency sometimes seems to be equated with treating as many patients as possible within a specified period of time, rather than taking time to consider all the possibilities of care. Both procedures and efficiency appear to demand a form of action which is closer to presumption or ritualistism than to experimental practice. The occupation structures within which much nursing, and teaching and other professions are conducted today seem to preclude the opportunity for reflective practice. Nursing is, therefore, faced with a dilemma — it wants to encourage reflective practice, even to claim that it has it but, like some other professions, the structures within which it is conducted seem to inhibit regular reflection in practice.

One might, therefore, ask how nursing can introduce the structures which encourage reflective practice. Two elements seem significant: firstly, nursing needs its own theory of practice and, secondly, it needs to train both mentors and managers to help students and qualified staff to take the time to question and to reflect upon their own practice. Clearly there are implications here — economic, political and others, that lie beyond the scope of this paper, but they do need to be recognised since all aspects of practice have wider implications. It is not the purpose of this paper to enter the political debate, but nursing does need to devise its own theory of practice so that it can present an alternative theory of practice to that which emphasises business efficiency. At the same time, this paper is not attacking the idea of an efficient service, only one which appears to have a limited concept of efficiency. One of the reasons why this approach has become prevalent is that there seems to be no alternative theory of practice to combat such claims.

However, it is no good seeking to make claims for nursing practice unless the structures are in place that encourage reflection in practice, and this is just as essential, maybe more so, than the external concerns. The structures of nursing should encourage nurses to reflect upon their practice, so that like the cabinetmaker's apprentice who has time and ability to respond to 'the shapes slumbering within the wood', nurses may respond to every aspect of their practice with the highest quality of professional care.

Conclusion

The purpose of this paper has been to address two questions — what is reflective practice and can it exist within a profession? Reflective practice is something more than thoughtful practice. It is that form of practice which seeks to problematise many situations of professional performance so that they can become potential learning situations and so the practitioners can continue to learn, grow and develop in and through their practice. Can this exist within a profession? What should exist are the structures within which this reflective practice can occur and is encouraged — trained and aware managers and mentors, educators who understand the relationship between theory and practice and who can assist practitioners to learn in practice, and the time and opportunity for practitioners to think. If these are all in place, then reflective practice may become a frequent occurrence.

References

Argyris C, Schön D (1974) *Theory in practice: increasing professional effectiveness*. Jossey Bass, San Francisco.

Berger P, Luckmann T (1961) *The social construction of reality*. Penguin, London.

Cervero R (1988) *Effective continuing education for professionals*. Jossey Bass, San Francisco.

Cheren M (1990) Promoting active learning in the workplace. In: R M Smith (ed) *Learning to learn across the lifespan*. Jossey Bass, San Francisco.

Freire P (1972) *Pedagogy of the oppressed*. Penguin, Harmondsworth.

Giddens A (1979) *Central problems in social theory*. Macmillan, London.

Goffman E (1959) *The presentation of self in everyday life*. Pelican, Harmondsworth.

Habermas J (1972) *Knowledge and human interests*. Heinemann, London.

Heller A (1984) *Everyday life*. Routledge and Kegan Paul, London.

Heidegger M (1968) *What is called thinking*. Harper and Row, New York.

Illich I *et al.* (1977) *Disabling professions*. Marian Boyars, London.

Jarvis P (1983) *Professional education*. Croom Helm, London.

Jarvis P (1987) *Adult learning in the social context*. Croom Helm, London.

Jarvis P (1992) Efficiency in practice: the role of the educator. *Nurse Education Today* 12, 1: 3–10.

Jarvis P (1992) *Paradoxes of learning*. Jossey Bass. San Francisco (In press).

Merton R K (1968) *Social theory and social structure*.

Mezirow (1981) A critical theory of adult learning and education. *Adult Education* 32, 1: 3–24.

Parsons T (1951) *The social system*. Routledge and Kegan Paul, London.

Parsons T (1954) *Essays in sociological theory*. The Free Press, New York.

Schön (1983) *The reflective practitioner*, Basic Books. New York.

Schutz A (1970) *On phenomenology and social relations.* University of Chicago Press, Chicago.

Schutz A (1972) *The phenomenology of the social world.* Heinemann, London.

Smith R M (ed) (1990) *Learning to learn across the lifespan.* Jossey Bass, San Francisco.

Wirth J (1979) *John Dewey as educator.* Robert Krieger, New York.

30. Preparing Professionals for the Demands of Practice

Donald A. Schön

The crisis of confidence in professional knowledge

In the varied topography of professional practice, there is a high, hard ground overlooking a swamp. On the high ground, manageable problems lend themselves to solution through the application of research-based theory and technique. In the swampy lowland, messy, confusing problems defy technical solution. The irony of this situation is that the problems of the high ground tend to be relatively unimportant to individuals or society at large, however great their technical interest may be, while in the swamp lie the problems of greatest human concern. The practitioner must choose. Shall he remain on the high ground where he can solve relatively unimportant problems according to prevailing standards of rigor, or shall he descend to the swamp of important problems and nonrigorous inquiry?

This dilemma has two sources: first, the prevailing idea of rigorous professional knowledge, based on technical rationality, and second, awareness of indeterminate, swampy zones of practice that lie beyond its canons.

Technical rationality is an epistemology of practice derived from positivist philosophy, built into the very foundations of the modern research university (Shils, 1978). Technical rationality holds that practitioners are instrumental problem solvers who elect technical means best suited to particular purposes. Rigorous professional practitioners solve well-formed instrumental problems by applying theory and technique derived from systematic, preferably scientific knowledge. Medicine, law, and business — Nathan Glazer's "major professions" (Glazer, 1974) — figure in this view as exemplars of professional practice.

But, as we have come to see with increasing clarity over the last twenty or so years, the problems of real-world practice do not present themselves to practitioners as well-formed structures. Indeed, they tend not to present themselves as problems at all but as messy, indeterminate situations. Civil engineers, for example, know how to build roads suited to the conditions of particular sites and specifications. They draw on their knowledge of soil conditions, materials, and construction technologies to define grades, surfaces, and dimensions. When they must decide *what* road to build, however, or whether to build it at all, their problem is not solvable by the application of technical knowledge, not even by the sophisticated techniques of decision theory. They face a complex and ill-defined mélange of topographical, financial, economic, environmental, and political factors. If they are to get a well-formed problem matched to their familiar theories and techniques, they must *construct* it from the materials of a situation that is, to use John Dewey's (1938) term, "problematic." And the problem of problem setting is not well formed.

When a practitioner sets a problem, he chooses and names the things he will notice. In his road-building situation, the civil engineer may see drainage, soil stability, and ease of maintenance; he may not see the differential effects of the road on the economies of the towns that lie along its route. Through complementary acts of naming and framing, the practitioner selects things for attention and organizes them, guided by an appreciation of the situation that gives it coherence and sets a direction for action. So problem setting is an ontological process — in Nelson Goodman's (1978) memorable word, a form of worldmaking.

Depending on our disciplinary backgrounds, organizational roles, past histories, interests, and political/economic perspectives, we frame problematic situations in different ways. A nutritionist, for example, may convert a vague worry about malnourishment among children in developing countries into the problem of selecting an optimal diet. But agronomists may frame the problem in terms of food production; epidemiologists may frame it in terms of diseases that increase the demand for nutrients or prevent their absorption; demographers tend to see it in terms of a rate of population growth that has outstripped agricultural activity; engineers, in terms of inadequate food storage and distribution; economists, in terms of insufficient purchasing power or the inequitable distribution of land or wealth. In the field of malnourishment, professional identities and political/economic perspectives determine how people see a problematic situation, and debates about malnourishment revolve around the construction of a problem to be solved. Debates involve conflicting frames, not easily resolvable — if resolvable at all — by appeal to data. Those who hold conflicting frames pay attention to different facts and make different sense of the facts they notice. It is not by technical problem solving that we convert problematic situations to well-formed problems; rather, it is through naming and framing that technical problem solving becomes possible.

Often, a problematic situation presents itself as a unique case. A physician recognizes a constellation of symptoms that she cannot associate with a known disease. A mechanical engineer encounters a structure for which he cannot, with the tools at his disposal, make a determinate analysis. A teacher of arithmetic, listening to a child's question, becomes aware of a kind of confusion and, at the same time, a kind of intuitive understanding, for which she has no readily available response. Because the unique case falls outside the categories of existing theory and technique, the practitioner cannot treat it as an instrumental problem to be solved by applying one of the rules in her store of professional knowledge. The case is not "in the book." If she is to deal with it competently, she must do so by a kind of improvisation, inventing and testing in the situation strategies of her own devising.

Some problematic situations are situations of conflict among values. Medical technologies such as kidney dialysis or tomography have created demands that stretch the nation's willingness to invest in medical services. How should physicians respond to the conflicting requirements of efficiency, equity, and quality of care? Engineering technologies, powerful and elegant when judged from a narrowly technical perspective, turn out to have unintended and unpredicted side effects that degrade the environment, generate unacceptable risk, or create excessive demands on scarce resources. How, in their actual designing, should engineers take such factors into account? When agronomists recommend efficient methods of soil cultivation that favor the use of large landholdings, they may undermine the viability of the small family farm on which peasant economies depend. How should their practice reflect their recognition of the risk? In such cases, competent practitioners must not only solve technical problems by selecting the means appropriate to clear and self-consistent ends; they must also reconcile, integrate, or choose among conflicting appreciations of a situation so as to construct a coherent problem worth solving.

Often, situations are problematic in several ways at once. A hydrologist, employed to advise officials of a water supply system about capital investment and pricing, may find the hydrological system unique. He may also experience uncertainty because he has no satisfactory model of the system. In addition, he may discover that his client is unwilling to listen to his attempts to describe the situation's uniqueness and uncertainty, insisting on an expert answer that specifies one right way. He will be caught, then, in a thicket of conflicting requirements: a wish to keep his job, a feeling of professional pride in his ability to give usable advice, and a keen sense of his obligation to keep his claims to certainty within the bounds of his actual understanding.

These indeterminate zones of practice — uncertainty, uniqueness, and value conflict — escape the canons of technical rationality. When a problematic situation is uncertain, technical problem solving depends on the prior construction of a well-formed problem — which is not itself a technical task. When a practitioner recognizes a situation as unique, she cannot handle it solely by applying theories or techniques derived from her store of professional knowledge. And in situations of value conflict, there are no clear and self-consistent ends to guide the technical selection of means.

It is just these indeterminate zones of practice, however, that practitioners and critical observers of the professions have come to see with increasing clarity over the past two decades as central to professional practice. And the growing awareness of them has figured prominently in recent controversies about the performance of the professions and their proper place in our society.

When professionals fail to recognize or respond to value conflicts, when they violate their own ethical standards, fall short of self-created expectations for expert performance, or seem blind to public problems they have helped to create, they are increasingly subject to expressions of disapproval and dissatisfaction. Radical critics like Ivan Illich (1970) take them to task for misappropriating and monopolizing knowledge, blithely disregarding social injustices, and mystifying their expertise. Professionals themselves argue that it is impossible to meet heightened societal expectations for their performance in an environment that combines increasing turbulence with increasing regulation of professional activity. They emphasize their lack of control over the larger systems for which they are unfairly held responsible. At the same time, they call attention to the mismatch between traditional divisions of labor and the shifting complexities of present-day society. They call for reforms in professional norms and structures.

In spite of these different emphases, public, radical, and professional critics voice a common complaint: that the most important areas of professional practice now lie beyond the conventional boundaries of professional competence.

The late Everett Hughes, a pioneering sociologist of the professions, once observed that the professions have struck a bargain with society. In return for access to their extraordinary knowledge in matters of great human importance, society has granted them a mandate for social control in their fields of specialization, a high degree of autonomy in their practice, and a license to determine who shall assume the mantle of professional authority (Hughes, 1959). But in the current climate of criticism, controversy, and dissatisfaction, the bargain is coming unstuck. When the professions' claim to extraordinary knowledge is so much in question, why should we continue to grant them extraordinary rights and privileges?

The crisis of confidence in professional education

The crisis of confidence in professional knowledge corresponds to a similar crisis in professional education. If professions are blamed for ineffectiveness and impropriety, their schools are blamed for failing to teach the rudiments of effective and ethical practice. Chief Justice Warren Burger criticizes the law schools, for example, because trial lawyers are not good at their jobs. In the present climate of dissatisfaction with public schools, schools of education are taken to task. Business schools become targets of criticism when their M.B.A.'s are seen as having failed to exercise responsible stewardship or rise adequately to the Japanese challenge. Schools of engineering lose credibility because they are seen as producing narrowly trained technicians deficient in capacity for design and wisdom to deal with dilemmas of technological development.

Underlying such criticisms is a version of the rigor-or-relevance dilemma. What aspiring practitioners need most to learn, professional schools seem least able to teach. And the schools' version of the dilemma is rooted, like the practitioners', in an underlying and largely unexamined epistemology of professional practice — a model of professional knowledge institutionally embedded in curriculum and arrangements for research and practice.

The professional schools of the modern research university are premised on technical rationality. Their normative curriculum, first adopted in the early decades of the twentieth century as the professions sought to gain prestige by establishing their schools in universities, still embodies the idea that practical competence becomes professional when its instrumental problem solving is grounded in systematic, preferably scientific knowledge. So the normative professional curriculum presents first the relevant basic science, then the relevant applied science, and finally, a practicum in which students are presumed to learn to apply research-based knowledge to the problems of everyday practice (Schein, 1973). And the prevailing view of the proper relationship between professional schools and schools of science and scholarship still conforms to the bargain enunciated many years ago by Thorstein Veblen (1918/1962): from the "lower" technical schools, their unsolved problems; from the "higher" schools, their useful knowledge.

As professional schools have sought to attain higher levels of academic rigor and status, they have oriented themselves toward an ideal most vividly represented by a particular view of medical education: physicians are thought to be trained as biotechnical problem solvers by immersion, first in medical science and then in supervised clinical practice where they learn to apply research-based techniques to diagnosis, treatment, and prevention. In this view of medical education, and its extension in the normative curriculum of other professional schools, there is a hierarchy of knowledge:

> Basic science
> Applied science
> Technical skills of day-to-day practice

The greater one's proximity to basic science, as a rule, the higher one's academic status. General, theoretical, propositional knowledge enjoys a privileged position. Even in the professions least equipped with a secure foundation of systematic professional knowledge — Nathan Glazer's (1974) "minor professions," such as social work, city planning, and education — yearning for the rigor of science-based knowledge and the power of science-based technique leads the schools to import scholars from neighboring departments of social science. And the relative status of the various professions is largely correlated with the extent to which they are able to present themselves as rigorous practitioners of a science-based professional knowledge and embody in their schools a version of the normative professional curriculum.

But, in the throes of external attack and internal self-doubt, the university-based schools of the professions are becoming increasingly aware of troubles in certain foundational assumptions on which they have traditionally depended for their credibility and legitimacy. They have assumed that academic research yields useful professional knowledge and that the professional knowledge taught in the schools prepares students for the demands of real-world practice. Both assumptions are coming increasingly into question.

In recent years there has been a growing perception that researchers, who are supposed to feed the professional schools with useful knowledge, have less and less to say that practitioners find useful. Teachers complain that cognitive psychologists have little of practical utility to teach them. Business managers and even some business school professors express a "nagging doubt that some research is getting too academic and that [we] may be neglecting to teach managers how to put into effect the strategies which they develop" (Lynton, 1984, p. 14). Policy makers and politicians express similar doubts about the utility of political science. Martin Rein and Sheldon White (1980) have recently observed that research not only is separate from professional practice but has been increasingly captured by its own agenda, divergent from the needs and interests of professional practitioners. And Joseph Gusfield (1979, pp. 22), addressing himself to sociology's failure to provide a firm and useful grounding for public policy, has written a passage that could have a much more general application: "The bright hope had been that sociology, by the logic of its theories and the power of its empirical findings, would provide insights and generalizations enabling governments to frame policies and professionals to engineer programs that could solve the exigent problems of the society and helping intellectuals to direct understanding and criticism. Our record has not been very good. In area after area — gerontology, crime, mental health, race relations, poverty — we have become doubtful that the technology claimed is adequate to the demand. . . . It is not that conflicting interests lead groups to ignore social science. It is rather that our belief in the legitimacy of our knowledge is itself in doubt."

At the same time, professional educators have voiced with increasing frequency their worries about the gap between the schools' prevailing conception of professional knowledge and the actual competencies required of practitioners in the field. An eminent professor of engineering, commenting on the neglect of engineering design in schools devoted to engineering science, observed nearly twenty years ago that, if the art of engineering design were known and constant, it could be taught — but it is not constant (Brooks, 1967). Another dean of an engineering school said, at about the same time, that "we know how to teach people how to build ships but not how to figure out what ships to build" (Alfred Kyle, personal communication, 1974). The dean of a well-known school of management observed a decade ago that "we need most to teach students how to make decisions under conditions of uncertainty, but this is just what we don't know how to teach" (William Pownes, personal communication, 1972). Law professors have been discussing for some time the need to teach "lawyering" and, especially, the competences to resolve disputes by other means than litigation. A major school of medicine is undertaking a pilot program one of whose goals is to help students learn to function competently in clinical situations where there are no right answers or standard procedures. In all these examples, educators express their dissatisfactions with a professional curriculum that cannot prepare students for competence in the indeterminate zones of practice.

Awareness of these two gaps, each contributing to and exacerbating the other, undermines the confidence of professional educators in their ability to fulfill their mandate. Nevertheless, many professional schools — certainly those of medicine, law, and business — continue to attract large numbers of students in search of the traditional rewards of status, security, and affluence. Self-doubt coexists with pressure to provide traditional services to students who seek traditional rewards.

Thoughtful practitioners of professional education have tended to see these problems in very different ways. Some, in the fields of medicine, management, and engineering, have focused attention on difficulties created for professional education by the rapidly changing and proliferating mass of knowledge relevant to professional practice. They see the problem as one of "keeping up with" and "integrating" into the professional curriculum the stream of potentially useful research results. Others, in law or architecture, for example, have focused on aspects of practice for which traditional professional education provides no formal preparation. They recommend such marginal additions to the standard curriculum as courses in professional ethics or professional/client relationships. Still others see the problem as a loosening of earlier standards of professional rigor and probity; they want to tighten up the curriculum in order to restore it to its former level of excellence.

These are patchwork approaches to problems seen as peripheral. But another group of critics, including some students, practitioners, and educators, raises a deeper question. Can the prevailing concepts of professional education ever yield a curriculum adequate to the complex, unstable, uncertain, and conflictual worlds of practice? A recent example of this school of thought is a book by Ernst Lynton (1985) that links the troubles of the professional schools to a multidimensional crisis of the university and calls for a fundamental reexamination of the nature and conduct of university education. Such commentaries trace the gaps between professional school and workplace, research and practice, to a flawed conception of professional competence and its relationship to scientific and scholarly research. In this view, if there is a crisis of confidence in the professions and their schools, it is rooted in the prevailing epistemology of practice.

Turning the problem upside down

It is striking that uneasiness about professional knowledge persists even though some practitioners do very well in the indeterminate zones whose importance we are learning to recognize. Some engineers are good at engineering design. Some lawyers are good at lawyering, competent at the skills of negotiation, mediation, and client relations that lie beyond the conventional boundaries of legal knowledge. Some business managers are manifestly better than others at making sense of confusing situations; and some policy makers are significantly endowed with the ability to work out useful integrations of conflicting views and interests.

Few critics of professional practice would deny these things, but few would take them as a source of insight into the crises of professional knowledge and education. The difficulty is not that critics fail to recognize some professional performances as superior to others — on this point there is surprisingly general agreement — but that they cannot assimilate what they recognize to their dominant model of professional knowledge. So outstanding practitioners are not said to have more professional knowledge than others but more "wisdom," "talent," "intuition," or "artistry."

Unfortunately, such terms as these serve not to open up inquiry but to close it off. They are used as junk categories, attaching names to phenomena that elude conventional strategies of explanation. So the dilemma of rigor or relevance here reasserts itself. On the basis of an underlying and largely unexamined epistemology of practice, we distance ourselves from the kinds of performance we need most to understand.

The question of the relationship between practice competence and professional knowledge needs to be turned upside down. We should start not by asking how to make better use of research-based knowledge but by asking what we can learn from a careful examination of artistry, that is, the competence by which practitioners actually handle indeterminate zones of practice — however that competence may relate to technical rationality.

This is the perspective of the present book, which starts from the following premises:

- Inherent in the practice of the professionals we recognize as unusually competent is a core of artistry.

329

- Artistry is an exercise of intelligence, a kind of knowing, though different in crucial respects from our standard model of professional knowledge. It is not inherently mysterious; it is rigorous in its own terms; and we can learn a great deal about it — within what limits, we should treat as an open question — by carefully studying the performance of unusually competent performers.

- In the terrain of professional practice, applied science and research-based technique occupy a critically important though limited territory, bounded on several sides by artistry. There are an art of problem framing, an art of implementation, and an art of improvisation — all necessary to mediate the use in practice of applied science and technique.

Not only the question of the relationship between competent practice and professional knowledge but also the question of professional education needs to be turned upside down. Just as we should inquire into the manifestations of professional artistry, so we should also examine the various ways in which people actually acquire it.

When, in the early decades of this century, the professions began to appropriate the prestige of the university by placing their schools within it, "professionalization" meant the replacement of artistry by systematic, preferably scientific, knowledge. As awareness of the crisis of confidence in professional knowledge has grown, however, educators have begun once again to see artistry as an essential component of professional competence, to ask whether the professional schools can or should do anything about it and, if so, how education for artistry can be made coherent with the professional curriculum's core of applied science and technique.

The debates surrounding these questions have taken different forms in different professions and schools. In an engineering curriculum organized mainly around engineering science, for example, how should students learn engineering design? How should students of such policy sciences as economics, decision theory, operations research, and statistical analysis learn the political and administrative skills of policy implementation?

Legal education has traditionally aimed at preparing students to "think like a lawyer." Law schools pioneered in the use of Christopher Langdell's case method to help students learn how to make legal arguments, clarify legal issues by adversarial process, and choose from among plausible judicial precedents the one most relevant to a particular question of legal interpretation. For some years, however, faculty members in some of the most eminent law schools have argued the need to develop competences that go beyond thinking like a lawyer — for example, skills in trial work, client relations, negotiation, advocacy, and legal ethics. In medical education, new programs have been devised to address the problems of preparing students not only for the biotechnical demands of clinical practice but also for family practice, management of the chronically ill, and the psychosocial dimensions of illness. Critics internal and external to the business schools now question the adequacy of the hallowed case method to the specific demands of management in particular industries as well as to the more general demands of responsible stewardship and management under conditions of uncertainty. In such fields as these, a professional curriculum organized around preparation for presumably generic competences of problem solving and decision making has begun to seem radically incomplete.

In some fields, the question of professional artistry has come up in the context of continuing education. Educators ask how mature professionals can be helped to renew themselves so as to avoid "burnout," how they can be helped to build their repertoires of skills and understandings on a continuing basis. Teacher education is an interesting example. Public awareness of the problems of schools has tended over the past thirty years to move in and out of focus, crystallizing from time to time around such issues as the quality of teaching and the in-service education of teachers. Teachers, who often resent becoming targets of blame for the perceived failures of public education, tend nevertheless to advocate their own versions of the need for professional development and renewal. Critics inside and outside the schools have argued in recent years that we must foster and reward development of the craft of teaching.

Where the core curriculum of professional education is relatively diffuse, unstable, and insecure, as in Nathan Glazer's "minor professions," the problem of education for artistry tends to take a different form. In social work, city planning, divinity, and educational administration, for example, educators tend to ask more open-endedly what competences ought to be acquired, through what methods, and in what domains of practice and even to wonder aloud whether what needs most to be learned can best be learned in a professional school. Here education for artistry becomes embroiled in the larger question of the legitimacy of professional education.

As we consider the artistry of extraordinary practitioners and explore the ways they actually acquire it, we are led inevitably to certain deviant traditions of education for practice — traditions that stand outside or alongside the normative curricula of the schools.

There are deviant traditions in the professional schools themselves. In medical schools and schools modeled at least in part on medicine, one often finds a dual curriculum. When interns and residents under the guidance of senior clinicians work with real patients on the wards, they learn more than application of medical science taught in the classroom. There is at least an implicit recognition that research-based models of diagnosis and treatment cannot be made to work until the students acquire an art that falls outside the models; and on this view, widely held by practicing physicians, the medical practicum is as much concerned with acquiring a quasi-autonomous art of clinical practice as with learning to apply research-based theory.

Beyond the confines of professional schools, there are other deviant traditions of education for practice. There are apprenticeships in industry and crafts. There is athletics coaching. And, perhaps most important, there are the conservatories of music and dance and the studios of the visual and plastic arts. The artistry of painters, sculptors, musicians, dancers, and designers bears a strong family resemblance to the artistry of extraordinary lawyers, physicians, managers, and teachers. It is no accident that professionals often refer to an "art" of teaching or management and use the term *artist* to refer to practitioners unusually adept at handling situations of uncertainty, uniqueness, and conflict.

331

In education for the fine arts, we find people learning to design, perform, and produce by engaging in design, performance, and production. Everything is practicum. Professional knowledge, in the sense of the propositional contents of applied science and scholarship, occupies a marginal place — if it is present at all — at the edges of the curriculum. Emphasis is placed on learning by doing, which John Dewey described long ago as the "primary or initial subject matter": "Recognition of the natural course of development . . . always sets out with situations which involve learning by doing. Arts and occupations form the initial stage of the curriculum, corresponding as they do to knowing how to go about the accomplishment of ends" (Dewey, 1974, p.364).

Students learn by practicing the making or performing at which they seek to become adept, and they are helped to do so by senior practitioners who — again, in Dewey's terms — initiate them into the traditions of practice: "The customs, methods, and *working* standards of the calling constitute a 'tradition,' and . . . initiation into the tradition is the means by which the powers of learners are released and directed" (1974, p.151).

The student cannot be *taught* what he needs to know, but he can be *coached*: "He has to *see* on his own behalf and in his own way the relations between means and methods employed and results achieved. Nobody else can see for him, and he can't see just by being 'told,' although the right kind of telling may guide his seeing and thus help him see what he needs to see" (1974, p.151).

Often, there is a powerful sense of mystery and magic in the atmosphere — the magic of great performers, the mystery of talent that falls capriciously, like divine grace, now on one individual, now on another. There are the great performers who symbolize it and the child prodigies whose occasional appearance gives evidence of its continual renewal. In this rather magical environment, the function of coaching is controversial. In the absence of talent, some coaches believe, there is little to be done; and if there is talent in abundance, it is best to keep out of the student's way. Others believe that talented students can learn, by a kind of contagion, from exposure to master practitioners. And still others frame learning by doing as a disciplined initiation into the setting and solving of problems of production and performance.

Perhaps, then, learning *all* forms of professional artistry depends, at least in part, on conditions similar to those created in the studios and conservatories: freedom to learn by doing in a setting relatively low in risk, with access to coaches who initiate students into the "traditions of the calling" and help them, by "the right kind of telling," to see on their own behalf and in their own way what they need most to see. We ought, then, to study the experience of learning by doing and the artistry of good coaching. We should base our study on the working assumption that both processes are intelligent and — within limits to be discovered — intelligible. And we ought to search for examples wherever we can find them — in the dual curricula of the schools, the apprenticeships and practicums that aspiring practitioners find or create for themselves, and the deviant traditions of studio and conservatory.

References

Brooks H (1967) Dilemmas of Engineering Education, *IEEE Spectrum*, pp. 89–91.

Dewey J (1938) *Logic: The Theory of Inquiry*. Holt, Rinehart and Winston, New York.

Dewey J (1974) *John Dewey on Education: Selected Writings*. (R D Archambault, ed), University of Chicago Press, Chicago.

Glazer N (1974) The Schools of the Minor Professions, *Minerva*, 12:(3): 346–363.

Goodman N (1978) *Ways of World Making*. Hackett, Indianapolis.

Gusfield J (1979) 'Buddy, Can You Paradigm?' The Crisis of Theory in the Welfare State. *Pacific Sociological Review*, 22(1): 3–22.

Hughes E (1959) The Study of Occupations. In: R K Merton, L Broom, L S Cottrell, Jr (eds), *Sociology Today*, Basic Books, New York.

Lynton E (1984) Universities in Crisis. Unpublished memorandum, Boston.

Lynton E (1985) *The Missing Connection Between Business and the Universities*, McGraw-Hill, New York.

Rein M, White S (1980) Knowledge for Practice: The Study of Knowledge in Context for the Practice of Social Work. Working paper, Division for Study and Research in Education, Massachusetts Institute of Technology.

Schein E (1973) *Professional Education*. McGraw-Hill, New York.

Shils E (1978) The Order of Learning in the United States from 1865 to 1920: The Ascendancy of the Universities. *Minerva*, 16(2): 159–195.

Veblen T (1962) *The Higher Learning in America*. Hill and Wang, New York. (Originally published 1918).

31. Barriers to Reflection on Experience
David Boud and David Walker

Having given quite explicit guidelines to our co-authors, we were confronted with the task of writing our chapter within the framework which we had provided. We had said to the others, 'write yourselves into your chapters, don't just treat experience as if it happened to other people. Tell the story of how you came to adopt your present perspective on learning from experience.'

Our plan was quite straightforward. We would use as our organizing theme an account of, and reflection on, our work together over the past decade. We decided to take our earlier model of reflection on learning (Boud *et al*. 1985) and work through it focusing on our collaborative activities. We would do this as a real exercise and we would follow wherever our reflections led us. This meant going back through our experience of collaboration, drawing out what we considered to be significant (*return to experience*); working with any feelings that had come out of it, that might help or hinder our reflection (*attending to feelings*); and then going on to reappraise the experience in the light of what had arisen (*re-evaluation*). This final stage involved singling out an aspect of the experience and relating it to previous experience and learning (*association*), integrating the new experience with previous learning (*integration*), testing its validity (validation) and making it our own (*appropriation*). We proceeded along these lines.

However, having done it, we were confronted with an unexpected experience in the light of the reactions of several colleagues to the draft that we had produced. They failed to see connections that were obvious to us. We reflected further. These reflections brought home to us the unpredictable nature of the process of learning from experience, led us to new ways of viewing our own experience, and clarified for us what was involved in using our model for reflection. We have incorporated this new learning into our chapter.

Return to experience

We met for the first time through being allocated to the same table in a workshop on self-directed learning which Malcolm Knowles conducted near Sydney in 1978. We had both heard of his work, had some sympathy for his outlook on learning and wanted to meet the famous man in person. Little of the workshop remains in mind, except for the tremendous impact of Knowles as workshop leader — he provided clear leadership, but essentially trusted us to look after our own learning. Perhaps it was this which prompted us into conversation, perhaps we would have talked about learning whatever the quality of the workshop. Regardless of causes, our continuing relationship emerged from our mutual interest in the role of experience in learning.

We visited each other's workplaces and discovered that our specific educational practices had more in common than we would ever have imagined; one of us was an

David Boud and David Walker: 'Barriers to Reflection on Experience' from David Boud, Ruth Cohen and David Walker (eds) *USING EXPERIENCE FOR LEARNING* (Open University Press, 1993), pp. 73–86.

academic with an interest in improving teaching in universities and the other was a priest who was committed to bringing spirituality into organized religion. Our involvement in the Australian Consortium on Experiential Education (ACEE) — a Sydney-based group of teachers and trainers involved in helping others learn through their experience — maintained our focus on the importance of experience, and developed our confidence in its central role in learning.

However, it was some time before we started to collaborate. The impetus was a move, within ACEE, to explore how experience leads to learning. Members of the organization conducted workshops in which were demonstrated various approaches to teaching and training. They provided a range of different experiences, techniques and strategies. However, organizing frameworks which transcended the particularities of any given method were absent and there was little explanation of how best to draw learning effectively from experience. While the workshops were highly stimulating, they ultimately left us feeling unsatisfied.

This dissatisfaction, together with our belief that we were engaged in very worthwhile activities, stimulated a group of us to undertake a more systematic study of factors which are important in facilitating learning from experience. The key factor which we identified for closer exploration was that of learners reflecting on their experience. Different descriptions were used for what we termed reflection: debriefing, processing, journal keeping, each with a characteristic flavour, but we took all to have a common core in which learners examined their experience and worked with it in some way leading to the possibility of new learning.

The outcome of the study was a book which described a variety of techniques relating to reflection. Together with our late colleague Rosemary Keogh, our role was to provide the conceptual glue which held the collection together. Little did we know at the beginning how difficult our task would be. None of the existing frameworks provided a satisfactory structure in which to place the rich and interesting techniques of experiential learning which were so ably described by others.

After many meetings in a smoke-filled corner of the government building in which Rosemary worked, and after many drafts and false starts, we finally arrived at a model with which we all felt comfortable. It didn't include everything which we had originally hoped for, but it did satisfy our basic criterion of simplicity and it did point to key ideas about which we were enthusiastic. In our efforts to understand experience further, we had moved from a focus on the experience itself, to working with that experience through systematic reflection.

While it took us twenty-three pages to describe (Boud *et al.* 1985), the essence of the model was that there were three key factors in reflecting on experience. The first was a return to the experience, in which the learner recalled the experience, in a descriptive way as it had apparently occurred, without judgement or evaluation. The second was to attend to feelings that arose out of the return to the experience. Obstructive feelings needed to be worked with so that reflection could take place constructively, and supportive feelings needed to be fostered to assist the process of reflection. The third factor was the re-evaluation of the experience, in which learners linked with this experience elements from their past experience (*association*), integrated this new experience with existing learning (*integration*), tested it in some way (*validation*) and made it their own (*appropriation*).

This model pointed to enough important features of reflection to enable us to help learners make a useful start on reflecting on their past experience. The framework was a generic one which could be readily translated into specific circumstances, e.g. in debriefing group activities, in keeping a learning journal or, as we are doing in this chapter, providing the structure for reviewing an entire sequence of activities. However, this did not seem enough. The model referred to a particular circumstance of reflection — what happens after the event — but what should occur at other times?

The stimulus and opportunity for the additional work needed to develop our ideas further came with the Second International Conference on Experiential Learning, held in Sydney in 1989. The ACEE was the joint sponsor and we became heavily involved in the organizing committee. Our work associated with the conference led us to focus again on the experience itself, to explore further the elements that were important within a learning event. We realized that we had not yet taken sufficient account of learners' prior experience, and their intent, on what and how they learn. These needed to be related to our reflection model. We saw, too, the need to focus on the opportunities which occur for reflection while the learner is still engaged in an activity. Our experience at the conference of trying to implement our views about experiential learning, alongside others which we felt to be incompatible, highlighted for us that reflection happens in the midst of action, not only in the calm light of recollection at leisure! We were also well aware of the fact that our model did not fully capture what we ourselves regarded as important in our own learning: the surprise of meeting the unexpected, the change of direction required as we confronted difficulties, and the importance of advance preparation to help address at least some of the challenges which may arise.

We devised a number of activities for conference participants to help them focus on their intents and their expectations of the conference. These included pre-conference correspondence, daily sheets of simple reflective exercises related to each stage of the conference (entering and departing from the experience, noticing and acting within it), a workshop which examined the framework we were using, and a final keynote workshop to help conference participants reflect on their learning from the week. These activities brought together our ideas and their personal experience of the conference. While we did not achieve all that we had hoped, we received enough encouragement from the participants who appreciated what we were doing to enable us to persist in the direction we were taking.

Following the conference, we entered a tortuous period in which we took some time to focus on the next stage of our research. In retrospect, we realize that we needed time to recover emotionally from the conference, but rather than fully debrief the experience we spent meeting after meeting with a whiteboard and pen trying to pick out ideas from among the feelings. At many points we felt that we had reached an understanding only to find that what seemed so clear when we talked, not surprisingly, did not translate into writing. While we were searching for expression of our thoughts, we received an invitation from Deakin University to write a monograph for a distance

337

education course they were designing about adult learning in the workplace. We proposed that we would write about our current thinking and they accepted. As it turned out, we were not able to write a monograph for students without including other material, thus reducing the space for our new thinking. So we worked in parallel on the monograph (Boud and Walker, 1991) and a paper (Boud and Walker, 1990).

Our reflection in the midst of this action focused enough on our feelings from the conference for us to reach beyond them and begin building our thinking anew. We reminded ourselves that what had brought us together was an interest in the role of experience in learning. We had begun to collaborate around the issue of reflection after the experience, and this had led us back to explore further the nature of experience. We had begun with a model for reflection, but now we were being drawn into a model of experience which included much more than reflection after the event.

We took up again two important concepts: *personal foundation of experience* and *intent*. We singled out two further aspects of experience which we had begun to work with earlier, but which now became the focus of our attention: *noticing* and *intervening*. We saw these two activities as part of the dynamics of reflection-in-action, which led us to apply our previous research on 'reflection after the event' to 'reflection which takes place during the event', and which is an important constituent of it. We also became more aware at this time of the need to prepare for the experience. We summarized our work diagrammatically (see Figure 1).

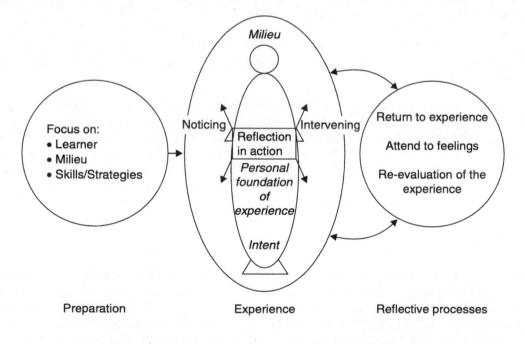

Figure 1   **Model of reflection processes in learning from experience**

338

We have written thus far mostly about the development of our concepts and the events which have been a catalyst to that development. However, there was also a very definite feeling dimension to this collaborative experience. It was a mixture of excitement and frustration, certainty and doubt, unity and discord. We experienced high excitement and certainty when we reached stages where we could look at what we had achieved and say, 'damn it, this really does make sense. It doesn't matter what anyone else thinks, what we have here is worthwhile just for us.' This often came after periods of doubt and what felt like wallowing in uncertainty. There was frustration as we tried to articulate our perceptions. Yet we had to make a statement and stick to it. We had to persist and not let our feelings of inadequacy hold us back. In our efforts, we were encouraged by feedback which made us feel at one with the on-going research being conducted by our colleagues. However, at times, there was a discordant note as comments and actions of colleagues made us feel somewhat apart from the mainstream.

As we looked back over our work together, we understood that we had tried to explore how to facilitate learning, and were offering our thoughts on how this could be done. However, there remained a discord. We recognized a tension between what we have understood and were satisfied with, and what is left out of our portrayal of the process of learning from experience.

In focusing on positive action around reflection, both after and in the midst of action, we had not explored sufficiently the many negative aspects which impede learning. It became glaringly obvious that we had not directly addressed the issues of barriers which inhibit working with experience. We had confronted our own barriers to learning as a result of our experience at the conference, but even then we had not been able to name them as barriers, even though we had experienced a strong sense of being blocked. We knew that barriers are strong and that many are not easily susceptible to removal or being circumvented. Some have indeed served an important purpose in our lives, for example, in protecting us from the degree of pain we would have had to face if we [had] not held back from jumping into a difficult situation from the deep end. It was this focus on barriers to learning, both conceptual and emotional, that emerged from our return to the experience of working together. However, before focusing on them further, we needed to proceed with the next stage of our model. These barriers became the focus of our further reflection.

Attending to feelings

The excitement and sense of achievement, which has been predominant, remains strong. We have fostered these supportive feelings by sharing our research with others, and attending to their feedback. Our mutual acknowledgment of the feeling provides further strength and helps the positive mutual interaction. Conversely, we have experienced a sense of frustration as to the adequacy of our expression. Are we presenting our ideas well and taking account of all the issues relevant to them? We sometimes doubt that we can do justice to our research within the space limitations of a chapter. There is the feeling, too, of academic caution, which sometimes can bring a paralysis that prevents publication. However, our challenge to — and support for —

each other helps to overcome these obstructions, and the desire to go on being creative is an effective antidote to them.

Building on the positive is an important part of our dynamic. At times, there was a shared feeling of 'pumping up' the mental adrenalin to generate enough enthusiasm and achievement to carry us through the often tedious task of writing it down in a way which would make sense to ourselves and, hopefully, other readers. This building of momentum was only noticeable in retrospect, but always included a clear sensation of the need to get far enough in one of our meetings to carry us through to the next.

Re-evaluation of the experience

Association

After we reviewed our experience together and explored the feeling dimension, we moved into a new phase. We turned to the whiteboard and spent an absorbing few hours engaged in an exercise which we have often used in our workshops. In the centre of the blank space, we wrote 'BARRIERS TO WORKING WITH EXPERIENCE' and sat back and pondered on that theme. At times we wrote furiously, at others we waited for associations to strike us as we trawled our consciousness and waited for our intuition to provide inspiration. As we wrote, we thought and discussed and attempted to articulate to each other what we were trying to express. We made no attempt to fit the fragments together and find patterns, just to associate whatever was in our consciousness relating to barriers to working with experience.

At the end, the board was packed with words, phrases and fragments of ideas, too messy and dense to reproduce here. However, to give the flavour, we list in Table 1 some of the associations which emerged from our own experience, and that of others, about barriers to working with experience. Although we had not only been thinking of ourselves during the generation phase, as we transcribed them and read through them individually, we recalled examples of each of them in our own lives: 'you're not allowed do that' (translated as: someone from your class/with your accent must be excluded from these privileges); 'I'm not bright enough to go to university'; 'I'm too frightened to try that again', etc.

Table 1   Our brainstormed list of barriers to working with experience

- Presuppositions about what is and is not possible for us to do.
- Not being in touch with one's own assumptions and what one is able to do.
- Past negative experiences.
- Expectations of others: society, peer group, figures of authority, family.
- Threats to the self, one's world view, or to ways of behaving.
- Lack of self-awareness of one's place in the world.
- Inadequate preparation.
- Hostile or impoverished environments.
- Lack of opportunity to step aside from tasks.
- Lack of time.
- External pressures and demands.

- Lack of support from others.
- Lack of skills: in noticing, intervening.
- Intent which is unclear or unfocused.
- Established patterns of thought and behaviour.
- Inability to conceive of the possibility of learning from experience: 'this is not learning', 'this is not possible'.
- Stereotypes about how we learn.
- Obstructive feelings: lack of confidence or self-esteem, fear of failure or the response of others, unexpressed grief about lost opportunities.

We were somewhat overwhelmed by the number and diversity of blocks to learning we had identified. Nevertheless, we were satisfied that we were beginning to come to grips with a very important issue to us and we pressed on to see if any *integration* of all this was possible.

Integration

In meetings following our session with the whiteboard, we played with the ideas generated and struggled to articulate some of the patterns which were emerging for us concerning barriers to learning. We returned again to some of our earlier thinking and came to a working definition: barriers are those factors which inhibit or block learners' preparedness for the experience, their active engagement in it, and their ability to reflect rationally on it with a view to learning from it. With this definition in mind, it was possible to bring together our ideas under a number of headings: understanding barriers to learning; their origins; their interaction with each other; how to deal with them; and how to work with them.

Understanding barriers to learning

Our working definition points to the fact that barriers can inhibit learning at each stage of our understanding of the learning process: the preparation, the experience itself and the reflection on it (Boud and Walker, 1990). In preparation they can inhibit learning by reducing the learning potential of the experience, by limiting the learner's awareness of the learning environment, failing to focus existing knowledge and skills in relationship to it, and creating a vague or ill-defined intent for entering the experience. Within the experience, they can limit the essential processes of noticing and intervening, thereby having an adverse affect on the learner's engagement in it. They can paralyse the reflection processes within the experience, and after it, so that the experience becomes non-reflective and is robbed of much of its learning potential. After the experience, these barriers can raise emotional factors which made reflection impossible or limit it; they can isolate and impoverish the new experience by making it difficult to relate the new experience to past experience; they can make it difficult to integrate new learning with past knowledge, and to make judgements and draw conclusions from it. They can also make it difficult for the learner to appropriate the new learning.

Looking at the barriers in terms of their origins in relation to the learner, some barriers are external impositions while others stem from ourselves. External barriers

341

can come from people, the learning environment, the larger personal situation and context of the learner, and social forces, such as stereotyping, cultural expectations, classism and so on. Internal barriers stem from the unique personal experience of the learner. They can include previous negative experiences, accepted presuppositions about what the learner can do or about what learning can take place, a lack of awareness of one's assumptions, the emotional state of the learner, established patterns of behaviour.

Classifying types of barriers in terms of whether they are external or internal to the learner raises the important point of the interaction between them. Many of the supposedly external barriers only begin to have real force when we take them on ourselves and think and act as if they were true. Often self-imposed censorship is more pernicious than anything imposed by others. The power that external forces have is in proportion to the degree to which we appropriate them. There is a strong dynamic whereby learners are tricked, or trick themselves, into thinking barriers are external when they are not — 'no-one from my background could possibly aspire to a job like that'.

A second realization was that personal distress mixed with the mostly unconscious oppressive behaviour of others underlies many of the barriers we identified. Although we experience barriers as internal — 'I can't possibly do that' or 'I don't want to do that' — they often arise from external influences which impacted on us at an earlier time and which left us feeling disempowered or de-skilled or inhibited. When we were treated as working-class boys who 'should' have low expectations of life, rather than as the particular individuals whom we were, we internalized the external oppression and censored our own aspirations.

Our own experience led us to the view that barriers to learning revolve around the individual learner, even when the key factors involved appear to be social or cultural. While some influences may impinge on many people, in the final instance, a barrier is only a barrier when a particular learner is impeded in learning. What may seem to be endemic, may not apply in a given case. This means that the real battleground for working with these barriers is the learner; the learner is the locus within which we need to situate barriers to learning. While it is in this individual context that barriers are revealed, and it is here that often one must address them, we cannot deny that social intervention on a broader front aimed at addressing endemic discriminatory practices is also necessary to achieve a learning society.

Discovering barriers to learning

We were not content to leave our considerations of barriers there. We wanted to make learning more effective, to change it, not just to understand it. We wanted to know how to help learners (ourselves included) work with the barriers and find ways of eliminating or circumventing them. Facilitation of learning is essentially about helping learners deal with their barriers to learning. Helping them to conceive of a barrier to learning as susceptible to influence rather than an inherent deficiency can be a personally empowering step. However, a key element in facilitation is raising awareness of the existence of barriers, and their origin and nature.

How does one notice a barrier? Comparing one's thoughts, feelings and behaviour with those of others can indicate that we are experiencing differently, which can prompt us to ask why. The feedback of others can also help us recognize inadequacies in our ability to work with experience, as can working through a common experience with a group. Exposure to others is one of the best ways of becoming aware of barriers to learning from experience. Hearing them tell their story, and telling our story to them, can help us to see ourselves and how we experience and learn.

Sometimes, it is necessary to cease being involved in a certain type of activity in order to become aware that it may not be fruitful in terms of learning. Action not only reinforces presuppositions, but sometimes obscures the assumptions from which it flows. Action of a different kind, exposure to new experiences, reaching beyond the confines of a limited set of experiences, can expose limitations, highlight barriers to learning, and give us a new appreciation of our learning capacities.

Our own personal awareness, our instinctive feelings, can also alert us to barriers. Heeding our own comfort level within a given situation can bring us to an awareness of our abilities, or lack of them, to work with experience as a source of learning. Being in touch with oneself within the experience is an important way to appreciate one's potential, or lack of it, to learn from the experience.

Working with barriers

Some barriers stem from the perception of the learner, and a transformation of that perception can lead to their diminishing or disappearing. Others, however, are more deep-seated. The barrier has been learned and the ability to respond has been impaired. Sometimes, this is an emotional impairment which has occluded the learner's capacity to learn anew. This can often require the learner to re-visit past experiences and examine them from their current, more powerful perspective. At times, more intensive therapeutic assistance may be required, which goes beyond the scope of the educational facilitator.

It is important to recognize whether the barriers can be altered or transformed with ease or with difficulty. Four useful steps emerged from our considerations on how to work with barriers. The first is to acknowledge that they may exist. An acceptance of their presence is the beginning of working with them. Secondly, having acknowledged them, they need to be named (Griffin, 1987). The more clearly we understand them and can describe them, the more easily we will be able to work with them. This clarifying and naming can come from our own reflection and experience or from the help and experience of others.

The third step is to identify how the barriers operate by examining their origins. A useful concept in this regard is that of critical reflection, which presupposes that our experience is substantially influenced by presuppositions we bring to it. These exist prior to experience as part of our personal foundation of experience. The forces that shape these presuppositions and fix us into certain patterns of behaviour, thought or feeling sometimes need to be recognized and challenged. Critical reflection is a useful instrument for recognizing these forces, both those which come from our own personal story and those which come from the social, cultural context in which we have developed. The enlightenment that comes through critical reflection helps us to understand the origins of barriers to learning from experience, and offers us new opportunities to overcome them, by clarifying how they operate and what needs to be done to counter them. As we reflected on this step, we became aware that the very model of reflection which is being illustrated in this chapter can have an important role to play in critical reflection.

The fourth step is to work with the barriers. Working with them can involve strategies which are confrontational or transformative. Re-examining past experiences from a current, more powerful situation, or reframing old experiences or concepts in the light of new understanding can lead to their transformation (Minsky, 1982; Bolman and Deal, 1991). The recognition of one's powerlessness or lack of awareness in past situations puts them in a new perspective and transforms our understanding and appropriation of them. Sometimes, confrontational strategies are appropriate. This involves taking a stance which contradicts the influence of the barrier in every respect. For example, a barrier which causes a learner to believe that they cannot do something, when there is no apparent external limitation present, can be contradicted by the learner acting as if they could undertake the task and dealing with the feelings that this stance provokes. One can find ways of contradicting former patterns of behaviour and substitute them for the former ways. One can enter into forbidding experiences with new awareness and knowledge and work through the issues as one is experiencing them.

Validation

Much needs to be done now to validate these ideas in terms of our own experience. To what extent does it help us make sense of our own experiences, the barriers we have encountered to learning and the way which we have been effective in dealing with these barriers in our own lives? We have done this implicitly to some extent in constructing the thinking we describe above, but we now need to extend this to other examples, ones we were not thinking of before. These thoughts also need to be checked against the experience of others. This occurred as others read this account in draft form and their comments helped to clarify and explicate our thinking about barriers.

One of the most significant points that emerged from our integration was the application of our reflection model to using critical reflection in dealing with barriers. It became the immediate focus of our research, and we set to working on a paper in which we relate our model of reflection to the exercise of critical reflection (Walker and Boud, 1992).

Appropriation

We cannot tell in advance what knowledge we will make our own. Having a theoretical framework in itself does not remove the barriers. The next step is to accept the challenge which our reflection has posed for us. Explaining a problem does not mean that we have dealt with it. We feel than we have made some progress, but this needs to be consolidated and made our own. What we have appropriated about barriers to learning from experience we will only be able to be identify in retrospect.

Second thoughts

We had shown a draft of the preceding sections to two of our colleagues. To our surprise, they found a massive discontinuity between the experience of collaboration we had described and the reflections on barriers which followed. They saw a huge leap from the account of the experience to the later reflection, which seemed unconnected, both in style and content, to the recount of the experience which led to them. Our immediate reaction was to protest that this couldn't possibly be the case — our experience was seamless, we moved from one section to the other without being at all conscious that we were doing anything other than continuing the natural course of our reflection. Our considered response led us to reconsider what we believed about learning from experience.

Re-reading our text, it was clear that the reference to barriers had emerged rather abruptly and unexpectedly from what had gone before. Yet we knew that it had come directly from our experience. In describing our experience, we had not captured something important. How on earth did we get from the stage of feeling good about writing together to that of confronting major barriers to learning from experience? It clearly did not come directly from our experience as we described it. What had led us to move from the reflection on our collaborative experience to a focus on barriers? As we reflected further, several possibilities emerged.

Our work together had been an exploration of learning about learning from experience, and a focus on the essential elements of it which could be developed to enhance learning. In presenting those elements of learning from experience, we tended to emphasize their positive contribution to learning. However, what we had presented could also have implications for impediments to learning. The focus on barriers which emerged was simply a development of our original thoughts, a consideration of our key points from a different point of view, i.e. how learning can be impaired. We needed to develop this aspect of our thoughts to appreciate the full significance of the elements we had been emphasizing. As we reflected in this way, the movement from our previous work to a consideration of barriers did not seem quite so abrupt. However, it did not explain why we had made the transition from one to the other. We searched further for some explanation.

A possible explanation for this related to the work in which we were concurrently engaged on critical reflection. We had received an earlier response to our model which had questioned its application to critical reflection. This had led us to begin to explore this area and, while working on this chapter, we were simultaneously working on the paper on critical reflection for the Third International Conference on Experiential Learning held at Pondicherry in India (Walker and Boud, 1992). It was an application of our model to critical reflection. We investigated the sources of the critical reflection movement, and found that they were very much concerned with the assumptions and presuppositions which limited the experiences of people and constrained their freedom. We could see how our current preoccupation with such limits and constraints could cause us to move from the positive aspects of the work we had been reflecting on for this chapter, to explore how learning from experience could be limited or impeded.

Two important realizations emerged from these reflections. The first was that our present preoccupations had deeply influenced our reflection on past experience. They had caused us to view our experience in a new light and open up areas that previously we had not noticed, or at least did not consider important enough to explore. This whole experience gave us another view about how our model for reflection could be used, and how, in using it, one needs to be aware of one's present situation and preoccupations.

This experience also brought home to us that our lived experience can never be fully transmitted to another person, even when we go to great lengths to describe that experience. Sometimes, important dynamics operate which seem so commonplace to us that we do not include them in our descriptions. Indeed, we may not even be aware that they exist. There are many stories we can tell about our experience. All may be 'true' to the teller, but they each reflect some part of the whole. Some will resonate more with the reader than others as they touch their sensibilities and have meaning for them. The more the reader learns, the more they can build a fuller picture; but this picture is always partial, large chunks are obscured and many meanings can be drawn from it.

Conclusion

This reflection on our collaborative work in the light of our model has been a more enriching experience than we had anticipated. It has given new meaning to our past experience and aspects of it that we had hitherto overlooked. It has enabled us to apply the model we had developed, and given us new ways of seeing how it can be used. Above all, it has given us some fascinating insights into the ways in which we create our own version of experience.

We had thought that we could end this chapter by making some useful remarks about barriers to learning and the importance of reflection. But we can no longer do this in the way we had anticipated. What we can say is that learning from experience is far more indirect than we often pretend it to be. It can be prompted by systematic reflection, but it can also be powerfully prompted by discrepancies or dilemmas which we are 'forced' to confront. It can be helped by 'naming' the process and admitting that there is an event which is unresolved. Other people can provide an invaluable means of identifying the discrepancy or dilemma; they can often see what may be obvious, but which is too close for us to notice. By supportively drawing it to our attention, they can help us learn from experience, even when they do not see themselves in that role.

Much as it can be convenient to break up our experience, to name the parts and to work intensively on some aspects of it, we have come now to recognize the importance of what some of our colleagues elsewhere in this book are emphasizing. Whatever else we do, we must always consider the whole. We must treat the whole of our experience as relevant and not be too surprised when connections are made which, previously, we had been unable to see. Much as we may enjoy the intellectual chase, we cannot neglect our full experience in the process. To do so is to fool ourselves into treating learning from experience as a simple rational process.

References

Bolman L, Deal T (1991) *Reframing Organisations*. Jossey Bass, San Francisco, CA.

Boud D, Walker D (1990) Making the most of experience. *Studies in Continuing Education*, 12(2): 61–80.

Boud D, Walker D (1991) *Experience and Learning: Reflection at Work*. Deakin University Press, Geelong, Victoria.

Boud D, Keogh R, Walker D (1985) Promoting reflection in learning: A model. In D J Boud, R Keogh, D Walker (eds) *Reflection: Turning Experience into Learning*, pp. 18–40. Kogan Page, London.

Griffin V (1987) Naming the processes. In D J Boud, V Griffin (eds) *Appreciating Adults Learning From the Learners' Perspective*, pp. 209–221. Kogan Page, London.

Minsky M (1982) *The Society of Mind*. Picador, London.

Walker D, Boud D (1992) Facilitating critical reflection: Opportunities and issues for group learning. In *Proceedings of the Third International Conference on Experiential Learning*, pp. 43–57. Pondicherry, Union Territory Administration, India.

Evaluation and Assessment

Assessment is a key role for anyone involved in facilitating learning. The focus for the extracts in this section is on assessment and evaluation of learning in the clinical environment and issues of formal theoretical assessment through examinations and assignments are not addressed in any significant way in the any of the extracts or articles provided.

Many definitions of assessment exist and lead to a general confusion about what it is and what it is not. Nicklin and Kenworthy (1995) provide a relatively simple yet unambiguous definition which might prove useful:

> 'Measurement that directly relates to the quality and quantity of learning and as such is concerned with student progress and attainment.'

> (Nicklin and Kenworthy, 1995: PG .69)

In nursing and midwifery education continuous assessment of practice is now the required strategy to ascertain whether a learner meets certain competencies which allow him/her to progress through his/her programme of study. Continuous assessment of practice integrates formative and summative assessment strategies which increases the chances of validity and reliability of the assessment strategy. It is a concept which embraces and integrates different assessment strategies into a unified approach and as such is arguably not an assessment strategy in its own right but rather a philosophy of assessment (Oliver and Endersby, 1994).

The English National Board (1986), define continuous assessment of practice as, "*a planned series of progressively updated measurements of student achievement and progress*". In England assessors are registered nurses who have undergone a short preparation for the role in accordance with guidelines from the English National Board (1990).

Rowntree (1992) and Jarvis (1985) are two key figures in the area of assessment. They suggest that the process of assessment carries with it a great deal of responsibility. Rowntree (1992) feels that assessment is about getting to know people and making judgements about their capabilities. Jarvis and Gibson (1985) contend that assessment is the gatekeeping mechanism through which people do, or do not, make progress in their chosen course or occupation.

Assessment is therefore an ethical activity (Milligan, 1996). There is a requirement to be as certain as possible about the accuracy of judgements made in assessment and to be able to actively support those judgements be they good or bad. There is an inescapable fact that, however sound the assessment strategy, the assessment of individuals in the ever changing context of clinical practice requires the exercise of professional judgement.

The purpose of evaluation is to learn from past educational events in the life of a student or course and adapt them appropriately to reflect future needs. Evaluation should be an integral part of the learning process and not an afterthought or an add on. Using the principles of reflective practice as a basis, evaluation provides an opportunity to reflect, to learn from the past and adapt for the future.

The learning organisation needs evaluation material of all kinds if it is going to continually adapt to new circumstances, events and avoid extinction (Nicklin and Kenworthy, 1996). All those involved within the learning organisation are also dependent on this information and require to be kept updated on all evaluation data.

Very often the reviewing of a student's learning experience in the clinical setting at the end of a placement becomes ritualised and, increasingly, comments and observations made by them serve no real purpose as no action arises from them (Bradshaw, 1989). Planned, systematic and focused evaluation if utilised appropriately serves both to enhance the educational experiences available to the students and to promote professional development of facilitators through a process of critical reflection.

References

Jarvis P, Gibson S (1985) *The teacher practitioner in nursing, midwifery and health visiting.* Croom Helm, London.

Nicklin P, Kenworthy N (1995) *Teaching and assessing in nursing practice*, 2nd edn. Scutari Press, London.

Oliver R, Endersby C (1994) *Teaching and assessing nurses: A handbook for preceptors.* Baillière Tindall, London.

Rowntree D (1992) *Assessing students — How should we know them?* Harper and Row, London.

32. The Process of Assessment
Robert Oliver and Colin Endersby

Introduction

The subject of assessment involves factors which relate to how an individual learns, how an individual puts his/her learning into practice and even the psychological and logistical factors involved in attempting to ascertain how much learning has taken place. On first inspection of the subject, assessment would appear to be quite simple, in that if learning has occurred then it must, in some way or another, stand up to some form of assessment. In reality, many questions need to be asked about the techniques used in assessment and the assumptions that underlie them, and this cannot be tackled in isolation from the assumptions which underlie the theories of learning used, experiences available and indeed the very philosophy of the curriculum.

Learning, as has already been discussed, is not an altogether straightforward process and, by implication, neither is assessment. For example, in trying to ascertain the degree of competence in communicating with a patient, attitudes, communication skills, environment and personality will all have an effect on the outcome. The central question that needs to be addressed is that of which factors can be assessed and which factors cannot. To return to our discussion in [an earlier chapter], the assessment strategy for a skills-based course would be rather different from that of a predominantly student-centred course where the learning outcomes are that much broader.

The trend away from periodic practice-based assessments to continuous assessment (ENB, 1988) to some extent reflects the complexities both of the learning process and of the nature of nursing itself. Conversely, the requirement that nurses should meet certain competencies will also add another dimension to the subject. As has already been mentioned, to follow one school of thought stringently with regard to the nature of learning is perhaps unwise, bearing in mind the vast array of competencies which need to be mastered. The types of assessment which can be used are varied and range from journal keeping to formal written examinations. The purposes of such assessments are naturally just as varied, but within our discussion, the general classifications of "Formative" and "Summative" will be explored.

Formative and summative assessments

The terms *formative* and *summative* are possibly the most widely used terms in assessment. There is a tendency to treat them as distinct entities and to classify assessments into one or the other accordingly. Broadly speaking, formative assessment refers to the process of ascertaining a student's progress during a course of study or experience, usually in an informal way. It is usually individually-based and will not

Robert Oliver and Colin Endersby: 'The Process of Assessment' from *TEACHING AND ASSESSING NURSES* (Baillière Tindall, 1996), pp. 102–112. Reprinted by permission of the publisher W B Saunders.

normally be counted towards a final mark or grade. It is reasonable to suggest that such assessments not only will lead to the student gaining an insight into their areas of strengths and weaknesses in a non-threatening manner, but also should guide further learning strategies. By implication, the outcome of formative assessments may occasionally direct both the student and the teacher to the conclusion that the student has little aptitude for the subject, and hence counselling may be required.

Summative assessment, on the other hand, involves the assessment of learning which has taken place and hopefully applied to practice and is most obviously typified by a final examination (usually written).

Both types of assessment have their roles to play. The formative assessment essentially allows us to "diagnose" difficulties and, with the student, to "prescribe" corrective action. The summative assessment is traditionally a far more decisive tool and will always have a strong bearing on the individual's future within that course of study. There is however, an alternative way of considering these two types of assessment. Instead of considering them as separate entities, it has been suggested (Rowntree, 1977) that they are opposite ends of a continuum with uniquely formative and summative assessments occurring relatively rarely. Most assessments therefore can be seen as having an element of each to some extent. For example, most formative assessments will therefore contribute towards decisions regarding the individual's future and most summative assessments, particularly if effective feedback is given, will act as a diagnostic tool which will direct further learning.

The assessment continuum can be depicted as follows:

Formative .... Summative

(Diagonal Line)

Rowntree (1977) further went on to identify other continuum to describe further types of assessment.

Informal	....	Formal
Process	....	Product
Divergent	....	Convergent
Idiographic	....	Nomothetic
Course Work	....	Examinations
Continuous	....	Terminal

Informal–formal. Formal assessment aims to gain knowledge about the student but essentially has no instructional value. Informal assessment, on the other hand, is diagnostic and should be unobtrusive. Rowntree describes formal assessment as "publicly satisfied purpose for public use" and informal as "privately specific purpose for private use". Individual formative tutorials are examples of an informal assessment.

Process–product. A process assessment through techniques such as projects, student-centred learning and contract learning, reveals how a student has learned, whereas a product assessment will merely reveal the end result of the process.

Divergent–convergent. Divergent assessment is, by necessity, individually tailored because it examines the individual's development in contrast to the convergent assessment (typically a final standard examination) which tells the assessor more about the similarities between students rather than the ways in which they diverge. Certain project work could be said to be divergent but only if the individual is allowed to explore and investigate in an individual manner.

Idiographic–nomothetic. Student-centred and self-assessment techniques can be said to be idiographic in so far as they attempt to discover the uniqueness of the individual. Nomothetic assessments are concerned with a more standardized form of data collection from the process, (marking, streaming, etc.).

Course work–exams. According to Rowntree a summative assessment at the end of the course cannot be justified without information regarding the work that has been completed throughout the course. Naturally both course work and examinations may take many forms and here the grey areas between formative and summative are most evident.

Continuous–terminal. Although continuous assessment is an admirable tool for formative aspects of the process, it will usually contribute to a final summative grade. Traditionally in nursing (ENB, 1987), a terminal examination is required although it could be argued that if an acceptable summative assessment could be compiled from the continuous assessment tool then terminal examination would not be necessary.

On examination of these various types of assessment, it is feasible that the items on the left-hand side are components of, and interact with, each other. For instance, a formative assessment could be said to be informal, process based, divergent, ideographic, continuous and established through course work. Conversely, a summative assessment could be said to be formal, product based, convergent, nomothetic, unique and concerned with terminal or periodic exams.

The discussion on formative and summative assessment is central to this chapter and will be revisited later in terms of assessment strategy and the guidelines within which they must operate. The next stage in the discussion will be centred upon the question of how far we can depend on the results of an assessment to give us the information we require accurately.

Validity

Validity can be said to be "an examination of the approximate truth or falsity of the propositions" (Cook and Campbell, 1979). Put more simply it is "a measure of the truth or accuracy of a claim" (Burns and Grove, 1987). In terms of assessment, it could be adjusted to ask the question: "Do we believe that the results reflect accurately what is purported to have been tested?" Many questions will surround the debate concerning validity and many of these questions have their foundation in learning theory. For instance, can the student actually carry out the nursing care that they have written about in the final examination or did they learn it by rote? Does the assessment reflect what the student actually does or will do or does it reflect their ability to take an assessment?

353

Broadly speaking, validity, as with research, can be divided into five categories:

1. *Face validity.* This type of validity is highly informal and to an extent instinctive in as far as it is concerned with whether the assessment looks as though it will reveal the relevant information. It is only possible realistically in the light of professional knowledge, expertise and an in-depth understanding of the other types of validity.

2. *Construct validity.* This refers to how the assessment is constructed in terms of pass/fail criteria, progression of knowledge, formative and summative components as well as procedural implications such as examination boards and regulations.

3. *Content validity.* This refers to what is actually being assessed and not only refers to items such as competencies but also addresses the question about whether items can realistically be assessed or not (e.g. attitudes).

4. *Concurrent validity.* Ideally, if an assessment is to reveal useful information we need to know to what extent this can be done. This is difficult with an entirely new assessment strategy and hence it needs to be based substantially on either the results of similar strategies elsewhere or the results of pilot schemes.

5. *Predictive validity.* Although the easiest to define, predictive validity is possibly the most difficult to achieve. Predictive validity refers to whether we can predict an individual's performance and behaviours based on the results of their assessments. Naturally, the more isolated the assessment events are (as with terminal examinations and practical testing), the less predictive validity can be said to exist. Generally speaking, the more continuous the process the greater the predictive validity.

Reliability

The reliability of an assessment is in some ways only a matter of degree. If for instance we devised a completely "reliable" assessment then a student would gain exactly the same result if they completed the assessment on more than one occasion. There are important factors outside the assessment strategy which will have a strong influence over this occurrence. The student's physical condition, mental state, environment, home circumstances, etc. will all affect their performance. Hence the reliability of an assessment is difficult to achieve. If however, a group of students of similar abilities and experiences undertake, a multiple choice question paper and achieve wildly differing results then it could be said with some certainty that this was an unreliable assessment. The use of pilot schemes to test the reliability of an assessment must involve large numbers of students in order to offset novel personal circumstances which may alter the results.

Continuous assessment

The use of periodic assessment, as has been discussed, will at the very least, provide us with very little reliability and questionable validity in assessment of any type. It is known that reliability will increase the longer the assessment is carried on. It makes sense, therefore, to redesign assessment strategies into a continuous format which integrates both formative and summative assessments. Continuous assessment is a concept which embraces and integrates different assessment strategies into a unified approach and as such is arguably not an assessment method in its own right, but rather a philosophy of assessment. In other words it can be defined as "a planned series of progressively up-dated measurements of student achievement and progress" (ENB, 1986).

The use of continuous assessment in nurse education has been a feature of nursing curricula since 1988 and according to the ENB (1988) must meet certain criteria. Apart from the legal requirements with regard to the Nurses, Midwives, Health Visitors Approval Order No. 873 1983 (19(1)(c)) which each strategy has to meet, it is also necessary that such a strategy reflects a curriculum in which theory and practice are related.

If it is assumed that in the curricula, theory reflects practice and *vice versa*; it should, and indeed is, feasible within a framework of continuous assessment to devise separate assessment strategies for each. As far as dividing the curricula for assessment purposes is concerned, this is usually looked at in terms of "parts" which comprise smaller units. Each part should have a set of component assessments which maximise validity and reliability, incorporate formative and summative assessment and reflect "the acquisition of knowledge, skills, attitudes and competencies of differing complexity and application" (ENB, 1988).

Profiles

Representing the data obtained from assessments, particularly if a continuous assessment strategy has been used, can present problems. In recent years, one way of overcoming this problem has been through the use of *profiles*. According to Frith and Macintosh (1984) "The term Profile is used to describe multidimensional methods of presenting information usually about individuals and their achievements, attributes or performances." The major differences between different profiles is not surprisingly their content and method of presentation but as Frith and Macintosh go on to point out, they should all have the following characteristics:

1. Lists of items such as skills, competencies, subjects and personal attributes.

2. Some way of indicating the level achieved.

3. A way of indicating what evidence supports the grades arrived at.

A profile is therefore a method of visually presenting information obtained through assessment either formatively or summatively and through a variety of strategies which may be mentor-, peer- or self-assessed. In its most basic form, a profile could just provide a list of marks obtained for various subjects throughout the curriculum as distinct from an overall mark. More commonly, however, the following profiles are used.

Numerical rating scale (Figure 1)

On the positive side, this design of profile is easy to use, but the example given is open to wide interpretation. Therefore alongside such a scale, clear guidelines would need to be given as to the meaning of each skill and each level of achievement. Consequently, a tool such as this which on first inspection appears easy to design and use may, in the long run be neither. Its major uses would be where the skills being assessed were not open to interpretation (e.g. resuscitation training) rather than where they deal with more complicated behaviour.

Topic: Communication

Circle the number most appropriate:

    1 = Needs further practice

    2 = Adequate level achieved

    3 = Shows aptitude

    4 = Excellent level of practice

					Comments
Listening skills:	1	2	3	4	
Information giving:	1	2	3	4	
Response to questions:	1	2	3	4	
Conveying messages:	1	2	3	4	

Figure 1   Numerical rating scale

Grid profile

The information contained on a grid profile gives more detail as to the different levels of competence which has been achieved and hence requires less subjective judgment. It may still, as with our example, be numerical in nature:

Communication	1	2	3	4
Conveying messages	Conveys the basic meaning of message			Conveys messages effectively

With these guidelines in mind, we now have to turn our attention towards the problem of how assessment will actually take place in the clinical setting and how the more theoretical components of assessment can be used in the clinical area.

Assessment strategies in nursing

Nursing, like virtually any other profession, has two readily identifiable components (theory and practice) which, in the learning environment, should become increasingly more indivisible as the student progresses through the course. The dilemma has, for some years, been how to overcome the problem of having separate assessment strategies for each. The final written examination and the continuous assessment of both practice and course work should complement each other so as to overcome these difficulties. The reader must naturally reach their own conclusions as to whether this goal has been achieved for students in their area.

Refinements have occurred in the last decade as we have progressed from a system of having isolated and unique practical assessments to continuous assessment

(ENB, 1987) and from central to devolved examination systems. These two policy changes have ensured that not only are national standards met but that they are also sensitive to local conditions and experiences. There is however, a certain degree of flexibility within guidelines issued which allow individual examination boards to develop their own formal assessments whilst ensuring that competencies are adequately assessed.

Taken that continuous assessment is the vehicle in which types of assessment must be placed and that further there must be a combination of formative and summative assessment, it now seems appropriate to examine some of the types of assessment which may be used.

Methods of assessment

There are many ways of classifying types of assessment. They could, for instance be said to be student centred or teacher centred, but this may be misleading because some types may incorporate both, such as with projects. We have already discussed earlier Rowntree's classification and seen that most assessments are a combination of approaches. The ENB (1987) has stated that a continuous assessment format "may be of a form that takes into account the students' needs and preferences", but at the same time it must demonstrate that a predetermined level of competence has been reached. For the purposes of our discussion, therefore, no attempt has been made to categorise the types of assessment into one category or another as this is dependent on so many differing factors (e.g. the personality and teaching style of the teacher) that it would be misleading.

Peer- and self-assessment

The concept that assessment can be carried out introspectively or with peers has gained momentum in recent years (e.g. Burnard, 1987). Its advantages are clear to see in as far as it tends to be less threatening to an individual to identify their own strengths and weaknesses either on their own or with their equals. The disadvantages are similarly immediately obvious, particularly in relation to its possibly threatening nature with regard to revealing weaknesses to a peer group. An outline of how peer- and self-assessment can be organised is given below (adapted from Burnard, 1987) and may serve as a foundation for setting up groups for this purpose.

1. Establish by consent a group of individuals who wish to be involved in this form of activity.

2. Establish confidentiality rules within the group in order that individuals will feel free to express themselves.

3. Set aside times for regular meetings and, if possible, give each meeting a function, e.g. to examine the rough drafts of a dissertation or project that everyone would have completed.

4. Each individual will have prepared not only their draft but will also have made notes about its strengths and weaknesses and perhaps even their thoughts for future work.

5. If common problems are found through informal discussions before the meetings, such as difficulty interpreting the criteria being used to assess the piece of work, then clarification should be sought from the relevant tutor.

6. At the meeting, each individual presents their work uninterrupted and with their own self-criticisms for a period of, e.g. 10 minutes.

7. Following this activity, the group then discusses the individual's work and comments before moving on to the next individual and repeating the process.

The inherent dangers will be largely overcome by each student having to present their work in turn although it has to be said that those students who the rest of the group consider as more advanced may present a threat to the others.

Portfolios

One particular vehicle for assessment, the *portfolio*, can be identified as predominantly student centred, and largely self-assessed in a formative sense. A portfolio can be loosely described as a collection of varied materials such as journals which by definition will include the individual's reflections (see below), profiles, project work, results of peer- and self-assessments.

Portfolios could be said to form "a loose and untested constellation of innovative projects" (Glen and Hight, 1992). The content of a portfolio is quite naturally a possible consequence of self-direction and hence will be largely subjective and therefore divorced from the curriculum. In terms of its ideal applications, as Glen and Hight point out, it is well suited to the adult learner. In assessment terms, unless rigid direction and guidelines are given, its principal uses will be formative and will focus on the characteristics given above for formative assessments.

Journals

The journal or diary as a method of self-assessment (Burnard, 1988) is seen as an integral part of the reflective process and hence enables students to complete at least a part of the learning cycle as described by Kolb (1984). As Burnard points out a journal or diary requires that entries are made on a weekly basis and could include the following, but may be adapted by the individual:

1. Problems encountered and the resolution of those problems.

2. Likes and dislikes of work experience.

3. New learning, including new references, skills, disorders, treatments, etc.

4. Application of learning to nursing.

5. Notes on self-development.

6. Other comments.

The use of journals for some students may be beneficial even in terms of a summative assessment (Scriven, 1967) in so far as individual criteria for the assessment of the journal may be worked out between the student and teacher. This would only fulfill some of the criteria for summative assessment, and if nomothetic and convergent aspects are to be assessed, then these have to be within broad areas of, for instance, referencing, writing style and other generalities which have little to do with the content. Some students, however, will not warm to the task and the journal may be of little use to them in any meaningful sense.

Formatively, the journal or diary is an immensely useful tool, considering as it does the progression from inexperience to experience, and it has the intrinsic value of being student centred; hence it provides a sensitive measurement of the individual's development.

Diaries or journals can on some courses be compulsory and by definition will be open to scrutiny if part of the assessment process is performed by anyone other than the person completing it. Its effectiveness as a truthful document and an accurate reflection of what is actually being felt and experienced must be called into question. To overcome this problem to some extent, a part of the journal needs to be identified as private and access restricted to the student.

The student's personal accounts of satisfying/unsatisfying experiences used in this case as part of a journal, can form part of a needs-assessment strategy (MacDonald and Grogin, 1991; Banfield, 1990). The journal can be used in this context to form a basis with which to identify the future learning needs of the student by analysing the gap between what is actually known and what needs to be known. Using it in this way, the use of contracts (see below) is arguably more relevant.

Case studies

Many of us who have taught students in the clinical area will be familiar (though perhaps not by name) with a strategy of teaching and assessment known as case studies. Traditionally descriptive case studies (care studies) have been used as a form of project work where the student will identify a patient or client and write about their problems and the care given. This may be of benefit for some students in terms of being able to integrate theory into practice. In education terms, case studies may have a much wider use and have almost certainly been encountered by most of us at some time or another. In this second context, a case study is a problem-solving and analysis exercise based on real or simulated scenarios and may be completed by an individual or a group.

Case studies may take several forms and may be designed to fit any level from, e.g. basic care to fairly complex management situations. Broadly speaking, the most applicable case studies to use in the clinical area are as follows.

Critical incidence case study

A series of incidents leading up to and including the penultimate event of a situation are described. The task of the student is to identify what they need to find out in order to complete the picture and to define the full circumstances, e.g.

> Mr Smith is admitted to the surgical unit for routine repair of hernia. He arrives at 0830 h with his wife, who departs a few minutes later. Upon his first contact with you, he appears nervous and agitated. He is due to go to theatre at 1000 h and despite the data obtained at admission not

identifying any obvious problems regarding his physical well-being, you are worried that either he is not psychologically prepared for surgery or that something else is causing him concern.

What additional information would you require in order to complete a more comprehensive assessment of Mr Smith's psychological state and how would you go about obtaining it?

Next-stage case study

With this case study, a series of events is revealed to the student and he/she are required to identify what is most likely to happen next. This will require a high degree of analysis and the ability to pull together information, e.g.

Mr Jones moved in with his daughter and family largely because, although fit, he was mentally unable to care for himself at home. His behaviour had always been described as strange by relatives and he had been living alone in squalid conditions since the death of his wife 10 years earlier. He was largely cared for by his daughter and her husband but this took the form of mental support and physical chores. The relationship between Mr Jones and the rest of the family, including three children, was not close. Five years ago Mr Jones developed a vascular disorder which led to gangrene for which he persistently refused the advised surgical treatment. He has been visited daily for the last five years by the community nursing team for the dressing to be changed.

Within the last year, both the son-in-law and daughter have visited the GP because they maintain that Mr Jones's mental state has deteriorated considerably. So far, social services, psychiatrist and community psychiatric nurse have all visited and identified that there is a problem, but stated that there is nothing they can do. It is obvious that all concerned in the family are under considerable pressure.

Given the above facts, what could be the possible consequences to this situation?

The live case study

As distinct from the next-stage case study, the live case study asks what should be done next rather than what will happen next. Taking the above example, it is easy to see that a different outcome to the scenario can be brought about by asking the question:

In the above situation what actions would you take to prevent this situation deteriorating further?

The use of case studies in the ways mentioned above is a common feature of many written examinations but they can be used very effectively in the clinical situation as an impromptu or planned method of assessing the student's ability to analyse, comprehend and, to an extent, deal with various situations.

Skills of the assessor

The interviews that take place between the student and mentor during and at the end of an experience should be seen as an important part of the education process. Students need to have regular discussions about their progress during an experience in order to make any changes to their practice that are required.

This process is commonly seen as one person making a judgment on the performance of another. This is fine when the student has performed well in the view of the teacher/mentor, but when placed in the position of having to be critical, many people find the process uncomfortable or even threatening. The reason for this is that they may feel that they are in the position of making a unilateral decision about the performance of the student, that the responsibility is all theirs, that these decisions may affect the whole future of that student and, in some instances, could lead to the end of the student's course. This commonly leads to the teacher/mentor not making a reasoned decision at all but marking the student as average.

By applying the concepts outlined in this chapter, it will be seen that the decision-making process is a shared one made by the student, the mentor, other trained staff who have worked with the student, the ward sister, the ward teacher, the student's course teacher and, in some instances, the course director. When viewed in this light, the decisions that have to be made become much easier and of course much more balanced.

The first step in this process is to look at the structure of the interviews that are to take place. Keeping in mind that this is an important part of the student's education process, i.e. the need to develop "self-appraisal skills", we need to consider that all students are individuals and accept that one structure may not be suitable for all of them.

Summary

The subject of assessment involves factors which relate to how an individual learns, how an individual puts their learning into practice and even the psychological and logistical factors involved in attempting to ascertain how much learning has taken place.

The trend away from periodic practice-based assessments to continuous assessment to some extent reflects the complexities both of the learning process and of the nature of nursing itself.

Broadly speaking, formative assessment refers to the process of ascertaining a student's progress during a course of study or experience in, usually, an informal way.

Summative assessment on the other hand involves the assessing of learning which has taken place and hopefully applied to practice and is most obviously typified by a final examination.

Validity can be said to be "an examination of the approximate truth or falsity of the propositions" (Cook and Campbell, 1979). Put more simply it is "a measure of the truth or accuracy of a claim" (Burns and Grove, 1987).

Continuous assessment can be defined as "a planned series of progressively up-dated measurements of student achievement and progress" (ENB, 1986).

A profile is a method of visually presenting information obtained through assessment either formatively or summatively and through a variety of strategies.

Assessment is a learning opportunity and can form a useful basis for further development.

References

Banfield V, Brooks E, Brown J *et al.* (1990) A strategy to identify the learning needs of staff nurses. *Journal of Continuing Education in Nursing*, 21(5), 209–211.

Burnard P (1987) Self and peer assessment. *Senior Nurse*, 6(5), 16–17.

Burnard P (1988) Journal as an assessment and evaluation tool in nurse education . . . journal or diary. *Nurse Education Today*, 8(2), 105–107.

Burns N, Grove S (1987) *The Practice of Nursing Research Conduct Critique and Utilisation*. W.B. Saunders, Philadelphia.

Cook T D, Campbell D T (1979) *Quasi experimentation: design and analysis for field settings.* Rand McNally College Publishing, Chicago. (In N. Burns and S. Grove *The Practice of Nursing Research Conduct Critique and Utilisation*. W.B. Saunders, Philadelphia.)

ENB (1986) Devolved final written examinations. (1986 /30/ ERDB.)

ENB (1987) Devolved continuous assessment for theory in first level nursing courses.

ENB (1988) Devolved continuous assessment.

Frith D S, Macintosh H G (1984) *A Teacher's Guide to Self-assessment*. Stanley Thornes, Cheltenham.

Glen S, Hight N (1992) Portfolios: an "affective" assessment strategy? *Nurse Education Today*, 12(6), 416–423.

Kilty J (1977) Self and peer assessment and peer audit human potential resource project. University of Surrey, Guilford.

Kolb D (1984) *Experiential Learning: Experience as a Source of Learning and Development*. Prentice Hall, Englewood Cliffs.

MacDonald R, Grogin E R (1991) Personal accounts of satisfying and unsatisfying nursing experiences as a needs assessment strategy. *Journal of Continuing Education in Nursing*, 22(1), 11–15.

Rowntree D (1977) *Assessing Students: How Shall We Know Them*. Harper and Row, London.

Scriven M (1967) The methodology of education. In R.O. Tyler, R.M. Gagne and M. Scriven (eds) *Perspective of Curriculum Evaluation*. AERA Monograph Series on Curriculum Evaluation No. 1. Rand McNally, Chicago.

33. What is Assessment?

Derek Rowntree

If we wish to discover the truth about an educational system, we must look into its assessment procedures. What student qualities and achievements are actively valued and rewarded by the system? How are its purposes and intentions realized? To what extent are the hopes and ideals, aims and objectives professed by the system ever truly perceived, valued and striven for by those who make their way within it? The answers to such questions are to be found in what the system requires students to *do* in order to survive and prosper. The spirit and style of student assessment defines the *de facto* curriculum.

A cause for concern

I was constantly reminded of the crucial nature of assessment during the writing of a previous book on curriculum development (Rowntree, 1974). There I found that in every chapter, whatever I was writing about — aims and objectives, the design of learning experiences, the sequencing and structuring of knowledge, the evaluation and improvement of teaching — questions of assessment kept rearing their heads and threatening to dominate the discussion.

If assessment is so crucial, one might expect the subject to have an extensive literature already. So why add to it? Indeed much has been written (see, e.g. Ebel, 1972; Gronlund, 1971; Hudson, 1973; Lewis, 1974; Pidgeon and Yates, 1969; Schofield, 1972; Terwilliger, 1971; Thorndike, 1972; Thyne, 1974; etc.) But, for the most part, the literature takes for granted the present nature of assessment and seeks improvement merely through increasing its efficiency. Thus, for example, it is easy to find writers concerned with how to produce better multiple-choice questions, how to handle test-results statistically, or how to compensate for the fact that different examiners respond differently to a given piece of student work. It is much less easy to find writers questioning the purposes of assessment, asking what qualities it does or should identify, examining its effects on the relationships between teachers and learners, or attempting to relate it to such concepts as truth, fairness, trust, humanity and social justice. Writers of the former preoccupation rarely give any indication of having considered questions of the latter kind. Insofar as they appear to regard assessment as non-problematic, their writings, though often extremely valuable in their way, gloss over more fundamental questions about whether what we are doing is the right thing and offer simply a technical prescription for doing it better. This James Thyne (1974) approvingly calls 'the goodness of examinations as technical instruments'. Even then, the implications of doing it 'better' are rarely pursued very far. In short, the literature addresses itself chiefly to the question 'How?' rather than the question 'Why?'. In this [book] I shall try to adjust the emphasis.

Derek Rowntree: 'What is Assessment?' from *ASSESSING STUDENTS: HOW SHALL WE KNOW THEM?* (Kogan Page Ltd, 1977; 1987), pp. 1–13.

The discontinuity between technical and philosophical considerations in assessment is not new and has long been recognized. Here is Kandel (1936) saying of examinations what I would wish to say of all forms of assessment:

> '. . . the problem of examinations is not primarily one of discovering more accurate scientific and technical methods of constructing and scoring examinations. The problem of examinations strikes at the very roots of the whole meaning and significance of education in society. . . . The essence of the problem is the validity of education.' (p. 151)

My hope is that this book will encourage colleagues in education (by which I mean students as well as teachers) to bring together the technical and the philosophical, and to examine assessment anew from a broader perspective. Teachers tend to be trapped in a time-vortex that inhibits them from giving too much thought to assessment that has happened previously, or will happen later, to their students in institutions other than their own. Awareness is greatest near the gateways between two stages in a student's career, e.g. top juniors, or 6th form, or first year at college. But, even then, attention tends to be restricted to the last or next gateway. My contention is that we can all learn much by considering how assessment operates in learning mileux other than the ones with which we are directly concerned. Thus the university teacher may gain substantial insights from thinking about assessment in the primary school, and so may the primary school teacher from thinking about assessment in higher education. Similarly, teachers in one country can learn from the practices of those in another country or another time. Hence I make no apology for including examples from all levels of education, and from other countries (especially the U.S.A.) and other times. Further, we should at least be aware that educational assessment has more than a family resemblance to many other forms of assessment prevalent in our society. To name but a few:

> everyday conversational dialogue;
> medical and psychiatric diagnosis;
> the writing of biography;
> forensic cross-examination;
> job-interviews and promotion appraisals;
> criticism of art and literature;
> 'refereeing' of books and of papers submitted for publication in scholarly journals.

Such forms of assessment will sometimes offer revealing parallels and contrasts with those common in education.

In recent years, writings and conferences debating basic aspects of student assessment have begun to occur more frequently. Extreme positions get taken up. People may be passionate apologists for the system as it is now held to exist. Or they may be equally passionate denouncers of assessment as a tyrannical means of persuasion, coercion and social control, enhancing the power of one group of people (the teachers, together perhaps with whatever others they may believe themselves to be representing — 'the discipline' or profession, parents, employers, 'society') over another group (the students). Not surprisingly then, debates on assessment can raise strong feelings. The clash of ideologies — in the Marxian sense of ideas being used as weapons in a struggle for dominance between groups with conflicting interests — can be more in evidence than honest reflection and rational analysis. Consequently, assessment debate is awash with hidden assumptions, unstated values, partial truths, confusions of ideas, false distinctions, and irrelevant emphases. It is also flooded with specialist terminology — jargon, even — which we will have to find our way around in the following pages.

The nature of assessment

Some of the confusions and false distinctions will become apparent as we begin exploring a working definition of assessment. Dictionary definitions tend to agree that to assess is to put a value on something, usually in financial terms. Such definitions are clearly not centred on educational assessment, although it is true that certain outcomes of educational assessment, e.g. a student's degree class, may well determine the salary he can expect. Again, such valuational definitions do chime in with what many teachers think of (erroneously, I would say) as essential components of assessment, *viz* the assigning of numerical marks or letter grades, and the ranking of students in order of preference or relative achievement.

More basically, assessment in education can be thought of as occurring whenever one person, in some kind of interaction, direct or indirect, with another, is conscious of obtaining and interpreting information about the knowledge and understanding, or abilities and attitudes of that other person. To some extent or other it is an attempt to *know* that person. In this light, assessment can be seen as human encounter. In education we are mainly conscious of this 'encounter' in the shape of teachers finding out about their students. But we must not forget that students also assess one another, especially when working together as co-operative teams. They also assess their teachers (see Miller, 1972; Page, 1974). Mutual assessment is perhaps what Nell Keddie (1971) has in mind when she refers to 'the ways in which teachers and pupils scan each other's activities in the classroom and attribute meaning to them' (see also Downey, 1977). Nor should we hesitate to turn the definition in upon itself and think of the person (student or teacher) finding out about *himself* —self-assessment.

Despite one of the assumptions commonly made in the literature, assessment is not obtained only, or even necessarily mainly, through tests and examinations. Finding out about a student's abilities and so on may not involve testing him or measuring his performance in any formal way. We can imagine a spectrum of assessment situations ranging from the very informal, almost casual, to the highly formal, perhaps even ritualistic. At the informal end of the spectrum we have, for instance, the continuous but unself-conscious assessment that takes place between partners in an everyday conversation where each is constantly responding to what he takes to be the emerging attitudes and understandings of the other as he decides what to say next in consequence. Compare this with the monologue of a platform speaker or with the programmed patter of the kind of door-to-door evangelist who steadfastly ignores all responses that might suggest he should depart from his 'script'.

In a classroom conversation, however, where the intentions of the participants may be rather more directed to specific tasks and goals, the assessment may be slightly more formal, or at least more self-conscious. When assessment becomes the purpose, even if unstated, of initiating a conversation, e.g. in asking the student what he knows or feels about an issue, the formality becomes yet greater. So too, as far as the teacher at least is concerned, when he unobtrusively observes the student in action in order to assess. The ultimate in formality, for both teacher and student, is reached when the student is required to perform in what is patently a test-situation — quiz, interview, practical test, written examination, or whatever.

But it is worth noting here that, despite another common confusion, all these shades of assessment can be practised without any kind of measurement that implies absolute standards; it may be enough simply to observe whether, for each student, some personal, even idiosyncratic, trait or ability appears discernible to greater or lesser extent than hitherto. There need be no requirement to compare the findings for one student with those for another, let alone arrange students in some kind of order as a result of any such comparisons. Joan Tough (1976, p. 32) makes the point very well in distinguishing between testing and 'appraisal':

> 'How does the child walk and run? What is the quality of his movement? What kind of control does the child have of fine and intricate manipulation and of movement that needs concentration of strength and effort? What is the child's general co-ordination of movements like? Is he awkward and ungainly or does he move easily and smoothly without apparent effort? Many of these qualities would defy measurement, and many would defy comparison with other children. But all could be appraised, i.e. described in terms which build up a picture of what the child is like.'

Again, despite many assumptions to the contrary, assessment is not the same thing as grading or marking. If you 'grade' or 'mark' a student (or his work — the distinction is often unclear both to students and teachers) you are attaching a letter or number that is meant somehow to symbolize the quality of the work and allow comparison with the work of other students. Such grading cannot take place without prior assessment — the nature and quality of the student's work must be determined before it can be labelled with a suitable symbol. But assessment can, and perhaps usually does, take place without being followed by grading. Assessment can be *descriptive* (e.g. 'Bob knows all his number bonds up to 20') without becoming *judgemental* (e.g. 'Bob is good at number bonds'). It may be that in secondary and higher education the only assessments that count are those which are, in fact, followed by grading. But in infant schools and, to a large extent, in junior schools (with the exception of those still preparing children for the 11-plus exam) developing skills are constantly being assessed without any apparent compulsion to label them with letter grades or numerical marks. Odd, then, that a colleague of mine, admittedly in higher education, should rebuff a suggestion that we abandon the grading of essays by saying 'No, we can't claim to be teaching properly unless we know how our students are progressing.'

Just as tests and examinations are possible means of assessment, so grades and marks are possible outcomes. But they are not the only ones possible. Assessment is also a necessary precondition for *diagnostic appraisal* — ascertaining the student's strengths and weaknesses, and identifying his emerging needs and interests. In truth it is the practice of diagnostic appraisal (not grading) that enables us to claim we are teaching. Given that the student has reached such-and-such a state, what can he or should he aim for next? What implications does this have for the ensuing learning experiences? Diagnostic appraisal does not involve grading. Nor need it necessarily be based on formal tests and measurements. It is dependent on some kind of assessment having taken place, however, together with pedagogic judgements as to what new learning experiences are possible, and value-judgements (the student's perhaps, as well as the teacher's) as to which are desirable.

There is a further useful distinction we can make between two words which, in everyday parlance, and indeed in most dictionaries, seem virtual synonyms — assessment and evaluation. In education, though, it is common in Britain to use the two words to refer to two rather different, though closely-related activities. If assessment tries to discover what the student is becoming or has accomplished, then evaluation tries to do the same for a course or learning experience or episode of teaching. Evaluation is an attempt to identify and explain the effects (and effectiveness) of the teaching. In such an attempt, assessment is clearly a necessary component. Assessment, whether formal or informal, reveals to us the most important class of 'effects' — the changes brought about in the knowledge and understanding, abilities and attitudes of our students. If students have not changed or have somehow changed for the worse, e.g. they may have learned to solve simultaneous equations but also to detest algebra, we suspect something is wrong with the teaching. But student assessment is only part of evaluation. A full evaluation will also need, for example, to consider the effects of the course on people other than students — on the teachers participating, on other teachers who have contact with the students, on parents, on employers, on other people in the community, and so on. Thus, data additional to the assessment data — gained perhaps through participant observation, discussions, interviewing, reading of local newspapers, internal memoranda, etc. — will be needed. Incidentally, in the U.S.A. the word 'assessment' is rarely used in this context at all; instead, the word 'evaluation' usually has to do duty for both the concepts described above. In scanning the American literature, one must know whether one is looking for evaluation (of students) or evaluation (of courses).

The American literature (Scriven, 1967) has, however, developed a distinction between types of evaluation (of courses) that is equally useful in thinking about assessment. Thus, *formative* evaluation is intended to develop and improve a piece of teaching until it is as effective as it possibly can be —a well-tested programmed textbook would be a prime example. *Summative* evaluation, on the other hand, is intended to establish the effectiveness of the teaching once it is fully developed and in regular use. The distinction is, in fact, rather hard to preserve in considering the evaluation of most kinds of teaching; but it is very descriptive of what goes on in student assessment. Diagnostic appraisal, directed towards developing the student and contributing to his growth, can be thought of as formative assessment. Summative assessment, on the other hand, is clearly represented by terminal tests and examinations coming at the end of the student's course, or indeed by any attempt to reach an overall description or judgement of the student (e.g. in an end-of-term report or a grade or class-rank). Peter Vandome and his colleagues (1973) recognize this distinction and remind us that each is generally used (though it need not be) for a different purpose, by labelling the former 'pedagogic' and the latter 'classificatory'. In formative (pedagogic) assessment the emphasis is on potential, while in summative (classificatory) assessment it is on actual achievement.

The dynamics of assessment

In Rowntree (1974) I considered how the concepts we have been talking about flow together in a teaching situation. Figure 1 illustrates the dynamic relationships between formative assessment, formative evaluation and summative assessment. At each stage in his teaching (T) the teacher makes an assessment (A) of the student's learning which, together perhaps with non-assessment data on the effects of the teaching (N), enables him to evaluate how successfully he has taught so far (E). The assessment also helps him to diagnose (D) the new needs of the student, and diagnosis and evaluation together go to determine the purpose and nature of the next stage of the teaching (T). This 'teachmg', which may be of a few seconds' or a few weeks' duration continues until further assessment gives rise to more evaluation and diagnostic appraisal. If these essentially formative assessments are translated into grades (G) for the student and some or all of these grades are to count towards an overall summative assessment, the system may be called 'continuous assessment'. Strictly speaking it might better be described as 'continuous grading'. The student may, in addition, be given a final summative assessment (big A), perhaps taking account of some or all of the previous formative assessments as well as a special end-of-course examination assessing what he has learned over the course as a whole. He may also be given a final, overall grade (big G), made up out of some or all the grades awarded so far.

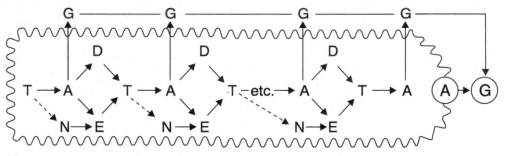

Key:

T = Teaching; A = Assessment of what the student has learned (essentially formative); N = Other data on effects of teaching; E = Evaluation of teaching effectiveness; D = Diagnostic appraisal of student's needs; G = Grade based on A; Ⓐ= Assessment of what the student has learned overall (summative); Ⓖ= Grade based on Ⓐ and previous Gs.

Figure 1   Assessment, evaluation, diagnosis, and grading

Clearly, then, the field of assessment is full of conceptual quagmires and terminological traps for the unwary or short-sighted. Further specimens will be identified later. But already we see the need for considerable circumspection when approaching the literature. We must keep asking ourselves, for instance, whether an author is talking about evaluation or assessment, informal assessment or formal, formative or summative, pedagogic or classificatory. And, if it is possible to tell which kind of assessment he is talking of, we must ask whether what he says really applies to that kind and to that kind only.

Questions of responsibility

Nor should we overlook, at a practical level, the conflict and ambivalence of purpose that can arise in a teacher as he decides what to do about the result of an assessment. Especially, he may be troubled as to how sensible it is both to evaluate the effectiveness of his own teaching and to grade the students according to what they have learned from it. Who or what is on trial? Who deserves the grade — the teacher or the student? If, in an extreme case, the teacher 'fails' his student, has the course indeed failed him or has the student failed the course? (Note, as a grim parallel, that many a terminally ill patient feels that he has 'failed' his surgeon.) Of course, when a student has been openly uninterested and has made no effort to learn, then it may be only in a weak sense that the responsibility can be laid upon the teacher rather than the student. But suppose the student has shown great interest and worked conscientiously, perhaps even learned a great deal, though not entirely what the teacher wanted him to learn, and gained personal satisfaction from his progress? Then the teacher who sees fit to penalize the student for having failed to satisfy teacher's requirements may in quite a strong sense be asked to consider that he has failed his student.

Does it matter who is 'to blame' for ineffective learning? Not much when assessment is used privately for diagnostic appraisal or evaluation and therefore benefits the student. More so, however, when assessment is done with public grading in view; for this is often not so much for the student's benefit (through discovering his learning needs and improving the teaching) as for the benefit of other people who will use it (with no thought of shared 'blame') to determine what the student's life-chances are to be.

The most casual browse through the literature of assessment is enough to establish that the vast bulk is concerned with how to use assessment for purposes of grading and ranking. Only a minuscule proportion considers how to use it to enhance the student's educational growth. This bias in the literature faithfully reflects the priorities of the education industry. As Donald McIntyre (1970) forthrightly says:

> '. . . although we spend an enormous amount of time and money on assessment, very little is obtained which helps teachers to teach. Instead, we give pupils marks or grades, that is, we concentrate on *judging* them, on saying how 'good' or 'bad' they are, on putting them in an 'order of merit'. Assessment of this . . . sort can make no contribution to effective teaching. Its function is to select pupils, gradually as they pass through our schools, for different positions in the socio-economic hierarchy of our society, positions for which we then proceed to train them.'

Such ideological interpretations can easily be attached to the grading decisions that arise out of assessment, but not so easily to diagnostic and evaluational decisions. Assessment itself can be a reasonably objective gathering of information; though, of course, some kind of subjective preference will inevitably be directing the assessor's attention to some things rather than others. But the form assessment takes, and the uses to which the gathered information is put, may vary with the assumptions that are being made about the division of responsibility in teaching and learning. Thus, 'grading' assumes that the teaching is essentially beyond reproach, and that the student is to be rewarded according to how well he has discharged his responsibility to learn from it, and that this will be revealed objectively and reliably by assessment. 'Diagnostic appraisal' makes no assumptions about the responsibility for teaching and learning; and its value-judgements about the student's apparent strengths and weaknesses and needs are not published as objective truths about the student. 'Evaluation' does tend to make assumptions about responsibility, however, and they may be quite the opposite of those made by 'grading'. Evaluation assumes that weaknesses in the student's learning may well be explicable by weaknesses in the teaching and that it is the responsibility of the teaching to change in such a way as to optimize the student's learning.

In educational practice, of course, these three attitudes to assessment often operate together. Clearly, different teachers within a teaching team may take up different stances. But even the teacher who is assessing with a view to ranking his students according to how much they have learned may be shocked into an evaluational stance if he discovers that scarcely any of them have learned anything. And, of course, a given teacher may intentionally operate with different assumptions at different times. If he slips unwittingly from one set of assumptions to another, or if he needs to co-operate with people whose assumptions he fails to recognize as being different from his, then confusion can arise.

Five dimensions of assessment

To provide a framework for our exploration of assessment, I have chosen to identify within it five dimensions. These five dimensions refer to five different kinds of mental activity among people who undertake assessment. Each kind of mental activity results in decisions being made and actions being taken. Naturally, the five dimensions correspond to what seem to me to be the key activities in the process of assessment. The questions underlying these five dimensions are as follows:

> *Why assess?* Deciding why assessment is to be carried out; what effects or outcomes it is expected to produce.

> *What to assess?* Deciding, realizing, or otherwise coming to an awareness of what one is looking for, or remarking upon, in the people one is assessing.

> *How to assess?* Selecting, from among all the means we have at our disposal for learning about people, those we regard as being most truthful and fair for various sorts of valued knowledge.

> *How to interpret?* Making sense of the outcomes of whatever observations or measurements or impressions we gather through whatever means we employ; explaining, appreciating, and attaching meaning to the raw 'events' of assessment.

How to respond? Finding appropriate ways of expressing our response to whatever has been assessed and of communicating it to the person concerned (and other people).

To put some flesh on that austere framework, let me give a couple of examples. An infants' teacher may wish to assess the developing self-confidence of a new child in her class with a view to helping him settle in; she may do this by observing the child in situations that he might see as threatening; she may interpret the behaviour she observes by comparing it with behaviour in similar situations in the past and considering what experiences have contributed to the child's growth; she may respond by encouraging the child, providing some 'growth experiences' for him, and perhaps by writing some brief diary comment. On the other hand, a secondary school mathematics teacher may wish to predict his students' chances in a public examination; he may therefore assess their ability to solve a range of problems under 'mock' examination conditions; he may interpret their performance by comparison with what he believes to be the standards of the examiners; he may respond by giving each student a grade for the examination as a whole and giving extra tuition to those students he feels are not yet ready to enter for the public examination. (He may also notice areas in which his previous teaching might have been improved.)

Some words of warning. I am not suggesting that the five dimensions will all be present in any given assessment situation — certainly not all consciously, or all in the mind of any one individual. Nor am I suggesting that those that do enter a person's mind will or should arrive in the sequence I followed in my list and examples. Nor, yet again, am I suggesting that the dimensions are clearly separable from one another or that any one of the mental activities can be carried out and 'completed' without either reference to one of the others or the need to return to it later with 'second thoughts'. In fact, as in most human information-processing, we start where our situation demands, putting the emphasis where we feel it is wanted and pursuing each activity as far as we need, returning if necessary more than once to re-cycle our earlier decisions. Thus, if a teacher is limited as to the assessment techniques he can choose among (as in the Open University where he cannot easily meet his students face-to-face), his decisions about what to assess will be highly dependent on prior decisions (and not necessarily his) about what techniques are available, rather than vice versa. But any teacher, once he has engaged with the problems of how to assess, how to interpret the outcomes and how to respond to them, is likely to see development in his views as to what should be assessed and why.

Interestingly, for the parallels between teaching and doctoring are always illuminating, the How to Assess / Interpret / Respond dimensions are very similar to what Michael Balint (1964, Preface) described as the successive phases of the *diagnostic* process in medicine — listening, understanding, and using the understanding so that it should have a therapeutic effect. That is, '"listening" provides the material which is then ordered into "understanding" . . . "using the understanding so that it should have a therapeutic effect" is tantamout to a demand for a more exacting form of diagnosis; the therapist is expected to predict with a fair amount of accuracy what sort of effect his envisaged interventions will have.' So too is the teacher.

But before we consider further the dynamics of assessment, we must consider why it is done at all. In the [next chapter] we'll examine some functions and purposes commonly ascribed to assessment. And in [the chapter after that] we'll consider some outcomes that are not so generally ascribed, or even admitted.

References

Balint M (1964) *The Doctor, his Patient and the Illness*. Pitman, London. (first published 1957).

Downey M E (1977) *Interpersonal Judgements in Education*. Harper and Row, London.

Ebel R (1972) *Essentials of Educational Measurement*. Prentice-Hall, Englewood Cliffs, New Jersey.

Gronlund N E (1971) *Measurement and Evaluation in Teaching*. Macmillan, London.

Hudson B B (1973) *Assessment Techniques*. Methuen, London.

Kandel I (1936) *Examinations and their Substitutes in the United States*. Carnegie Foundation for the Advancement of Teaching, Bulletin 28, New York.

Keddie N (1971) Classroom knowledge. In: M F D Young (ed) *Knowledge and Control*. Collier-Macmillan, London.

Lewis D G (1974) *Assessment in Education*. University of London Press, London.

McIntyre D (1970) Assessment and teaching. In: D Rubinstein and C Stoneman (eds) *Education for Democracy*, second edition, Penguin, London.

Miller R (1972) *Evaluating Faculty Performance*. Jossey-Bass, San Francisco.

Page C F (1974) *Student Evaluation of Teaching: The American Experience*. Society for Research into Higher Education, London.

Pidgeon D, Yates A (1969) *An Introduction to Educational Measurement*. Routledge and Kegan Paul, London.

Rowntree D (1974) *Educational Technology in Curriculum Development*. Harper and Row, London. (Second edition published 1982).

Schofield H (1972) *Assessment and Testing: an introduction*. Allen and Unwin, London.

Scriven M (1967) The methodology of evaluation. In: R W Tyler *et al.* (eds) *Perspectives of Curriculum Evaluation*. Rand McNally, Chicago.

Terwilliger J S (1971) *Assigning Grades to Students*. Scott, Foresman, Glenview, Illinois.

Thorndike R L (ed) (1972) *Educational Measurement* (2nd edition). American Council on Education, Washington, DC.

Thyne J M (1974) *Principles of Examining*. University of London Press, London.

Tough J (1976) *Listening to Children Talking*. Ward Lock, London.

Vandome P *et al.* (1973) Why assessment? A paper given limited circulation in the University of Edinburgh.

34. The Purposes of Assessment
Derek Rowntree

Already we have seen that assessment has several purposes — diagnosis, evaluation, grading. But these are not ends in themselves, of course. They are means towards further ends. What are those over-arching purposes? In this chapter we shall consider why assessment is carried out at all. How is it justified? (Later we must ask what else is achieved that may not be explicitly claimed for it or even welcomed by the people involved.) More ominously, we can ask the question so often posed by the sleuth in old-fashioned crime-stories when considering whom to suspect of the murder: 'Who benefits?'

In general, the beneficiaries can be seen to be the student, his teacher and 'other people' (often referred to as 'society' — chiefly comprising parents, teachers and administrators in other educational institutions, and employers). Who benefits in particular instances depends on the nature and purpose of the assessment, e.g. formal or informal, formative or summative, pedagogic or classificatory, etc. Brian Klug (1974, p. 5), in what he says 'is undoubtedly an incomplete list', has gathered together thirty-two reasons for formal assessment. Here I shall concentrate on what I see as the six main reasons commonly advanced.

1. Selection by assessment

One very common purpose of assessment is the *selection* of candidates for various kinds of educational opportunity or career. In some parts of Britain, children are still assessed at the age of '11-plus' to decide for them whether they should have a grammar school education aiming towards university and the professional life, or some other sort. Again, at 16-plus, another batch of examinations or other assessment devices acts effectively to select some students for 6th-form education, some for other less prestigious further education, and some for the world of work. The '18-plus' controls entry to university and the professions and, of course, the universities and professional bodies have their own tests to select those students who are to be awarded degrees or professional standing. Even when he is well into his working life, a person's progress is still dependent on assessment. Whether by formal interviews or less formal observation and reporting by his boss, or by the appraisal of his peers, he is selected for advancement or redundancy. Such assessment always involves some kind of grading and the putting of people into categories, even if 'Pass' and 'Fail' are the only two used.

Selection tests are probably what most people think of when they talk about assessment. Actually, it is often somewhat euphemistic to call them 'selection' tests. For the majority of candidates many such tests function rather as *rejection* tests. Thus, the 11-plus rarely selected more than 20% of the children in an area to attend the local grammar school, and thereby rejected 80%. In the U.S.A., where selection testing,

Derek Rowntree: 'The Purposes of Assessment' from *ASSESSING STUDENTS: HOW SHALL WE KNOW THEM?* (Kogan Page Ltd, 1977; 1987), pp. 15–33.

especially for college entrance, is big business and heavily bureaucraticized, Hillell Black (1963) minced no words when he called his book on the subject *They Shall Not Pass*.

Selection (and rejection) is necessary because no country believes it can afford to give every citizen all he might desire in the way of education. A basic minimum may be available for everyone, e.g. ten years of normal schooling; but anyone who wants access to additional resources may have to prove that his need, or ability to benefit, is greater than that of others. We usually identify this competition for extra resources with the scramble for places in college and university. But, at the other end of the age-range, places in 'special schools' for children with learning difficulties are also limited: not every child whose parents and teachers believe he could profit from their more costly facilities will be selected. In many developing countries, places are in short supply even for secondary education and most children will fail to be selected.

One of the assumptions implicit in selection tests for advanced education is that only the brightest, most promising, and patently talented should be funded to continue. Now it is not logically obvious that extra educational resources should go to students who are already highly accomplished rather than to those with more ground to make up. However, advanced education is largely financed in the expectation that it will produce sufficient numbers of people capable of carrying out complex tasks in society — doctors, lawyers, engineers, etc. — and with the minimum investment of resources. To select students by lottery from among all interested candidates would clearly be egalitarian, and many students might gain entry and do well who would, at present, be considered too weak for selection. But such students might also make disproportionate demands on the teaching resources available, causing a reduction in the total number of 'capable persons' that could be produced.

Selection of 'students most likely to succeed' usually depends on public examinations. Since the Chinese invented them (before Europe had even evolved the feudal system) they have done something (though far less than as is usually assumed) to preserve some opportunities for talented children from poor families that might otherwise go to less promising children from richer homes. Essentially, selectors assume that the students who perform best in current examinations are those who would become most capable as a result of further educational investment. This is open to question, however: 'Correlation between GCE examinations and University examinations are, in general, low. . . . Whatever may be the value of the GCE 'A'-level examination as a school-leaving examination, as a basis for student selection for the University it has serious shortcomings' (Nicholson and Galambos, 1960). Comparisons of 'A'-level grades and degree class have rarely shown much of a correlation: see, for example, Petch (1961), Barnett and Lewis (1963), Nisbet and Welsh (1966), and UCCA (1969) which reports correlation coefficients between final degree and three 'A'-level results of between $r=0.33$ (engineering) and $r=0.17$ (social sciences). Such low correlations would suggest that less than 11% of the variation in university success can be 'explained' by variation in academic attainment at the time of entry. Perhaps such factors as personality and motivation may have as much or more influence on success in higher education (see Holland, 1960; Wankowski, 1970). For instance, medical students with poorer entry qualifications but with concern and empathy for ordinary people may emerge as better general practitioners than academic high-fliers who may feel they have failed if they do not get to be specialists or researchers. Of course every profession needs some reasonable level of academic performance from its would-be entrants. But there is little doubt that this level could, without detriment, be significantly lower than it is today if more serious attempts were made to assess interests and motivation and other personal qualities in applicants.

Assessment results are also used in selection for job and career opportunities. This is especially true of summative assessments at the end of a student's school or college career, or at the end of a period of professional training. In the absence of any thorough research, our knowledge of how employers actually use this assessment data is patchy and impressionistic (see Cox and Collins, 1975). Clearly, many use it as a screening device. That is, a candidate won't be looked at or even encouraged to apply unless he can offer a degree, or two 'A'-levels, or five 'O'-levels (including maths and English), or whatever is the going rate. This may be administratively convenient in cutting down the number of applicants. Again there may be a superstitious belief that the required qualifications betoken some kind of general quality of mind or spirit that will be useful to the employer. He may unconsciously be echoing the assumptions made by Lord Macaulay in defending the use of academic examinations to select administrators for the India Civil Service:

> 'Whatever be the languages — whatever be the sciences, which it is, in any age or country, the fashion to teach, those who become the greatest proficients in those languages and those sciences, will generally be the flower of youth — the most acute — the most industrious — the most ambitious of honourable distinctions.' (quoted in Keith, 1961, pp. 252–3)

Admittedly, a reverse tendency may sometimes operate here among many employers, perhaps based on more than superstition, to view 'the flower of youth' as being *less* useful in that they may think they 'know it all' and so object to undergoing further training.

As a pamphlet produced jointly by Army personnel staff and British Airways Staff College points out, there is a tendency to use examination results, so conveniently and effortlessly available, 'without due regard to their relevance. It is a safe bet that most entry qualifications expressed in terms of exam performance are the result of armchair deliberations rather than empirical investigation' (Kilcross and Bates, 1975). Even within education itself the respect paid by employers to qualifications (and other previous experience) is arbitrary and often capricious. Thus English schoolteachers start higher up the salary scale and enjoy better promotion prospects if they have a degree, regardless of the subject studied and whether or not it has any bearing on their work with children.

Again, too, universities are sometimes accused of encouraging 'qualifications for qualifications' sake' — perhaps as a means of ensuring a continuing market for their 'product'. Here the critic might point at the 'academic inflation' that results when universities begin to encourage their graduates to take up work that was not formerly done by graduates, and then infiltrate more and more graduates into that area until it eventually becomes spoken of as a 'graduate profession' and a degree becomes an *essential* entry qualification. Business management and accountancy and law appear to be heading in this direction. Ronald Dore (1976) gives many further examples. Having examined numerous career guides published since the beginning of the century, he sees their emphasis 'slowly shifting from personal aptitudes to quantitatively measurable educational achievement' (p. 24). The 'institutionalizing' of professional education has resulted in fewer and fewer opportunities for young people to work their way up from artisan to professional status (e.g. as an engineer) by 'learning on the job'. Consequently, employers are having to put more and more faith in certificates and diplomas awarded on the basis of other people's assessments.

Clearly there is no way of comparing the success in a job of people with qualifications and people without them if, in fact, the latter group were rejected as candidates. However, there is little evidence of a close connection between high educational qualifications and success in later life. In the U.S.A., for example, Donald Hoyt (1965) reviewed 46 studies of the relationship between college grades and subsequent achievement, only to conclude that 'present evidence strongly suggests that college grades bear little or no relationship to any measures of adult achievement'. Even medical school grades appear not to predict future proficiency as a general practitioner (see Taylor *et al*, 1965). The statistical investigations of Ivar Berg (1973) confirm that the variety of academic achievement among people doing the same job and earning the same rewards is as great as it is between people doing different jobs; and in some cases, selling insurance for instance, people with least education but most experience perform best. Fewer such studies have been carried out in Britain, but Liam Hudson (1966a) examined the degree-class gained by each of a large sample of distinguished scientists, politicians and judges, concluding that 'there was evidence of some slight relation between eminence and degree-class, but it was far from clear-cut and there were many striking exceptions'. For instance, more than half of High Court judges, and a third of Fellows of the Royal Society, had gained only second-, third- or fourth-class degrees. Is it the case that a person's job experience and achievements *since* gaining his qualifications generally assume far more relevance and significance in selection for later career opportunities? The suggestion made in recent years that a degree should carry an expiry-date, with the warning that its validity is not guaranteed beyond that time, would then be almost superfluous.

Nevertheless, most people still do need the ritual assessment 'qualifications' if they are to get started at all. It is not their fault if selectors place more trust than is justified in such credentials and then ludicrously over-generalize in ascribing qualities and special status to the possessor. Although Dave and Hill (1974)are talking about effects of school-leaving examinations in a developing country, India, are things so different in the West?

> 'A person's standing in the examinations affects many aspects of his life. Not only is it a basis of his economic success, but it affects his prestige in his family and his (or her) value in the 'marriage market'. The examinations thus form the basis of a kind of educational caste system, superimposed on the traditional caste system of the country.'

2. Maintaining standards

Closely related to the selection-purpose is this second purpose, but it has a life of its own. Teachers would probably still feel obliged to assess for this purpose even if they thought it immoral or impolitic to disclose individual results to outsiders. The clientele is broadly the same — employers and the 'invisible college' of academics in other institutions who must be assured that some form of 'quality-control' is in operation and that the people being certified this year are of pretty much the same standard as those certified last year and five years ago, and so on. Standards-oriented assessment can also be of interest to any administrators who want to 'keep tabs' on teachers.

As with purpose 1, the student is a secondary beneficiary insofar as he wants to be assured of the acceptability, almost literally 'the value' of his certificate. As one science student put it, rather more extremely than most would, in a debate reported by Ellsworth-Jones (1974): 'What matters to me is the job I get when I leave here. When I get a degree I want to know that employers will think it's worth something.'

Many difficulties attend the attempt to maintain standards. It is difficult enough to get teachers to agree on what the standard is or should be — whether, for example, the criterion is to be content covered, skills acquired, original knowledge created, attitudes expressed, none of these, or some of these and others in variously contested proportions. Discussions of standards easily degenerate into cliches, stereotypes and confident half-truths like 'the first-class mind proclaims itself'. Certainly one cannot judge the standard of, say, an examination paper simply by looking at the questions. One also needs to know what the markers accept as a satisfactory response. (For example, the spoof question-paper printed on [p. 136] may appear quite stiff; but for all we know the candidate has merely to write his name correctly on the answer-paper to score the 85% pass-mark). When the argument does come down to cases, in the analysis of a student's work, there is typically considerable disagreement (though surmountable by consent) among any group of assessors as to just what standard the student has attained.

The difficulties are compounded when the content of the curriculum is changing. This year's students may be assessed on areas of knowledge quite different from those of a year or so ago, even though the 'subject' is nominally the same. Inevitably then, it is quite impossible to establish the equivalence of standards between subjects and institutions. It makes no sense to ask whether the standard reached by physicists labelled 'second-class' in a given university or school is 'really' the same as that reached by 'second-class' historians, mathematicians and musicologists in the same institution in the same year, let alone in other institutions in other years. In fact, one simply has to take it as axiomatic that the 'quality-controllers' in various subject areas will be equally stringent in bestowing their approval on students. (Though one might still speculate as to what happens in universities to result in subjects like law and mathematics 'approving' (i.e. producing) a much smaller proportion of 'good' degrees than subjects like psychology and zoology, despite the fact that they start off with a far higher proportion of students entering with particularly high 'A'-level grades.) Whatever it means in terms of standards, the approval bestowed tends to operate, as Jonathan Warren (1971) has suggested, 'like a set of recommendations to an exclusive club written by long-term members who know the kind of people the other club-members prefer'.

Even within a subject, the standards being maintained are more probably standard assessment procedures rather than standard attainments. Indeed, there is a distinct possibility that standard procedures — especially if they include awarding a *fixed* proportion of As, Bs, etc. — may fail to acknowledge changes in level of attainment. Stuart Miller (1967) quotes statistics showing that even though the quality of students entering the University of California at Berkeley increased considerably between 1947 and 1960 (as measured by three different pre-entry criteria) their grade-point-averages in university remained precisely the same. Nearer home, in a letter to *The Times* (October 9th, 1972), Professor I. H. Mills argues that 'what we demand for "A"-level examinations in many subjects today is the same standard that was expected for final degree examinations thirty years ago'. Nor have the higher standards required of entrants to British universities in recent years been reflected in a proportionate increase in the 'good degrees' awarded. The standard of 'output' is maintained *despite* an apparent improvement in the standard of 'input'.

3. Motivation of students

After two assessment purposes whose benefits appear to be mainly administrative and go chiefly to people outside the immediate teacher-student relationship, this third purpose seems to be more educational and more related to the present needs of the student. With motivation we are talking of using assessment — e.g. homework assignments, weekly quizzes, classroom questioning, project reports, examinations, etc. — in order to encourage the student to learn. Many students would endorse this purpose. For instance, the male undergraduate quoted by Gerda Siann and Kate French (1975):

> 'The idea of Edinburgh University becoming a three-year holiday camp, all expenses paid, galls me, and I am reactionary enough to believe that the 'threat' of exams (i.e. the inherent threat of failure and becoming an outcast) is the only reason that the library doormats are cleaned.'

Though it must be noted that for every student who confesses himself in need of a constant prod from assessment there will be another who claims to be distracted and enervated by it. Whether we believe that such students are to be confirmed in these attitudes — or whether the former should be 'educated' to get on by himself without such constant stimulus and the latter 'educated' to come to terms with the need to periodically review his progress through others' eyes — may affect how we classify the use of assessment in particular cases.

However, we must also recognize that 'motivational' assessment could be used to benefit the teacher rather than the student. In effect, by structuring the student's allocation of time and effort, by legitimizing certain kinds of activity and outlawing others, by indicating what is to count as knowledge worth having and what is not, 'motivational assessment' can define the reality of academic life for the student and give the teacher control over his perceptions and behaviour. To be blunt, assessment can be used as an instrument of coercion, as a means of getting students to do something they might not otherwise be inclined to do — especially if unfavourable assessments can have unpleasant consequences. Thus, R. L. Bowley (1967) gives teachers a tip for a practice that sounds alarmingly like extortion:

> 'Occasionally it may be desirable to ask a class to make an especially hard effort when tackling a set piece of work. A simple but useful device to encourage this is to raise the total out of which the work is to be marked and inform the class accordingly beforehand. For example, if it is customary to mark out of a total of twenty, the raising of this figure to thirty will often have the desired effect.' (p. 116)

Some teachers consider it as much a necessary part of their duties to supply students with motivation as it is to supply them with objectives and structured lessons. Even though they may believe it to be in the students' long-term interest to achieve the objectives, they believe the students cannot be expected to recognize this and so provide self-motivation. Thus, assessment (in the form of quizzes, exams, etc.) may be used as one side of a carrot-stick inducement-system (the other side being represented by 'trying to make it as interesting as possible', audio-visual 'treats', etc.). The fervour with which this particular stick is waved can perhaps be seen as gradually increasing after the student's infant school years and reaching its peak in his later secondary school and college years.

But the line between coercion and encouragement is hard to draw. Much must depend on the intentions and perceptions of teacher and student and the relationship between them. Consider the teacher whose aim is for the student to become autonomous enough to develop his *own* goals and learning strategies. Even he may feel that the student's motivation will be all the better for some external stimulus from assessment. After all, many such a teacher, while valuing his own freedom to decide how he spends his time, will admit how the occasional deadline or external stimulus, like the imminent need to deliver a lecture, or prepare a report for a committee, or finish the next chapter of a book he is writing with a colleague, can concentrate and energize his activities. So too he is likely to encourage his students to work towards targets and deadlines, and public commitments — preferably ones they have identified and thought through themselves before agreeing them in discussion with him.

4. Feedback to students

It is necessary to distinguish between the motivating effect of knowing that you are to be assessed and the quite different sort of motivation resulting from knowing how you performed on the assessment exercise. The latter is much more clearly perceivable by students as being meant to help them learn. The student stands to benefit educationally from his tutor's response to what he has produced. In his study of the reactions of San Francisco teenage gang members to assessment, Carl Werthman (1963) quotes a student describing how he worked at getting more helpful feedback than is contained in a grade:

> 'After we got our compositions back I went up to him you know. I asked him about my composition. I got a D over F and I ask him what I did wrong. He told me that he could tell by the way I write that I could do

379

better than what I did. And he explained it to me and he showed me what I need to improve. And he showed me, if I correct my paper, I would get a D, a straight D instead of that F. O.K. And I got the D for half the work. But any way he showed me how I could get a regular D and pass his class. I mean I feel like that teacher was helping me.'

Feedback, or 'knowledge of results', is the life-blood of learning. Having said or done something of significance — whether a physical action, a comment in conversation, or an essay in an examination — the student wants to know how it is received. He wishes to know whether he communicated what he intended to communicate, whether what he said seemed right or wrong, appropriate or inappropriate, useful or irrelevant to his audience. And he may need a response fairly rapidly if it is to confirm or modify his present understanding or approach. Effective feedback enables the student to identify his strengths and weaknesses and shows him how to improve where weak or build upon what he does best.

Feedback from assessment comes in many forms, of varying degrees of usefulness (see Sassenrath and Garverick, 1965). In its least useful form it comes as a mark or grade. The student may be told his work has earned a C or 55% or 6 out of 10. This may give him some hint as to whether or not his teacher thinks he is making progress. That is, he may be able to compare this grade or mark with those he has earned on similar assessment previously. But, of course, it is very non-specific. It tells him neither what he has done to merit such a mark nor what he could do to earn a better one. Such non-specific feedback becomes increasingly useless to the student as the size and diversity of the performance being assessed increases. Thus a grade for a single essay gives little enough information, but to be given merely an overall grade for, say, an examination in which several essays were written leaves the student uncertain even whether he did equally well on all essays or whether some were thought atrocious and some brilliant.

Institutions often find it administratively convenient not to give students feedback about individual answers in an examination. Very often the marked papers are not even returned to students. Only a few years ago, Hilda Himmelweit (1967) reported that 'In the University of London, the teacher is even *forbidden* to inform the student of his performance in the different subjects in Part I, at the very time when he has to select his major subjects for Part II.' This may save a lot of arguments about the fairness or otherwise of the marking, but it is also to neglect a valuable educational opportunity. Even in continuous assessment, feedback on answers may be withheld, as sometimes happens in the Open University, so as to economize on question-writing by using the same questions again on subsequent students. Inadequate feedback can indicate that the assessment is serving the interests of people other than the students.

Another kind of feedback the student may obtain, sometimes instead of a grade or mark, is knowledge of whether he has passed or failed. Or, more widely, whether or not he has reached some standard. If he has some conception of what knowledge or skill is required to meet this standard, then a pass will tell him that he has achieved them. It will not tell him how or in what way he may have over-achieved, of course. Similarly, to be told he has failed will not tell him what particular aspects of the required performance he is deficient in. Interestingly enough, people who fail a driving test are given more information about their faults and where improvement is needed than are students who do poorly in the educational examinations (CSE or GCE) at the end of their school careers.

Again, whether instead of marks or grades or as well as, a student may be given a rank. He may be told that his performance puts him third from top of the class or into the bottom 10% of his age group. The student can gain little from this sort of feedback: unless he knows what sort of performance the reference group has put up, he won't be able to judge his own either. Is he third-best of a bad bunch or is he in the bottom 10% of an excelling group? More generally, merely to be told he is better or worse than certain others tells him nothing at all about whether he is better or worse than he himself has been or would wish to be, let alone in which particulars.

Feedback from assessment only begins to be useful when it includes *verbal comments*. The teacher who has made the assessment needs to verbalize his reactions to the student's performance, saying which aspects strike him as strong, weak, or simply interesting. Ideally, he should give whatever suggestions he can to help the student improve. This kind of feedback flows out from diagnostic appraisal. Even the briefest of comments, e.g. 'A well-argued essay in the main, but what evidence are your third and fourth conclusions based on?', can be more helpful to the student than a C or a 65% if we want him to learn from considering his performance again in the light of our reaction. Research has confirmed (see Page, 1958) that students who are given individualized verbal comments on their work, incorporating suggestions for improvement, do tend to 'improve' significantly more than students who are given standard comments (e.g. 'poor', 'average', 'good, 'excellent') or grades.

Robert Birney (1964) found that college students were agreeable to frequent assessment — so long as it was 'in language they understand'. That is, not in grades or marks, which told them nothing specific about their strengths and weaknesses, but in detailed verbal commentary. If the information fed back is really intended to contribute to the student's growth it must tell him either that he has already achieved what he was trying to achieve or else must enable him to take some further action towards achieving it. Even in the former case it may be able to indicate possible *new* objectives and ways of approaching them. Useful feedback then is more to be expected from formative assessment than from summative. However, apart from the demands of common courtesy, any examiners who subscribe to the ideal of 'continuing education' should ponder the waste of not giving the student a detailed analysis of how he has performed at the climax of his formal education. They might consider also the ethics of involving the student in what may be a nerve-racking assessment experience that yet leaves him no wiser as to who he is and what he can do. It is in such a milieu that the student can be asked, 'What did you get out of this course?', and reply in all seriousness, 'I got a B' (see Kirchenbaum *et al.*, 1971).

Of course, feedback need not be supplied directly by a teacher. For many students, their first experience of sustained feedback has come from programmed texts. In such texts, the author can weave into his line of argument occasional questions requiring the student to use the ideas that have been introduced so far. Having come up with his own answer to these self-assessment questions, the student reads on to compare it with the answer given and explained by the author. Thus the student is constantly informed as to how well he is learning and the assessment comes frequently enough for him to correct any significant misunderstandings as soon as they occur.

But nor does feedback have to be verbal. The teacher's smiles or scowls, the colleague's mirth or laudatory silences can have a shaping influence on the student's behaviour. Sometimes the student will get his feedback from pictures, e.g. when drawing graphs or envisaging the landscape depicted by a map. Sometimes real events will provide the feedback, e.g. when the screaming of his car's gears tells the driver that he has not got the feel of the clutch or when the smell from the test-tube indicates that the student has applied too much heat.

Such indirect kinds of assessment can be seen as steps towards *self*-assessment. Increasingly, if the student is to become capable of learning to work for his own satisfaction rather than for the approval of his teacher, he must assume responsibility for providing his own feedback. He must be weaned off dependence on others for knowledge of how well he is doing. This demands that he be encouraged to recognize and internalize rules and standards and strategies whereby he may test the validity of his own responses.

5. Feedback to the teacher

Just as assessment may give the student feedback as to how well he has learned, so too it may give the teacher feedback as to how well he has taught. This is how assessment contributes to course evaluation. Insofar as the assessment data reveal strengths and weaknesses in the student's learning, the teacher may be able to identify where he has failed to explain a new concept, confused an issue, given insufficient practice, and so on. Knowing where and how his students have had difficulty may enable him now to teach so as to remedy the situation.

At times, however, e.g. in end-of-course examinations, the teacher may get this feedback too late for him to be able to use it for the educational benefit of the students who provided it. He may use it, instead, to report on their achievements. He may also use it to modify his teaching for the benefit of *subsequent* students. Thus, some assessment can have as its purpose feedback to the teacher but without feedback to the student also being intended.

One of the great weaknesses of externally marked examinations like GCE is that the teacher normally gets no feedback as to the strengths and weaknesses demonstrated by his students. He thus has no means of knowing which of his prior teaching interventions have borne fruit and which have not. Were this evidence available, it might enable him to improve as a teacher.

6. Preparation for life

Some teachers would wish to justify assessment on the grounds that it reflects, and therefore prepares students for, 'real life'. Let us note, in passing, how odd it is to imply a distinction between the student's educational career and his real life. Education is *part* of his life, and an increasingly large part. Unavoidably, it may also in some sense prepare him for that part of real life which it is not. But this does not imply that education, or, to be exact, the people who control aims and objectives in education, should take the predicted real life for granted and merely train the student to 'cope'. Educationally, it would be equally valid, perhaps more so, to provide a counter-curriculum that might enable the student to challenge or ignore the pressures of 'real life'. Such an argument can be heard, for example, from teachers concerned about the power of commercial pop-culture.

How far is educational assessment a preparation? Certainly much of the *informal* assessment that goes on in school and college is related to the mainly informal assessment that goes on in the rest of life. Approbation and criticism (verbal or non-verbal) from teachers and fellow-students are not dissimilar to what the student will meet from parents, workmates and friends. But it is probably not this informal kind of assessment that teachers see as the life-preparer. Those who do see assessment as a preparation are most likely thinking of the competitive system of public examination, grading, and ranking. Such experience is thought to prepare students for the life-struggle in general and career advancement in particular. The thoughts of Luther Evans (1942, p. 59) are representative: 'A student who completes a programme of higher education without facing the rigorous evaluations of a grading system has missed one great chance to learn the helpful lesson that life is full of tests and trials.' An even more emphatic statement has been made by the 'Black Papers' author, Brian Cox (1971): 'All life depends on passing exams. . . . To create an education system without examinations is to fail to prepare children and students for the realities of adult life.' Let's hope they are not thinking of the 'rigorous evaluations' and 'realities' evoked by Norman Russell's poem:

End of a Semester

This is the week of tests the season of fear
everywhere the running the typing the scritch scratch
shuffling of papers the door and the people
coming going looking for the symbols
looking for the little symbols written on the papers
stuck with tape to doors and walls
this is the week of the fearhope swallowed in the stomach
a time of livingdying a time of cominggoing
a time of inbetween the things one cannot grasp
too fast too fast we never sleep
we only keep ongoing.

and somewhere someone in a great office
pushing buttons marking papers calling telephones
we think a devil who we cannot see is laughing

and all the things we knew were true
will never do will never do
we all are weak we all are strong
the days are long the days are long

this is the week of tests the season of fear
somewhere we think a devil who we cannot see is laughing.

Norman Russell (1966)

Fortunately, life outside education is not really like that. With the exception perhaps of the civil service and the armed forces, most people seldom ever again meet the experience of being tested or examined on prescribed syllabuses for the purpose of being graded and ranked and chosen. Assessment in industry and the professions is generally informal, diffuse, *ad hoc* and continuous. It is based largely on the person's 'track record' over a *period* of time and in fulfilling his duties rather than on what he can write about something at a given *point* in time. Nor is such assessment quantitative in any simple way. The candidate for, say, a high academic post may be chagrined to find that his thirty published papers do not win him preferment over another candidate whose output is thought more significant even though his papers number only three!

As things are now, competitive public assessment does prepare for future job-competition — in the sense that success in previous competitions is normally demanded as an entry qualification for further competition. But this is an artefact of the system and, even if such competition were regarded as reasonable (e.g. on the grounds of greater efficiency, maximization of output, etc.), we have no means of knowing whether people excluded at earlier stages might not have proved 'winners' if allowed to 'work their way up' through the lower reaches of their chosen profession (see Dore, 1976). There is, of course, enough evidence of 'late developers', and of people unexpectedly 'finding themselves' in a situation where they were called upon to draw on unsuspected powers and grow into the job, to make us suspect the efficiency as well as the ethics of competitive elimination from further competition. But even if such people are held to be exceptions, there is still reason to doubt whether any but the winners benefit from preparation. The losers, through loss of self-respect and reduced optimism may be *less* prepared to face up confidently to subsequent life-struggles. Even with dogs, as Scott (1972) observes: 'In a test set up so that one dog can do it and another can barely succeed, the initial difference in hereditary ability may not be great. However, the dog which fails soon stops trying, while the one which succeeds becomes more highly motivated with each success. It keeps on trying and succeeding at more and more complicated problems so that in the end the hereditary difference has been immensely magnified' (p. 132).

There is a growing feeling among teachers that education should no longer meekly accept that society must necessarily be competitive. Many recognize the emerging need for people to share and collaborate rather than seek maximum personal and material advantage. They would not see eliminative assessment as a preparation for this kind of co-operative living. Nevertheless, it might still be argued that people will always be competing, if not with somebody then with some*thing* — the soil, the weather, disease, poor housing — and so on. Some such competition, together with the attendant storm and stress, might widely be agreed to be an inescapable component of 'real life'. But one could accept that education could reasonably be expected to help students prepare for it, without accepting that the appropriate means must be to promote interpersonal competition in school.

Naturally, teachers who see the student's future in terms of his being externally assessed in competition with others rarely extol the preparatory virtues of *self*-assessment. Insofar as schooling does give the student opportunities to develop criteria for assessing himself and encourages him to take decisions based on his assessments, it will be 'preparing' him for a life in which he expects to have some control over his own destiny. There is considerable lip-service paid to the ideal of self-assessment, but the practice very often belies or trivializes the intent. Students may, for example, be 'trusted' to mark their own work — but using teacher's criteria as to what counts as 'good' work. They may be asked to assess their own progress during a term or over a course using whatever criteria seem appropriate to them — but their assessments are not allowed to influence the overall report that is given them. They are asked to choose which subjects to specialize in (e.g. Arts vs. Sciences) at an early age, without ever having been helped to develop relevant criteria for assessing their own strengths and weakness in relation to the various courses of action open to them. Obviously, self-assessment cannot be a preparation for anything, not even for further self-assessment, unless it is supported by open access to relevant information, unless the results of the assessment are regarded as significant and actionable, and unless the person assessing himself is to be allowed responsibility for the outcomes of his own judgements and decisions.

Balancing the purposes

I have outlined six broad categories of purpose in educational assessment. They are not entirely without overlap and we might possibly need a seventh 'miscellaneous' category to catch a few more purposes that are less commonly spoken of. Even so, we have seen more than enough to suggest that the teacher who pauses to ask why he is assessing has plenty to think about. How does he, in fact, thread his way through the various potentially conflicting purposes and what determines his personal intentions?

The teacher's use of assessment will be heavily influenced by the expectations of the teaching system within which he is working. But his attitudes to assessment will largely depend on his ideas as to what teaching and learning and knowledge and education are all about. That is, on his professional world-view, or what some sociologists (see Esland, 1972) call his *pedagogic paradigm*. Different teachers can be seen, for instance, as taking up different positions along a continuum whose opposite extremes are labelled by writers using such terms as closed vs. open (Bernstein, 1971); manipulative vs. facilitative (Rowntree, 1975); or transmission vs. interpretation (Barnes, 1976).

To put it crudely, one end of the continuum tends to attract the teacher whose first loyalty is to a public corpus of pre-existing knowledge on expertise (which he knows everyone ought to acquire) and the need to 'get it across' to a succession of students who learn, as far as their limited capacity and motivation will allow, by absorbing and reproducing the products of other people's experience. The other end of the continuum attracts the teacher who distrusts generalizations about what everyone ought to know, and who, believing people to have unlimited potential for growth unless 'discouraged', gives his first loyalty to individual students and encourages them to exercise their own developing motivation and sense of purpose in mastering cognitive and affective capacities, making their own meaning and creating new knowledge out of their own ideas and experiences. The paradigm with which a particular teacher operates will rarely be so extreme, of course. Although most of his or her paradigm may consist of beliefs and assumptions from one end of the continuum, it is likely to be tempered with more moderate beliefs. Of the two extreme paradigms indicated, the former is more likely to be found in secondary schools, the latter in infant schools; perhaps also the latter paradigm is more typical of arts-based subjects than science-based subjects, and more typical of women than men.

In the paragraph above, I mentioned only a few of the kinds of belief and assumption that go to make up a teacher's pedagogic paradigm. What if we go on to consider beliefs relevant to student assessment? We may decide that teachers attracted towards one end of the continuum may be more inclined to see assessment as an objective and accurate means of determining a student's present achievement and future potential, thus legitimizing selection and special treatment; and, insofar as students are aware that many are called but few are chosen, as a powerful device for reinforcing teacher's control over the wayward and idle. Conversely, teachers attracted to the other end of the continuum may tend to see assessment primarily as a means of developing the relationship between the student, themselves and the subject matter, by giving both the student and themselves more information about the present state of the student's understandings; but as incapable of providing valid information about the student to outside parties or about his long-term potential to anyone at all. Various belief-systems and attitudes will emerge as we push deep into the undergrowth of assessment. As I have indicated, we can look for them to tie in and be consistent with other aspects of the way the teacher sees education — his pedagogic paradigm.

Looking back over this chapter, it would appear that the 'purposes' I have discussed are those ascribed to assessment by the actions of *teachers*. Perhaps this is not surprising. It is, after all, teachers rather than students who develop the rules of the game and tell us what it is supposed to be achieving. Maybe in the [next chapter], where we look at some of the *unintended* effects of assessment, we shall catch a glimpse of the purposes that *students* ascribe to assessment by the ways they use it.

References

Barnes D (1976) *From Communication to Curriculum*. Penguin, London.

Barnett V D, Lewis T (1963) A study of the relationship between GCE and degree results. In: *Journal of the Royal Statistical Society*, 126: Series A (General), pp. 187–226.

Berg I (1973) *Education and Jobs: The Great Training Robbery* (first published 1970). Penguin, London.

Bernstein B (1971) Open schools, open society. In: Cosin B R *et al.* (eds) *School and Society: A Sociological Reader*. Routledge and Kegan Paul, London.

Black H (1963) *They Shall Not Pass*. Morrow. New York.

Bowley R L (1967) *Teaching Without Tears*. Centaur, London.

Cox C B (1971) In praise of examinations. In: C B Cox and A E Dyson (eds) *The Black Papers on Education*, pp. 71–77. Davis-Poynter, London.

Cox G, Collins H (1975) 'Arts assessment: who cheats and who cares?' In: *Assessment in Higher Education*, pp. 13–34, Vol. 1, No. 1, September 1975.

Dave R H, Hill W H (1974) Educational and social dynamics of the examination system in India. In: *Comparative Education Review*, pp. 24–38, Vol. 18, No. 1, February 1974.

Dore R (1976) *The Diploma Disease*. Allen and Unwin, London.

Ellsworth-Jones W (1974) How to fail an exam and become a martyr. In: *The Sunday Times*, 3 November 1974.

Esland G *et al.* (1972) *The Social Organization of Teaching and Learning*, Units 5–8 in Course E282, Open University Press, Bletchley, England.

Evans L D (1942) *The Essentials of Liberal Education*. Ginn, Boston.

Himmelweit H (1967) Towards a rationalization of examination procedures. In: *Universities Quarterly*, pp. 359–372, June 1967.

Holland J L (1960) The prediction of college grades from personality and aptitude variables. In: *Journal of Educational Psychology*, pp. 245–254, Vol. 51, October 1960.

Hoyt D P (1965) *The Relationship Between College Grades and Adult Achievement*. American College Testing Program, Iowa City.

Hudson I (1970) *Frames of Mind*. Penguin, London.

Keith A B (1961) *Speeches and Documents on Indian Policy 1750–1921*. Oxford University Press, Oxford.

Kilcross M C, Bates W T G (1975) *Selecting the Younger Trainee*. HMSO, London.

Kirchenbaum H, Napier R, Simon S (1971) *Wad-ja-get? The Grading Game in American Education*. Hart, New York.

Klug B (1974) *Pro Profiles*. NUS Publications, London.

Miller S (1967) *Measure, Number and Weight: A Polemical Statement of the College Grading Problem*, Learning Research Center, University of Tennessee.

Nicholson R J, Galambos P (1960) *Performance in GCE A-Level Exams and University Exams*. Occasional papers of the Institute of Education, University of Hull.

Nisbet J, Welsh J (1966) Predicting student performance. In: *Universities Quarterly*, 20 September 1966.

Petch J A (1961) *GCE and Degree*. Joint Matriculation Board, Manchester.

Rowntree D (1975) Two styles of communication and their implications for learning. In: J Baggaley *et al.* (eds) *Aspects of Educational Technology*, pp. 281–293, VIII. Pitman, London.

Russell N H (1966) End of a semester. In: *American Association of University Professors Bulletin*, p. 414, Winter 1966.

Sassenrath J M, Garverick C M (1965) Effects of differential feedback from examinations on retention and transfer. In: *Journal of Educational Psychology*, pp. 259–263, Vol. 56, No. 5.

Siann G, French K (1975) Edinburgh students' views on continuous assessment. In: *Durham Research Review*, pp. 1064–1070, 7, Autumn 1975.

Taylor C G, Price P B, Richards J M, Jacobsen T L (1965) An investigation of the criterion problem for a group of medical general practitioners. In: *Journal of Applied Psychology*, pp. 399–406, 49(6).

UCCA (1969) *The Sixth Report: Statistical Supplement 1967–68*. Universities Central Council on Admissions, Cheltenham.

Wankowski J A (1920) *GCEs and Degrees*. University of Birmingham.

Warren E J (1971) *College Grading Practices: An Overview*. ERIC Clearning House on Higher Education, Washington, DC.

Werthman C (1963) Delinquents in schools: a test for the legitimacy of authority. Reprinted in Cosin B R *et al*. (1971) *School and Society*, Routledge and Kegan Paul, London.

35. Assessment of Competence in Clinical Practice — A Review of the Literature

Elizabeth A. Girot

Continuous practical assessments for those programmes leading to registration began to be introduced in the UK in the late 1970s and were generally hailed, certainly by educationalists, as being a much more valid, reliable and realistic method of assessment (Quinn, 1989). However, now, with the increasing pressures on the role of the ward manager, the introduction of supernumerary status for learner nurses and shorter clinical placements, it could be argued that continuous practical assessment is in great danger of becoming no assessment at all. The extent to which experienced nurses are able to supervise and give the continued feedback on learners' progress that was considered such a significant improvement on the previous systems of assessments is questioned.

On examination of the literature, consideration will be given to how experienced nurses measure and help others measure performance. The tools practitioners use to assist them in forming their judgements need to be examined. Are practitioners concerned with students' successful completion of tasks or do they rely on intuitive judgements in the complexity of the 'real life' situation? If intuitive judgements are involved, do they have any foundations, or are they concerned with mere random form completion and personality measures?

In particular examination will be made of the various measurement tools available and different approaches to the assessment of competency in the 'real world' of nursing practice. Since the United Kingdom Central Council (UKCC) formally introduced the Nurses' Rules (Nurses, Midwives and Health Visitors Act 1979) in 1983, all courses throughout the UK, leading to registration had to begin to formally prepare students to work towards the achievement of the identified competencies. A 'competent practitioner' began to become the focus of assessment in nurse education (Quinn, 1989). This begs the question of what is meant by the term competence and how it can be assessed, especially at different levels of development.

Competency

The literature in relation to the term competency, certainly appears confusing and contradictory, the term being described as overdefined rather than ill defined. Furthermore, the uncertainty about definition seems to have been heightened by the growing concern to find ways of assessing it (Runciman, 1990). Miller *et al.* (1988) suggest two senses in which competence can be defined. Firstly, competence equating with performance, describing the ability to perform nursing tasks, and competence as a 'psychological construct' evaluating students' abilities to integrate cognitive,

Elizabeth A. Girot: 'Assessment of Competence in Clinical Practice — A Review of the Literature' in *NURSE EDUCATION TODAY* (1993), 13, pp. 83–90. Reprinted by permission of the publisher Churchill Livingstone.

affective and psychomotor skills when delivering nursing care. Whilst Runciman (1990) recognises the difficulty in observing this psychological construct, she suggests that it can be seen through the individual's competent performance. Therefore, the two senses are not mutually exclusive. The level of the students' performance is dependent on the development of their psychological construct (Miller *et al.* 1988).

Evaluation of student performance indeed seems a complex one. However, the literature suggests that, in the past, the assessment of practice has been offered little priority by those assessing and can be irrelevant to and estranged from practice (Darbyshire, 1990). Now, with a move towards preparing all first level nurses to either diploma or graduate status, in order to acquire CNAA validation, clear criteria and standards for clinical assessment must be set by the academic validating body in collaboration with employers (Runciman, 1990).

From a fragmented system of assessment throughout the UK before 1983, the UKCC competency statements, enabled the UK to work as a whole towards similar achievements. However, these statements are broad and appear to relate to the development of problem-solving skills and do not address the question of different levels of competence. In the USA, Benner (1984) defines levels of practice from novice or beginner nurses, to experts who have a deep background understanding and an intuitive grasp of situations. Competence, for Benner, consists of conscious, deliberate planning, where the nurse sets priorities and is efficient and effective in routine situations. The different levels and expectations are clearly defined by Benner, although the words competency and proficiency are often used synonymously in the literature. In many clinical areas where there are a number of different levels of nurses in training, practitioners need to have a clear understanding of the meaning of competency and how they assess it at different levels of preparation.

If competence is concerned with the ability to coordinate cognitive, affective and psychomotor skills, in the carrying out of nursing activities, all three elements of learning need to be addressed in the process of assessment. However, tools to ascertain competence in the cognitive domain seem to have been far more extensively developed than those in the affective and psychomotor domain (Kenworthy & Nicklin, 1989). Nevertheless, it could be argued that even in the cognitive domain, empirical or scientific knowledge as described by Carper (1978) or propositional knowledge as noted by Burnard (1987) have been given more emphasis than other aspects of knowledge. Ultimately, however, if we consider Polyani's (1966) notion of tacit knowledge 'we know more than we can tell', it would be appropriate to examine existing measurement tools to identify whether practitioners are being enabled to express themselves in relation to bridging the gap between knowing and telling in documenting all elements of a learner's performance.

Measurement tools

The problems inherent in the measurement of clinical competence and the limited number of clinical performance measures are quickly evident as the literature is reviewed (Ross *et al.* 1988). Whilst Ross *et al.* support Benner (1982) in the importance of assessing clinical competence in the context of the 'real situation', there has been great difficulty in finding an effective measurement tool.

According to Runciman (1990), many studies in the 1960s and 1970s in the USA were prompted by the goal of measurable learning outcomes and resulted in the development of rating scales and performance checklists. Among these is the Slater nursing competencies rating scale, and although still widely referred to in the literature, 'such techniques have been described as too detailed, dated and culture-bound' (Runciman, 1990, p. 18).

Competency-based education, and in particular evaluating competency, has been a focus in the American nursing literature for the past 10 years (Benedum et al. 1990). In the UK, since the introduction of the statutory competencies in 1983, education programmes and subsequently assessment schemes, are beginning to develop around these competencies. There still remains, however, the potential conflict of the profession's responsibility to produce a safe practitioner, and the elusive nature of what competence means in relation to these very broad statutory competency statements. This notion is supported by Pottinger (1975) and Benner (1982) in the USA.

Approaches to the use of continuous assessment tools appear to be widely documented, but few in the UK relate to the use of competencies. However, Aggleton et al. (1987) produced an approach where competencies are assessed around a problem-solving and skills based approach where learners either achieve or do not achieve the various activities identified. Shearer (1989) and Mather (1983) identify a list of competency statements supported by a four- and six-point rating scale, respectively. However, the use of rating scales alone has been highly criticised in the literature (Fletcher, 1985) and, in particular, Bondy (1983) recognised that whether using a scale from A–D, 5–1, or superior-weak, they were open to different interpretation and so lacked reliability. However, using the descriptive statements for each behaviour at each level in addition to the rating scales as above, Bondy recognises as time-consuming to write, producing a lengthy assessment tool.

In the assessment of qualities used by psychiatric students, Novak (1988) recognised a number of difficulties. She refers to Lewis (1976):

> 'If a quality cannot be itemized . . . we will have denied the difference between the nurse who has only the procedural skills and the one who is also personally and socially perceptive.' (Novak, 1988, p. 83)

Benner (1982) supports this, where competency-based assessment arises from an approach that analyses the functional aspects of the job, rather than considering the demands of the whole situation. She identifies that there is a great danger of reducing 'our concepts, descriptions, and vision to conform to our testing capability (which) is to have ordered our priorities perversely' (p. 309). She further emphasises the danger of overestimating the power of competency-based testing which will cause an undesirable reductionism in nursing, 'That is, the definition of practice will be reduced to the capabilities of the measurement tools' (Benner, 1982, p. 309).

Whilst the use of competency rating scales in the assessment of student progress is considered by some to provide a comprehensive approach to ensuring competency (Battenfield, 1986; Benedum et al. 1990), Benner (1982) retains her reservations, supporting the need to assess learners in the 'real life' practice situation. However, according to Runciman (1990), 'such assessments are open to scrutiny on grounds of being context-bound, subjective and lacking in comparability' (p. 14).

Since the 1960s however, there have been many attempts to reach the goal of a more objective clinical evaluation. A number of techniques have been tested including simulated exercises and group video testing, critical incident technique, and the use of the computer for clinical evaluation (Fivers and Gosnell, 1966; Matthews, 1988; Miller et al. 1988; Ross et al. 1988). Boreham (1978) however, points out the validity problems of not assessing the 'real life' situation does still present its own problems according to the study undertaken by Long (1976). He identified that ward sisters carrying out assessment found little time to complete the assessment forms and final interviews, they were open to influence by factors other than the student's ability, they spent little time with the students in practice, and the statements were difficult to understand. Much of this is supported recently by Darbyshire (1990).

In an attempt to move away from a task-orientated approach in the UK, Dunn (1986) devised a tool to measure the development of nursing skill, using the opinions of qualified staff, supported by ward sisters. A similar study was made by Llewellyn-Thomas et al. (1989) when both students and qualified nurses were asked to identify and weight the attributes of an 'exemplary' nurse in clinical practice, and use this strategy in the assessment of competence. From two further studies in the USA, McClosky and McCain (1988) classified the observable behaviours of recent graduates and experienced nurses to identify which behaviours nurses are best at and those that require further preparation to improve both basic and continuing education programmes. The value of this methodology of identifying nurses' perception of learner and qualified staff's behaviour has been recognised as a basis for a variety of different studies and in particular the assessment of clinical competence (Llewellyn-Thomas, 1989).

The importance of both self and peer assessment is becoming increasingly recognised (Cox, 1987; Sigsworth & Heslop, 1988; Underwood & Reed, 1990). Sigsworth and Heslop suggest that through self assessment the students felt more supported, part of the team and through the establishment of good relationships, felt safe during discussion of their progress.

The literature identifies many who recognise the need to continue the development of assessment schemes in nursing (Ross et al. 1988) and Benner (1982) emphasises the need for this to be based in the context of the 'real world'. She recognises that as the learner gains expertise, 'her actions become much more situationally determined and, therefore, much less formalizable' (Benner, 1982, p. 309). She also recognised that competency-based testing arose out of the need to move away from assessments based on individual's opinions, rather than on observation, description, and analysis of what nurses actually do. However, much of her work puts value on nurses' expert opinion supporting the notion that expert nurses are able to take account of the many factors that make up the 'real life' situation. It is felt that this should be explored more fully in relation to the assessment of learners' practice.

Expert opinion

Hepworth (1989) recognises that the process of critically assessing learner nurses, clinically, involves making judgements about an individual's ability in an essentially unique situation. This, she suggests, will involve the assessor in numerous professional judgements and the such judgements will be based on the complex interplay of a number of factors. Hepworth in nurse education, based her beliefs on the work of others, in particular Schön (1983), in general education. Schön argues that professional judgement in such intricate situations arise not from scientific analysis, but from 'knowledge-in-action'. He believes that this knowledge-in-action is the ability to consider and make decisions/judgements in unique situations as and when they present. Knowledge-in-action he considers as the type of knowledge only revealed in action, or the doing of the task, similar to Carper's (1978) aesthetic and personal knowledge and Burnard's (1987) experiential knowledge. According to Schön, there is no reason to expect the performer to be able to capture and make it into 'knowledge-in-action' (which can be acquired from books). He believes that the knowledge is based on the protracted and unique personal experience of the person concerned, and only exists in that individual's professional actions. In relation to the expression of this knowledge, there are parallels with Polyani's (1966) notion of tacit knowledge, where he believes: 'We can know more than we can tell' (p. 4).

This work has enormous implications both for those assessing clinical nurses' practice, in term of justifying their judgements of others and for those being assessed in the justification of their actions.

Alternatively, Hammond (1978) developed the Cognitive Continuum Theory where intuitive judgements and scientific experiments are the poles of a continuum of the many types of thinking (modes of inquiry/practice) which can be used in various situations, where most thinking lies in between the two. The less structured an activity, the more intuition is used as the way of thinking, whilst the better structured it is, the more assessors will use scientific analysis (Dowie & Elstein, 1988).

This in fact supports Benner (1982), where she postulates that competency-based testing seemed limited to the less situational, less interactional areas of patient care where the behaviour can be well-defined and patient and nurse variation do not alter the performance criteria.

According to Hammond, those who assess clinical competence operate at a mainly intuitive level (Hepworth, 1989). Eddy (1988) in relation to medical decision making, is not so impressed with this intuitive judgement and identifies the enormous variations in the decision making of doctors. In the same way, student nurse assessment by expert clinicians varies considerably, in spite of having specific criteria from which to measure their performance. Eddy shows little belief in the quality of professional judgement, in particular that of the highest experts.

However, on the contrary, Schön (1983) has great respect for what has traditionally been referred to as the artistic, or intuitive aspect of clinical practice. This belief is reflected in Dreyfus' assertion used by Benner (1982) in nursing that 'better thinking is done intuitively, because experts, who think better, think intuitively (Dowie &

Elstein, 1988, p. 99). With the ever changing situation in clinical nursing, Benner *et al.* using the Dreyfus model, judges that it is right that expert practitioners do use their expert intuition in clinical practice (Benner & Tanner, 1987). They further emphasise that, 'intuitive knowledge and analytic reasoning are not in an either/or opposition; they can — and do — work together (p. 31).

However, unfortunately, it is difficult to see any way of empirically testing such a proposition and the question of whether a valid independent and objective evaluation of expert performance in the clinical professions is possible. Nevertheless, it is important to distinguish between intuitive judgement based on the complexity of a number of factors and that which is based on the whim of personality.

Perhaps one way of marrying the two together, that is, intuitive knowledge and analytic reasoning, is through the use of critical reflection of practice. Some consideration will therefore be given to the value of this notion of critical reflection.

The value of reflection

'Within nursing the provision of care, the doing, is given greater significance than consideration of what is being done . . . The pressure to action tends to result in the perpetuation of traditional ways of giving nursing care, and because of this pressure there is little opportunity for nurses of any grade to reflect on what they are doing.' (Hughes, 1985, p. 18)

Accepting the belief that nurses view action as all important, it is necessary to recognise that the emphasis in assessment is not upon the action or experience per se, but upon the nature of the learning derived from that experience (Runciman, 1990). Evans (1988) suggests that the identification of learning comes through systematic reflection which involves collecting evidence to support statements of what has been learned. Only then, Evans proposes, 'can there be assessment for accreditation' (p. 7). Boyd and Fales (1983) are in no doubt about the value of reflective learning. They recognise that

'the bringing to consciousness of what is done naturally — is a significant aid to the use of reflective learning . . . once aware of their own process, people spontaneously gain greater conscious control over it and seek guidance for even more effective use of it.' (Boyd & Fales, 1983, p. 113)

This critically reflective learner according to Marsick (1987) portrays the vision of the 'knowledgeable doer' as described in Project 2000. Furthermore, Aggleton *et al.* (1987) support that continuous assessment provides opportunities for both trained staff and learners to reflect upon and monitor their own progress. There has been little work done in nursing in the UK, relating to this reflective practitioner. However, recently Powell's (1989) small study on whether clinical nurses use reflection-in-action in their daily work, found that they tended to separate theory from practice and that some were relatively unable to learn from their work. It is clear that if clinical nurses are involved in the assessment of learners, now more appropriately to diploma level, then the skills required to facilitate reflective learning will need to be learned. Runciman

(1990) supports this and emphasises the significant contribution that critical reflection can make both to learning and assessment in practice.

The role of the assessor

According to the ENB (1989) the role of the assessor/supervisor in the context of Project 2000 is a formal one. They should be first level nurses, and should have undertaken a course of preparation to enable them to facilitate students developing competence by overseeing and assessing their level of attainment.

This is the first time that nursing's governing body has identified the need for qualified staff to be formally prepared in relation to continuous assessment schemes. The quality of this preparation has not been identified and varies nationally. From the learner's perspective, Gott (1982) recognised that learners will perform differently in different learning situations, and the quality of their learning environment. Although a number of studies have recognised the need to involve all qualified staff in the teaching of nurses (Alexander, 1983; Marson, 1984), the role of the ward sister is the key to controlling the learning environment (Fretwell, 1980; Ogier, 1981; Orton, 1981). However, whilst many ward sisters in the UK do not appear to equate with Benner's (1984) 'expert' practitioner in terms of their 'enormous background of experience' subsequently possessing an 'intuitive grasp of each situation', they are in UK hospital nursing, the most senior clinical nurse in most clinical areas. They are in a powerful position according to Marson (1984) and it is from this position that change in the education development of learner nurses will come. Ward sisters therefore need to take the lead in guiding others to assess effectively for competency in the 'real world' of practice. They should therefore be targeted for preparation to oversee and assess students at each level of attainment considering all elements of learning and develop new skills in relation to reflection in practice. However, Kenworthy and Nicklin (1989) make an analogy between continuous assessment and a number of 'snapshots' with a camera. It is questionable however, as to how many snapshots need to be taken, and from how many directions, before the picture is complete, or indeed complete enough to make any effective decisions about performance.

Lelean's (1973) work would offer little foundation on which to build assessment by the ward sister. Since Lelean's study has been completed, the work of the ward sister seems only to have increased in complexity.

Validity and reliability

Of the numerous tools available, it is possible find support for almost any way of evaluating practice. However, there appears to be much in the literature that questions both validity and reliability (Bradley, 1986; Gallagher, 1983; Squier, 1981). Runciman (1990) suggests from the literature that a combination of approaches may be appropriate to identify and validate competency in practice. This was acknowledged some years ago by Wooley (1977), who suggested the use of subjective judgement based on intuitive knowledge and scientific measurement.

In summary, the number of tools available to assess students in practice are numerous and varied though few relate to the use of competencies, or to the different levels of attainment. It appears however, that in an attempt to enable practitioners to express themselves, the tools are made more specific. Subsequently, practitioners become more reductionist in their measurement and focus towards assessment of tasks rather than the psychological construct as noted by Miller *et al.* (1988). In spite of the subjective nature of the intuitive approaches identified by Runciman (1990), there seems much to commend intuitive assessment/expert opinion of experienced clinical nurses in the 'real world' of practice where these opinions are based on the unique experience of these practitioners. It has been identified that there is a need to marry intuitive knowledge and scientific reasoning (Benner & Tanner, 1987; Wooley, 1977) perhaps through skilled reflection in practice by all those assessing learners to identify this 'psychological construct'.

Not only do the tools used need to be further developed to enable practitioners to assess in the 'real world' of practice, and in all areas of learning, practitioners need to be prepared more effectively to gain skills in reflection and examine all areas of learning to both facilitate students' learning and evaluate their practice and express these effectively at each level of attainment.

References

Aggleton P, Allen M, Montgomery S (1987) Developing system for the continuous assessment of practical nursing skills. *Nurse Education Today* 7: 158–164.

Alexander M (1983) *Learning to nurse: integrating theory and practice*. Churchill Livingstone, Edinburgh.

Battenfield B L (1986) *Designing clinical evaluation tools: the state of the art*. National League for Nursing Publication, USA.

Benedum E, Kalup A, Freed D (1990) A competency achievement program for direct caregivers. *Nursing Management* 21 (5): 32–46.

Benner P (1982) Issues in competency-based testing. *Nursing Outlook* (May): 303–309.

Benner P (1984) *From novice to expert: excellence and power in clinical nursing practice*. Addison Wesley, Menlo Park.

Benner P, Tanner C (1987) How expert nurses use intuition. *American Journal of Nursing* (January): 23–31.

Bondy K N (1983) Criterion-referenced definitions for rating scales in clinical evaluation. *Journal of Nursing Education* 22 (9): 376–382.

Boreham N C (1978) Test-skill interaction errors in the assessment of nurses' clinical proficiency. *Journal of Occupational Psychology* 51: 249–258.

Boyd E, Fales A (1983) Reflective learning. *Journal of Humanistic Psychology* 23 (2): 99–117.

Bradley J (1986) Personality or performance? *Nursing Times* (May 14): 45–46.

Burnard P (1987) Towards an epistemiological basis for experiential learning in nurse education. *Journal Advanced Nursing* 12: 189–193.

Carper B (1978) Fundamental patterns of knowing in nursing. *Advances in Nursing Science* 1(v): 13–23.

Cox S (1987) Peer and self-assessment. *Nursing Times* (33): 62–64.

Darbyshire P, Stewart B, Jamieson L, Tongue C (1990) New domains in nursing. *Nursing Times* 86 (27): 73–75.

Dowie J, Elstein A, (eds) (1988) *Professional judgement: a reader in clinical decision making.* Cambridge University Press, Cambridge.

Dunn D (1986) Assessing the development of clinical nursing skills. *Nurse Education Today* 6: 28–35.

Eddy D (1988) In: J Dowie, A Elstein (eds) *Professional judgement: a reader in clinical decision making.* Cambridge University Press, Cambridge.

Evans N (1988) The assessment of prior experiential learning. CNAA Development Services. Publication No. 17, In: P Runciman (ed) (1990) *Competence-based education and the assessment and accreditation of workbased learning in the context of project 2000 programmes of nurse education: a literature review.* pp. 29–59. The National Board for Nursing, Midwifery and Health Visiting for Scotland.

Fivers G, Gosnell D (1966) *Nursing evaluation: the problem and the progress. The critical incident technique.* Macmillan, New York.

Fletcher C (1985) Means of assessment. *Nursing Times* (July 3): 24–26.

Fretwell J (1980) An inquiry into the ward learning environment. *Nursing Times* Occasional Papers 76 (16): 69–75.

Gallagher P (1983) Why do we fail them? *Nursing Mirror* (February 2): 16.

Gott M (1982) Theories of learning and the teaching of nursing. *Nursing Times* Occasional Papers 78 (11): 41–44.

Hammond K R (1978) *Toward increasing competence of thought in public policy formation.* Boulder, CO.

Hepworth S (1989) Professional judgement and nurse education. *Nurse Education Today* 9: 408–412.

Hughes F (1985) What do nurses do? *Senior Nurse* 2 (4): 19.

Kenworthy N, Nicklin P (1989) *Teaching and assessing in nursing practice: an experiental approach.* Scutari Press, London.

Llewellyn-Thomas HA, Sims-Jones N, Sutherland R N (1989) Measuring perceptions of the exemplary nurse. *Journal of Nursing Education* 28 (8): 366–371.

Lelean S (1973) *Ready for report nurse?* Royal College of Nursing, London.

Lewis E P (1976) Quantifying the unquantifiable (editorial) *Nursing Outlook* 24: 147. In: S Novak (ed) An effective clinical evaluation tool. *Journal of Nursing Education* 28 (8): 366–371.

Long P (1976) Judging and reporting on student nurse clinical performance: some problems for the ward sister. *International Journal of Nursing Studies* 13: 115–121.

Marsick V J (1987) *Learning in the workplace.* Croom Helm, London.

Marson S (1984) Developing the 'teaching' role of the ward sister. *Nurse Education Today* 4: 13–16.

Mather C (1983) The X-Y syndrome. *Nursing Mirror* (Sept 14): 35–37.

Matthews R, Viens D (1988) Evaluating basic nursing skills through group video testing. *Journal of Nursing Education* 27 (1): 44–46.

McClosky J, McCain B (1988) Nurse performance: strengths and weaknesses. *Nursing Research* 37 (5): 308–313.

Miller *et al.* (1988) Credit where credit's due. The report of the accreditation of work-based learning project. SCOTVEC.

Novak S (1988) An effective clinical evaluation tool. *Journal of Nursing Education* 27 (2): 83–84.

Ogier M (1981) Ward sisters and their influence upon nurse learners. *Nursing Times* Occasional Papers 77 (11): 41–43.

Orton H (1981) Ward learning climate and student nurse response. *Nursing Times* Occasional Papers 77 (17): 65–67.

Polyani M (1966) *The tacit dimension.* Routledge and Kegan Paul, London.

Pottinger P (1975) Comments and guidelines for research in competency identification, definition and measurement, prepared for the Education Policy Research Center, Syracuse University (ERIC Document ED 134541) (unpublished). In: P Benner (ed) (1982): Issues in competency-based testing. *Nursing Outlook* (May): 303–339.

Powell J (1989) The reflective practitioner in nursing. *Journal of Advanced Nursing* 14: 824–832.

Quinn F (1988) *The principles and practice of nurse education.* Croom Helm, London.

Ross M, Carroll G, Knight J, Chamberlain M, Forthergill-Bourbonnais F, Linton J (1988) Using the OSCE to measure clinical skills performance in nursing. *Journal of Advanced Nursing* 13: 45–56.

Runciman P (1990) Competency-based education and the assessment and accreditation of work-based learning in the context of project 2000 programmes of nurse education: a literature review. The National Board for Nursing, Midwifery and Health Visiting for Scotland (January).

Schön D (1983) The reflective practitioner: how professionals think in action. Temple Smith, London.

Shearer M (1989) Progressing nicely. *Nursing Times* 85 (3): 60–61.

Sigsworth J, Heslop A (1988) Self-assessment and the student nurse. *Senior Nurse* 8 (5): 14–16.

Squier R W (1981) The reliability and validity of rating scales in assessing the clinical progress of psychiatric nursing students. *International Journal of Nursing Studies* 18 (3): 157–169.

Underwood I, Reed S (1990) A strategy for continuous assessment of theory and practice in first level nursing courses. *Nurse Education Today* 10: 307–317.

Wooley A (1977) The long and tortured history of clinical evaluation. *Nursing Outlook* 25: 308–315.

36. The Use of Criteria-based Grading Profiles in Formative and Summative Assessment

Frank Milligan

This article outlines the development and use of criteria-based grading profiles for formative and summative assessment. The profiles were developed in 1991 in an attempt to improve assessment validity, inter-marker and inter-course reliability and student feedback within the Faculty of Health Care and Social Studies. Important underlying aspects of assessment theory are examined and it is argued that assessment should be conceptualised as an ethical activity requiring clarification for students of expectations through specification of criteria. It is concluded that the profiles have proved useful in guiding both lecturer and students in the completion and marking of assessed work and that further study and debate needs to take place in relation to the effectiveness and potential disadvantages of such profiles.

Introduction

In an attempt to assure the satisfactory marking and grading of both formative and summative work, a system of Grading Profiles was developed within the Department of Community and Mental Health Care, University of Luton. These have proved extremely useful to both lecturers and students. This article describes the development of these profiles, the assessment theory that underpins them, and debates the advantages and possible drawbacks of this type of assessment feedback. It is hoped that the article will stimulate further educational debate on the use of such explicit criteria and the most effective structural means by which they can be used.

Some of the arguments put forward within this article are specific to nurse education although the profiles themselves are used on courses and modules that non-nurses attend. Academic levels 1, 2, and 3 are referred to (certificate, diploma and degree respectively).

Development of the profiles

As part of my responsibilities on joining the University in 1993 I was asked to continue development of the Grading Profiles described here. Original development of the profiles started in 1991 as a response to several needs. Firstly, it was felt by some lecturers that a more innovative form of assessment criteria presentation could be developed that would benefit both students and lecturers. Secondly, with the broad range of activities undertaken within the Faculty of Health Care and Social Studies there was a need to maximise continuity and intermarker reliability with regard to the

Frank Milligan: 'The Use of Criteria-based Grading Profiles in Formative and Summative Assessment' in *NURSE EDUCATION TODAY* (1996), 16, pp. 413–418. Reprinted by permission of the publisher Churchill Livingstone.

marking of various assignments across different courses yet which were at the same academic level.

Although subject to ongoing development the profiles were comprehensively reviewed in the late summer of 1994 and it is this version of these documents that is discussed here.

The responsibilities of assessment

Rowntree (1992) and Jarvis (1985) are two influential authors with regard to assessment both in general and in nursing education. They make it clear that the process of assessment carries with it a great deal of responsibility. In a broad sense, assessment is about getting to know people (Rowntree, 1992) and making judgements about their abilities. It is essentially a gate keeping mechanism through which people do, or do not, make progress in their chosen course or occupation (Jarvis, 1985). Further judgements about their success or otherwise within the spheres beyond those gates will also be made. Assessment is then, when practised with the due care and attention required of such responsibilities, an ethical activity. We need to be reasonably certain of the accuracy of our judgements, essentially that we are right and that we can actively support the judgements made.

It follows from this that accountability on the part of the person/s charged with the grading of student work should extend to clarification of the criteria upon which the student was judged. If such clarification is not given or the punitive weapon of unsubstantiated professional judgement is the only, or most important criteria used, then the assessor is possibly left with little credibility and fails to meet the standard stated here of acting ethically in assessment matters. There is also a significant risk that norm referencing is taking place in that students are only being compared with their peers and not some pre-determined standard (Rowntree, 1992). Although there is some value in such comparison its use, as it will be shown, should be limited and always considered carefully.

The demonstration of accountability through an assessment process which makes its criteria open to the student has distinct advantages for nurse education. Many argue that we need to be consistent in our educational methods with that which we seek of our students as potential practitioners (Burnard, 1991; Cohen, 1993). To put it simply, we should mirror the values we hope to see from students (future practitioners) in the practice environment in our own practice as educators. For example, *The Code of Professional Conduct* (UKCC, 1992) asks that practitioners work in 'an open and co-operative manner with patients, clients and their families'. It seems reasonable to ask educationalists to mirror this in assessment and clearly defined criteria offer one method of achieving this.

Criterion referencing

Rowntree (1992) defines criterion referencing as the process through which 'we judge the student according to how well he (sic) has done by comparison with some predetermined criterion'. Similarly, Shepard (1983) notes that they help to locate students at a particular learning level: 'The distinguishing characteristics criterion-referenced tests is the care taken in explicating and representing the intended behavioural domain'. It is clear from Shepard and Rowntree that a good deal of interest was shown in criterion-referenced assessment in the 1970s. The type of language used also indicates that the work was frequently done within a reductionist/behaviourist paradigm. This point will be returned to in the conclusion.

The advantages of criterion-referencing over norm referencing, situations in which criteria are implicit or simple comparisons are made to grade students, are clear in terms of the arguments put forward here and in relation to the important question, i.e. how influential should the performance of other students be in judging an individual in relation to the requirements of a course? Rowntree (1992) describes situations in which assessors 'lost their nerve' when a large number of students passed or failed when criteria were carefully used and adhered to in assessment. The problem is that such a situation is perceived as a problem because the numbers doing very well, or failing, or performing in an average manner are seen in the light of a normal distribution curve. Failure to achieve such normal distribution (sic) is seen as a dilemma, and Jarvis (1985) confirms that such normative pressures are very much part of education. However, a group of students may be unusually strong or weak, or have students from both these extremes when measured against the criteria of a course, yet normal distribution (sic) of marks may still be sought. It seems that we need to constantly guard against those habits of rank ordering and comparison of individuals (Aronson, 1984) and be prepared to adhere to criteria, even if the numbers of students passing and failing do not look normal. The performance of other students then is of limited relevance in assessment of individuals as part of the process of achieving nurse registration.

A possible counter argument to this is the notion that norms create pressures that are then represented in stated criteria (Shepard, 1983). For example, the frequent use of reflective practice in nursing at this point in time may explain its inclusion in many courses criteria. Similarly, pressures exerted on students to submit typed assignments is something that was not so widely expected 10 years ago.

Bearing these points in mind the clarification of criteria, to both students and educators, based upon the standards and requirements that are set by the statutory instruments (Nurses Act 1989) and the English National Board (1990) seems an important task. Similarly, the criteria here achieve an important educational aim in that the academic level being sought is also clarified.

Clear identification of criteria helps to open the assessment process up for scrutiny by those being measured by it. For example, a low mark given in these profiles in written expression requires explanation. This clarity helps to ensure that lecturers have rationale for the mark allocated as it is clear to students where marks have been gained and lost.

The criteria described here were largely intuitively derived from lecturers' expectations of the necessary content of various assignments with reference to higher education literature on progression across academic levels. Bloom and others (1979; Krathwohol *et al.* 1973) work on a taxonomy of educational objectives was also influential as can be seen from some of the concepts used within the profiles. Progression across concepts such as description, analysis, synthesis and evaluation can be seen (Appendix 1). However, there are inconsistencies in Bloom's work that need to be considered when applied to nursing. For example, the identification of knowledge as a first level skill in Bloom's taxonomy is arguably problematic and inconsistent with the work of authors such as Benner (1984) and Chinn and Kramer (1991) who see nursing knowledge and its generation as deriving, in part at least, from practice and therefore as a complex phenomena not a low level skill. The article by Stephenson (1985), which explores the content of academic essays from the perspective of the skills and qualities required of different academic levels, does not clearly address this problem but gives further guidance on how the work of Bloom *et al.* could be interpreted for use within the profiles. Stephenson helps to clarify what is meant by the various levels present in Bloom's hierarchy of the cognitive domain and how they might be represented in essays.

Structure of the profiles

The profiles basically consist of a number of criteria with their descriptors divided into boxes that show the progression of marks from a fail to an A+ grade (Appendix 1).

Assessment criteria are devised on forms that outline their progression from level 1 to level 3. An example is shown in Appendix 2. It can be seen that descriptors are created that describe the parameters to be met if a mark within that particular range is to be given. For example, for the student to achieve a mark within the A range (A–, A or A+) at level 1 under the criteria for 'Focus on the task set', the following needs to be demonstrated: 'Has focused on the task set in a structured manner'. Similarly, at level 3, to achieve a mark in the same range: 'Has clearly focused on the task set in an insightful, creative and critical manner' (see Appendix 2). Through such forms the progression, in terms of the quality of work required at different academic levels, can easily be seen.

It is important that a reasonable and consistent progression across the descriptors is achieved if the criteria are to be considered valid and reliable. Valid, in that the criteria descriptors examine what is intended to be examined by the criteria in question and in the sense that it is an appropriate task, with appropriate progression, for the academic level in question. This latter point also carries an element of reliability as it is important that different educationalists look for similar performance at each academic level (Frith and Macintosh, 1988). Clarification of the criteria, as shown on the profiles, assists reliability as markers are aware of expectations and progression across academic levels 1, 2 and 3.

Once specific criteria headings are decided upon it is the descriptor element of the profile that tends to generate the most debate. Those that you see here evolved over 3 years of dialogue on the most effective wording. Once completed the different criteria are combined to form grading profiles for different courses and modules.

Where it has been feasible, standard grading profiles have been constructed to aid consistently across courses. These include profiles for: Learning Contracts, Seminar Presentations, Contract Evidence/Essay, Essay with Reflection, Projects and Practical Teaching. If lecturers wish, other criteria can be added to standard grading profiles tailoring them to the needs of particular courses/modules. A criterion commonly required is that of reflective practice and this has been added as and when necessary.

With the construction of a bank of criteria (Box 1) it has been possible to create a grading profile from scratch, if necessary, to meet the needs of a new course, module or assessment. This flexibility is a strength, although caution is required as the combination of criteria needs to be considered carefully if duplication or other problems are to be avoided. The overall validity of the grading profile is reliant upon suitable criteria being used within it for the chosen assessment (Frith and Macintosh, 1988). For example, omission of the criteria 'Use of literature and referencing' from a level 2 essay profile would arguably reduce the validity of the profile as they are essential items for most, if not all such work.

Box 1   **Criteria available for use within the profiles**

Analysis of learning needs (learning contracts)
Focus on the task set
Group/individual involvement
Handling results
Identifying resources and strategies (learning contracts)
Issue handling
Outlining evidence of learning (learning contracts)
Reflection
Relevance to practice
Spoken expression
Study method and structure
Use of current specific knowledge
Use of literature and referencing
Use of supportive educational rationale
Use of teaching aids (synopsis)
Written expression

Other specific criteria can be created if necessary. We are at present working on criteria for Poster Presentations which are used as assessment on some courses. Some of the criteria in Box 1 will be used in combination with new ones devised specifically for the task.

Columns are provided on the profiles (Appendix 1) for self and assessor assessment, weighting and formative or summative use. The forms contain two academic levels so that students can clearly see the progression required across academic levels. Weighting can be adjusted to allow emphasis to be given to criteria seen by lecturers as being of particular importance. As it will be seen, students are encouraged to self assess. For administrative purposes the profiles also clearly outline information that identifies the student, the assignment, and the course or module they are undertaking.

Uses

The profiles are used across a wide variety of courses within the Faculty. These include the modular Enhancement Health Care degree programme which enables health care professionals to 'top up' to an honours degree, the Dip HE Nursing Studies (Project 2000), the enrolled nurse conversion course and various English National Board courses including the ENB 997/8 (Teaching and Assessing) and the Diploma in Professional Practice. Profiles have also been devised for the AP(E)L process in an attempt to ensure that consistent and reliable credit is given to candidates, and for academic work with the Police Force and Social Services.

Advantages

One of the most positive aspects of the profiles is that they increase the amount of formative feedback given to the student. Reading the criteria descriptors clarifies where they lost marks and what their strengths are. Comparisons of individual criteria over a period of time also helps to gauge their personal progress; a measure of Rowntree's (1992) third criteria, how well they have done in comparison with themselves. Further written feedback is given on the back of the profile as it is made clear to lecturers that the forms are not intended to replace written feedback.

The profiles also act as a guide for the students informing them from the start of work on assignments what the requirements of the assessment are. Unused to such assistance, students often fail to see the value of this until it is made clear by a lecturer, or another student.

From the lecturers' viewpoint several advantages have been noted. It is generally agreed that reliability across different courses and modules has improved with the use of these documents and this has been confirmed by several different external examiners. Common expectations have been achieved through use of the profiles. Just as they act as a guide to students, so they structure lecturer analysis of assignments, a notoriously difficult area in terms of achieving reliability (Rowntree, 1992). However, this claim needs to be supported through research.

Self assessment is encouraged on the grounds that it also enhances the quality of formative information gained through the assessment. Marked discrepancies between student and lecturer interpretations of abilities become clear and can be discussed. Our experience shows that students will often be conservative in their marking, a point supported by Wondrak and Goble (1992), although occasionally high marks have been seen that are inconsistent with the quality of the work. Whether this tends to draw the lecturer into giving a higher mark needs to be considered and investigated.

The profiles are seen as only one part of the assessment process. They are reliant upon effective assessment guidelines, inter-marker agreement of what is sought from assignments and effective moderation to name but three other parts of that process.

What is missing?

Perhaps one of the important issues that work on the profiles has shown is the lack of a broad base of supportive literature and research upon which to found decisions about criterion referenced work. The literature that is available includes the document by

Hounsell (1994) which describes a wide variety of feedback methods for assessed work. Criteria are described in the document but there is no in-depth analysis of issues of reliability or validity, or discussion on the effectiveness or otherwise of the materials and criteria cited. The article by Wondrak and Goble (1992) explores reliability across student, peer and lecturer assessment of the same work when the criteria were devised by the student group. However, the criteria are not described, and therefore not analysed in the article.

Snyder (cited in Allen and Jolley, 1987) points to the importance of assessment in determining issues that potentially become 'hidden curriculum'. Specifically, Snyder noted that aspects of the curriculum that are not summatively assessed potentially carry less value and are revised less by students; an inadvertent consequence of assessment design. As an analogy, this may also hold true for these profiles. If this is so we as educationalists need to ask, what might be missing from these criteria and are they constructed in the most effective manner?

With regard to the former, other literature on marking and the use of criteria tends to concentrate on essay writing (Wilson, 1991; Downie and Basford, 1991) and propositional forms of knowledge (Downie and Basford, 1991). Although a common concern in assessment, there are other forms of knowledge that are important in nursing such as experiential, practical (Burnard, 1991) and intuitive (Belenky et al. 1986; Benner, 1984). We have attempted to embrace such ideas within the profiles but the assessment of practical knowledge is very much reliant upon students' abilities in the practice/clinical environment (assessment of practice, except indirectly, does not fall within the remit of these profiles), and intuitive knowledge, due to its abstract nature, possess even tougher problems. Reflective practice appears to offer the most fruitful path with regard to assessment of this form of knowledge (Powell, 1989). The latter point, with regard to structure, has not been resolvable through literature.

Conclusion

Although there is a good deal of debate over the issue of andragogy, its existence as a theory and its relevance to the education of nurses (for examples of differing views on this argument see Darbyshire, 1993 and Milligan, 1995), it is a truism that students have played a more central role in the educational process of nursing in the last 10–15 years. In terms of assessment, students can arguably be empowered by making clear to them the criteria upon which they will be assessed. This is not a major innovation, although upon reflection many people can recall times at which they have been assessed when the criteria upon which the assessment was made was not clear to them. However, an achievement of these profiles is the clear statement of explicit marking criteria to the student and lecturer. They clarify for both parties the criteria against which the work will be measured. They offer a convenient framework through which criteria can be constructed and combined to offer an innovative and reliable (this needs to be confirmed through research) system of assessment. They are flexible in that they can be used for formative and summative assessment and weighting of criteria can be specified. They are also consistent with some of the values we hope our students will mirror in their own practice.

The lack of more recent substantive research on the issue of marking criteria reduces the depth of analysis made here but there is little doubt that they have been well received by students and lecturers alike and they have improved inter-marker reliability, although room for further improvement remains. Descriptive guidelines for each criteria will be devised to further improve inter-marker reliability. Also, a more thorough evaluatory analysis of the profiles will be undertaken in the near future to substantiate these claims.

Further consideration needs to be given to the seemingly reductionist philosophy that underlies a great deal of the literature written on criterion-referencing in the 1970s (Shepard, 1983). Do the profiles, as a potential hidden curriculum issue convey a message suggesting that all knowledge is identifiable and measurable? Will they reduce opportunities for students to devise their own criteria. They could of course do this within the forms described here.

To conclude, what is missing from these profiles? Are there criteria that have been omitted? This is an especially important question when more abstract forms of knowledge, other than propositional, are considered (Belenky *et al.* 1986). Although generally viewed a strength, is the structure created a disadvantage in that it may discourage innovation beyond the issues described on the profile? Finally, if the system described here does (or can be adopted to) meet these criticisms then where should their use stop; should we have grading profiles for doctorate work?

Acknowledgements

A wide range of the University staff, both past and present, have contributed to the development of these profiles and the author of this article acknowledges their significant, important and helpful contribution. The original idea was very much the work of Merideth Wall, a former senior lecturer with the Department of Community and Mental Health Care.

References

Aronson E (1983) *The social animal.* W.H. Freeman and Company, USA.

Allen P, Jolley M (1987) *The curriculum in nursing.* Croom Helm, London.

Benner P (1984) *From novice to expert: excellence and power in clinical nursing practice.* Addison-Wesley, Menlo Park.

Belenky M F, Clinchy B M, Goldberger N R, Tarule J M (1986) *Women's ways of knowing.* Basic Books, USA.

Bloom B S (ed) (1979) *Taxonomy of educational objectives: the classification of educational goals handbook 1, Cognitive domain.* Longman, USA.

Burnard P (1991) *Learning human skills,* 2nd edn. Butterworth Heinemann, Guildford.

Chinn P L, Kramer M K (1991) *Theory of nursing,* 3rd edn. Mosby Year Book, USA.

Cohen J A (1993) Caring perspectives in nursing education: liberation, transformation and meaning. *Journal of Advanced Nursing* 18: 621–626.

Darbyshire P (1993) In defence of pedagogy: a critique of the notion of andragogy. *Nurse Education Today* 13: 328–335.

Downie C, Basford P (1991) How to devise and use a marking plan. *Nursing Times* May 1st 87 (18): 59.

ENB (1990) *Regulations and guidelines for the approval of institutions and courses 1993.* English National Board, Southend.

Frith D S, Macintosh H G (1988) *A teacher's guide to assessment.* Stanley Thornes, Glasgow.

Jarvis P (1985) *The sociology of adult and continuing education.* Routledge, London.

Krathwohl D R, Bloom B S, Masia B B (1973) *Taxonomy of educational objectives: the classification of educational goals. Handbook 2: Affective domain.* Longman, USA.

Hounsell D (1994) *Structured feedback. Some examples of current practice and commenting on students' essays, poster and seminar presentations, practicals, projects, problem-solving and group work.* TLA Centre.

Milligan F J (1995) In defence of andragogy. *Nurse Education Today* 15 (1): 22–27.

Nurses, midwives and health visitors approval order statutory instrument (1989) The nurses, midwives and health visitors (Registered fever nurses amendment rules and training amendment rules) approval order 1989. Statutory Instrument No. 1456. HMSO, London.

Powell J H (1989) The reflective practitioner in nursing. *Journal of Advanced Nursing* 14: 824–823.

Rowntree D (1992) *Assessing students: how shall we know them?* 2nd edn. Kogan Page, London.

Shepard L A (1983) Standards for placement and certification. In: S B Anderson, J S Helmick (eds) (1983) *On educational testing; intelligence, performance standards, test anxiety, and latent traits,* Jossey-Bass, USA.

Stephenson P M (1985) Content of academic essays. *Nurse Education Today* 5: 81–87.

United Kingdom Central Council for Nursing, Midwifery and Health Visiting (1992) Code of professional conduct, 3rd edn. UKCC, London.

Wilson D M (1991) Improving feedback on student papers: a quantitative method which aids marking and gives valid feedback. *Nurse Education Today* 11: 53–56.

Wondrak R, Goble J (1992) An investigation into self, peer and tutor assessment of student psychiatric nurse's written work assignments. *Nurse Education Today* 12: 61–64.

Appendix 1

The University of
Luton
Faculty of Health Care
and Social Studies

Title of work

Grading Profile Level 1/2
Essay, contract evidence

© Department of Community and Mental Health Care 1994

Form code = 6/94
1 of 1 1 of 2

Weighting Formative/ Summative	Criteria	Level 1 — Fail 0 1 F 23 E4	Level 2 — Fail 0 1 F 23 E4	D- 5 D6 D+ 7	C- 8 C9 C+ 10	B- 11 B12 B+ 13	A- 14 A 15 A+ 16	Points (A = Assessor, S = Self) A | S
	Issue handling	The selected issues are of little relevance and are handled in a very superficial manner	The relevance of the selected issues is superficial and limited comprehension is demonstrated	Some relevant issues are described and used in a superficial manner	Relevant issues are discussed and some evidence of analysis of them occurs	Relevant issues are selected with evidence of analysis and some synthesis	Issues are handled in a competent manner showing skills of analysis and synthesis	
	Written expression	Meaning very vague with poor written expression	Meaning vague and does not get to the point	Meaning clear, but disjointed not always getting to the point	Gets to the point and meaning reasonably clear — evidence of logical style	Meaning clear and fluent in a logical manner	Meaning clear and fluent with an articulate style	
	Use of literature and referencing	Fails to access relevant literature	Accesses some relevant literature but fails to demonstrate understanding. Poor referencing	Accesses some relevant lit' demonstrating limited understanding. Some accurate references	Accesses relevant literature demonstrating understanding but in a descriptive manner	Evidence of analysis and some synthesis of the literature cited. Consistent correct use of referencing	The analysis of the literature shows evidence of synthesis and some evaluation	
	Use of current specific knowledge	No evidence of relevant theoretical background	Little evidence of theoretical background and supporting rationale	Some evidence of theoretical background but limited in terms of supporting rationale	Supporting rationale given for the knowledge base cited demonstrating some understanding	Clear understanding of the knowledge base demonstrated through analysis within the rationale	Some evidence of evaluation of the relevant knowledge base and the supportive rationale	
	Focus on the task set	Clearly failed to address the task set	Has only addressed the task set in a superficial manner that lacks a clear focus	Begins to address the task with some evidence of focus	Has focused on the task set in a descriptive manner	Has focused on the task set in a structured manner	Has clearly focused on the task set in a structured manner with evidence of some creativity	

Name	Module			Self assessed mean score	Assessor mean score
See reverse for comments	Date of submission	Attempt			
Markers name	Marked at level 1, 2				

Appendix 2

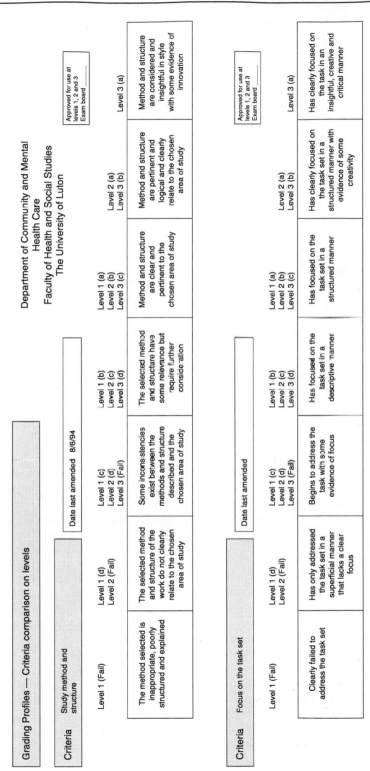

Grading Profiles — Criteria comparison on levels

Department of Community and Mental Health Care
Faculty of Health and Social Studies
The University of Luton

Criteria — Study method and structure

Date last amended 8/6/94

Approved for use at levels 1, 2 and 3
Exam board ____

Level 1 (Fail)	Level 1 (d) Level 2 (Fail)	Level 1 (c) Level 2 (d) Level 3 (Fail)	Level 1 (b) Level 2 (c) Level 3 (d)	Level 1 (a) Level 2 (b) Level 3 (c)	Level 2 (a) Level 3 (b)	Level 3 (a)
The method selected is inappropriate, poorly structured and explained	The selected method and structure of the work do not clearly relate to the chosen area of study	Some inconsistencies exist between the methods and structure described and the chosen area of study	The selected method and structure have some relevance but require further consideration	Method and structure are clear and pertinent to the chosen area of study	Method and structure are pertinent and logical and clearly relate to the chosen area of study	Method and structure are considered and insightful in style with some evidence of innovation

Criteria — Focus on the task set

Date last amended

Approved for use at levels 1, 2 and 3
Exam board ____

Level 1 (Fail)	Level 1 (d) Level 2 (Fail)	Level 1 (c) Level 2 (d) Level 3 (Fail)	Level 1 (b) Level 2 (c) Leve 3 (d)	Level 1 (a) Level 2 (b) Level 3 (c)	Level 2 (a) Level 3 (b)	Level 3 (a)
Clearly failed to address the task set	Has only addressed the task set in a superficial manner that lacks a clear focus	Begins to address the task with some evidence of focus	Has focused on the task set in a descriptive manner	Has focused on the task set in a structured manner	Has clearly focused on the task set in a structured manner with evidence of some creativity	Has clearly focused on the task in an insightful, creative and critical manner

37. Assessment of Clinical and Communication Skills: Operationalizing Benner's Model

Margaret J. Nicol, Andrea Fox-Hiley, Carol J. Bavin and Rosemary Sheng

The introduction of ward-based clinical assessment of nursing skills in the 1970s meant a more realistic method of assessment, but still essentially a 'snapshot' of the student's practical abilities. This is now being replaced by continuous clinical assessment which requires that student nurses meet the expected level of competence in a range of nursing skills in each clinical placement.

Benner's (1984) model of skill acquisition is currently receiving considerable attention by nurse educationalists and is providing the framework for many curricula (English, 1993). The model identifies five stages of development in nursing: novice; advanced beginner; competent; proficient; and expert. What is needed, however, is a more detailed description of what those stages mean in terms of the component parts of nursing, especially the clinical and communication skills.

This paper describes a framework for the assessment of clinical and communication skills, a framework which seeks to operationalize Benner's model by defining the level of performance expected in clinical and communication skills at each stage.

Introduction

Assessment of clinical skills continues to be a concern for all involved in the education of nurses. Woolley (1977) identifies that the skills controversy is a constant thread in nurse education and that it is essential to develop a working consensus on three major issues: the importance attached to skills acquisition; the level of competence expected; and whether, and if so in what way, student performance should be graded.

Quinn (1989) documents the development of the assessment of clinical skills and identifies the shift in the 1970s from the periodic use of checklists to continuous clinical assessment. The introduction of continuous clinical assessment was generally believed to offer a more valid, reliable and more realistic form of assessment (Quinn, 1989).

As Girot (1993) notes, however, in the past, clinical assessment has been offered little priority compared to assessment of academic ability. Furthermore, the introduction of new curricula in the light of the Project 2000 proposals (UKCC, 1986) has meant that student nurses spend more time in college and community-based activities. Clinical placements are now more varied and as a result experience is less predictable. As Girot

Margaret J. Nicol, Andrea Fox-Hiley, Carol J. Bavin and Rosemary Sheng: 'Assessment of Clinical and Communication Skills: Operationalizing Benner's Model' in *NURSE EDUCATION TODAY* (1996), 16, pp. 175–179. Reprinted by permission of the publisher Churchill Livingstone.

(1993) comments, with increasing pressures on clinical nursing staff, shorter clinical placements and supernumerary status, '. . . continuous clinical assessment is in danger of becoming no assessment at all' (1993, p. 83).

Nursing is a practice-based discipline and the assessment of clinical practice is essential. In order to facilitate meaningful assessment in the practice environment, it is necessary to develop a clear understanding of exactly what is to be assessed, and how. The introduction of rule 18 (Nurses, Midwives and Health Visitors Act 1979) has meant that all nursing courses in the UK leading to registration must prepare students to achieve stated competencies, and the issue of 'competence' has become the focus for assessment.

Miller *et al.* (1988) suggest two senses in which competence may be defined: the ability to perform nursing tasks; and the ability to integrate the cognitive, affective and psychomotor skills needed to deliver nursing care. What is needed however, is a detailed description of what this means in terms of performance, especially the meaning of the term 'competent'.

This paper describes our attempts to identify what is required for competent practice, and the development of a framework which provides an overview of the development of nursing skills throughout our pre-registration programme.

Benner's (1984) model of skill acquisition underpins the Project 2000 curriculum in our college. The model is based on the work of Dreyfus & Dreyfus (1980) and describes five stages of development in nursing: novice; advanced beginner; competent; proficient; and expert. Each stage is associated with discrete capabilities and development through the stages is dependent on increasing clinical experience of nursing (English, 1993).

Benner's (1984) model provides a logical framework for nurse education, with students entering as Novices, and reaching the level of Advanced Beginner by the end of the Common Foundation Programme. The level, Competent, is achieved by the end of the chosen branch programme. Proficient, and ultimately Expert, status is reached only after many years of experience in one clinical area and may not be achieved by all nurses.

Our problems arose when we tried to apply these levels to the development of the separate components of nursing, specifically the clinical and communication skills. Benner (1984) is referring to stages of development in *nursing*, however; as nurse teachers we are concerned with helping the student to develop the component skills which when put together become *nursing*. Thus, at the end of the Common Foundation Programme, the student who is considered to be an Advanced Beginner in *nursing* will in fact be Competent in some clinical and communication skills and a Novice in others. This led us to develop the Schedule of Skills Development (Table 1) which enables us to indicate clearly what we mean by each of Benner's (1984) levels in terms of individual clinical and communication skills.

412

Schedule of skills development

The Schedule of Skills Development is a list of the clinical and communication skills considered necessary as a Registered Nurse. Table 1 illustrates examples of skill acquisition during the Adult Nursing branch. Each branch programme will have its own schedule although clearly the content of the Common Foundation Programme will be the same. Against each skill, the stages of development as the student progresses through the course are plotted, providing a clear overview of the course. The achievement of the various skills will be included in the learning outcomes for the clinical placements.

Table 1   Schedule of skills development

Skill	Common foundation programme Terms						Adult branch Terms					Registration	
	1	2	3	4	5	6	7	8	9	10	11	3Yr	Precept
Recording blood pressure		A	B/C					D		E			
Recording temperature		A	B/C			D				E			
Hand washing	A		B/C			D	E						
Drug administration (oral)				A		B/C						D	E

Abbreviations

A: Foundation level
B: Safe and accurate performance under direct supervision in the skills centre
C: Safe and accurate performance under direct supervision in the care setting
D: Safe and accurate performance with indirect supervision in the care setting
E: Skill mastery
3Yr: End of preregistration programme
Precept: End of period of preceptorship

In order to do this, it was necessary to be clear about the expected level of performance at each stage. Reilly & Oermann (1985) describe a psychomotor taxonomy with five levels of attainment: imitation; manipulation; precision; articulation; and naturalization. These levels were adopted by Alavi et al. (1991), who subdivided the Precision level to distinguish between performance in the skills laboratory, and performance at this level within a care setting. As described in an earlier paper (Studdy et al. 1994), these levels were initially incorporated into our approach to skills teaching. However, difficulties were encountered because they refer only to the psychomotor aspects of the skill. We were concerned that emphasis on only the psychomotor aspects of nursing skills might lead to a fragmentation and a perception of nursing as merely a series of tasks.

Our approach to skills teaching is based on an integrated skills teaching model (Studdy et al. 1994), in which skills are not taught in isolation but set in context, and the relationship of other aspects of the curriculum are emphasized. Thus the term 'nursing

---

Box 1   Levels of clinical skill development

E: Skill mastery
Psychomotor components of the skill no longer require conscious thought
Cognitive and affective components are highly developed and an integral part of every nursing intervention
Performance, based on increasing knowledge and experience, is confident, efficient and responsive to situational cues
Reflection is central to practice at this level

D: Safe and accurate performance with indirect supervision in the care setting
Performance of the skill will be accurate, coordinated, effective and affective
The student is able to adapt his or her performance in response to changes in the care situation
Cognitive and affective components of the skill are integrated
The student is aware of his or her limitations and seeks help and advice as appropriate
Performance at this level is 'competent'

C: Safe and accurate performance under direct supervision in the care setting
The student is able to demonstrate accuracy in the skill, but not necessarily speed
Psychomotor dexterity is demonstrated
Cognitive and affective components of the skill are evident

B: Safe and accurate performance in the skills centre
The student is able to demonstrate accuracy in the skill, but not necessarily speed
Psychomotor dexterity is demonstrated
Awareness of the cognitive and affective components of the skill is demonstrated

A: Foundation
The student is able to demonstrate psychomotor components of the skill by following instruction
Performance is slow and lacks coordination
The student is able to identify the cognitive and affective components of the skill

---

skill' refers to more than just the performance of a task, it refers to the integration of the cognitive, affective and psychomotor domains (Bloom, 1968). A literature search failed to identity any suitable tool and so the Levels of Skills Acquisition were developed. Initially these focused on practical nursing skills (Box 1) but this was quickly expanded to include communication skills (Box 2).

Box 2   Levels of communication skill development

E: Skill mastery

Communication skills are a natural part of every professional interaction

Cognitive, affective and psychomotor components are highly developed and less subject to interference from other ongoing activities

Performance, based on increasing knowledge and experience, is confident, efficient and responsive to situational cues

Reflection is central to practice at this level

D: Safe and accurate performance with indirect supervision in the care setting

The student is able to use an appropriate blend of communication skills, in a coordinated and effective manner

The student is aware of his or her limitations and seeks help and advice as appropriate

The student is able to adapt his or her performance in response to changes in the care situation

Performance at this level is 'competent'

C: Safe and accurate performance under direct supervision in the care setting

The student is able to utilize and blend communication skills together

The communication skills chosen are appropriate to the patient/client and the situation

The skills are executed smoothly and appear natural

B: Safe and accurate performance in the skills centre

The student is able to utilize and blend communication skills together

The communication skills chosen are appropriate to the patient/client and the situation

The skills are executed smoothly and appear natural

A: Foundation

The student is able to identify the rationale for use of the skill, although tends to reiterate text book explanations

The student is able to state when use of the skill is appropriate, and to what degree

Performance of the skill is awkward and the student may appear self-conscious

---

The levels of skills acquisition

The Levels of Skills Acquisition are designed to complement our approach to teaching and the development of a Skills Centre (Studdy *et al.* 1994). Each level refers to development of not only the psychomotor but also the cognitive and affective domains of the skill. In the early stages of performance, practise inevitably focuses on the psychomotor domain. However, as the student becomes more practised, the psychomotor domain becomes increasingly autonomous, less directly subject to

415

cognitive control and less subject to interference from other ongoing activities (Fitts & Posner, 1967). As a result, the student is increasingly able to develop and integrate the cognitive and affective domains of the skill.

Level A (foundation) refers to the initial exposure to the skill, usually the first teaching session, where the student knows what he or she is required to do but needs practise.

Level B (safe and accurate performance in the skills centre). Currently practise is gained during clinical placements, but the Skills Centre will mean that students are increasingly able to reach Level B before using their skills on or with real patients. The Skills Centre will also enable self-directed practise by students so that they are able to develop at their own pace in an environment in which the 'threat to self' described by Rogers (1969) is minimized.

Level C (safe and accurate performance under direct supervision in the care setting) refers to the stage when the student is able to perform the skill, but is not yet able to cope with the complex and potentially unpredictable nature of the care setting. Under direct supervision the student is able to perform safely because the supervisor is able to take control should the need arise.

Level D (safe and accurate performance with indirect supervision in the care setting). The student is considered to be 'competent'. He or she is able to perform the skill safely and accurately, integrating the cognitive, affective and psychomotor domains in an effective way to deliver nursing care. Only indirect supervision is required with the student seeking help and advice as necessary. Being aware of his or her own limitations is vital to safe performance at this level. This is the level of performance that will be expected in most skills by the end of the branch programme or period of preceptorship.

Level E indicates skill mastery. Increasing knowledge and experience will enable development to the level of mastery, however this is not an automatic progression and some nurses may never achieve this in all skills. Experience alone is not the key, skill mastery results only if experience is accompanied by increasing knowledge and development of the skill through reflection. This level will probably be difficult to assess in any objective way, because breaking it into its component parts is likely to destroy the very thing, the high level of integration of all the domains, that we are trying to assess. We have attempted to identify the key aspects of performance at this level because despite the potential difficulties in assessing it, we 'know it when we see it'.

We felt that although the framework is primarily concerned with assessment of skills, it is important to include a level beyond 'competent' to which student nurses may aspire.

To illustrate the levels, let us take for example the development of the skill of recording blood pressure.

At level A, the student can state (with much probing and prompting!) the physiology of blood pressure, can identify factors which may affect the blood pressure and relate this to when and why it may be recorded. The student will be aware of the communication skills involved, especially body language. Performance will be slow and lacking in dexterity, with the student clearly having to think consciously through each stage. He or she may take several attempts to obtain a reading and lacks the confidence to know that it is correct.

At level B, the student is now more practised in the psychomotor aspects of the skill and is able with accuracy to apply the cuff and position the stethoscope. The reading is performed smoothly, letting the mercury column fall at an even, controlled rate. The student is more confident about the accuracy of the reading, and checks this by reinflating the cuff during the reading to confirm the systolic or diastolic pressure, rather than repeating the whole procedure. The student is able to perform accurately a blood pressure reading in a controlled setting and record this on an observation chart.

At level C, the student now transfers the skills of blood pressure recording to the clinical care setting under the direct supervision of an experienced nurse. The student now has to think about where to position the sphygmomanometer and consider whether it is necessary to remove clothing from the patient/client's arm to place the cuff accurately. They also have to contend with the extraneous noises of the clinical environment during the recording, and the fact that the blood pressure may be outside the normal range or less audible than that of a healthy colleague. The student now has to cope with his or her own anxieties and use communication skills, particularly their body language to reassure and not alarm the patient/client.

At level D, the student is no longer overwhelmed by the clinical situation. He or she is able to perform the recording in a smooth and efficient way and is confident that it is correct. Clinical staff do not need to check the recording as they know that the student will seek help if uncertain. The student is able to control his or her body language and use communication skills to reassure the patient/client if an abnormal reading is discovered, and immediately reports this to the nurse in charge. The student utilizes relevant knowledge to initiate nursing action, e.g. lying the patient flat if a very low blood pressure has been recorded. The student is now considered 'competent'.

At level E, all the actions which contribute to the recording of the blood pressure are spontaneous and skilfully executed. The nurse's knowledge of the factors which may result in blood pressure variation mean that recordings are only made appropriately and not unnecessarily. He or she will be able to support his or her actions with sound reasoning.

Discussion

The Levels of Skills Acquisition have been developed in order to provide a clearer picture of what Benner's (1984) levels in nursing mean in terms of the individual clinical and communication skills. By 'operationalizing' Benner's model in this way, we are able to provide those involved in the education of student nurses, and the students themselves, with a clear overview of what is expected, and the way in which their skills will develop over the pre-registration programme and beyond.

Darbyshire *et al.* (1990) argue that a concentration on the assessment of learning outcomes and behavioural changes may be to the detriment of the process component of student learning. Our approach seeks to prevent this by emphasising integration and it is the increasing ability to integrate the three domains which reflect development of the skill towards mastery. Darbyshire *et al.* (1990) are also concerned that the behaviourist approach may lead to a fragmentation of nursing into a series of tasks. We feel that our integrated approach will discourage this, but at the same time recognize that nursing cannot be learnt as a single entity, it has to be broken down into manageable pieces for the student to learn. What is important is to ensure that students have the skills necessary to put all the pieces together and gradually build up the picture that is nursing.

This framework has been developed for our new Project 2000 curriculum and so is as yet untested. However, the response from clinical colleagues thus far has been encouraging and we are confident that we have the beginnings of a comprehensive framework which will help to clarify the thorny issue of the assessment of clinical skills in nursing.

References

Alavi C, Loh S H, Reilly D (1991) Reality basis for teaching psychmotor skills in a tertiary nursing curriculum. *Journal of Advanced Nursing* 16: 957–965.

Benner P (1984) *From novice to expert: excellence and power in clinical nursing practice.* Addison-Wesley, Menlo Park, CA.

Bloom B (1968) Learning for mastery. In: F Quinn (1989) *Principles and practice of nurse education.* Chapman Hall, London.

Darbyshire P, Stewart B, Jamieson L, Tongue C (1990) New domains in nursing. *Nursing Times* 86 (27): 73–75.

Dreyfus H L, Dreyfus S (1980) A five-stage model of the mental activities involved in direct skill acquisition. Cited in: P Benner (1984) *From novice to expert; excellence and power in clinical nursing practice.* Addison-Wesley, Menlo Park, CA.

English I (1993) Intuition as a function of the expert nurse: a critique of Benner's novice to expert model. *Journal of Advanced Nursing* 18: 387–393.

Fitts P, Posner M (1967) *Human Performance.* Prentice Hall, Englewood Cliffs, NJ.

Girot E A (1993) Assessment of competence in clinical practice — a review of the literature. *Nurse Education Today* 13: 83–90.

Miller *et al.* (1988) Credit where credit's due: Cited in: E A Girot (1993) Assessment of competence in clinical practice — a review of the literature. *Nurse Education Today* 13: 83–90.

Reilly D E, Oermann M M (1985) *The clinical field; its use in nursing education.* Appleton-Century-Croft, Norwalk, CT.

Rogers C (1969) *Freedom to learn.* Merrill, Ohio.

Studdy S, Nicol M J, Fox-Hiley A (1994) The developement of multidisciplinary skills centre. *Nurse Education Today* 14: 177–193.

Quinn F (1989) *The principles and practice of nurse education.* Chapman Hall, London.

United Kingdom Central Council (1986) *Project 2000 — a preparation for practice.* UKCC, London.

Wooley A S (1977) The long and tortured history of clinical evaluation. *Nursing Outlook* 25: 308–315.

38. Evaluation of Tools to Assess Clinical Competence

Vivien E. Coates and Mary Chambers

Assessment of student nurses' clinical skills is an important issue in nurse education. However suitable instruments are difficult to locate, and also to design. In the course of this article the need for scientifically designed and tested assessment instruments is discussed. The thoroughness with which 11 clinical assessment documents were developed was evaluated using specific criteria. It was found that in the majority of cases use of a systematic research process to guide development was not evident. However it must be noted that the assessment documents were only evaluated via their presentation in journal articles. Full details of the entire project had perhaps not been published. The implications of the results, some of the difficulties inherent in instrument design and the limitations of this small review are considered.

Introduction

In order for student nurses to qualify as nursing practitioners they must demonstrate that an acceptable standard of clinical competence has been achieved. The need to have a certain standard of expertise is common to all health professionals and is important to protect the public, to ensure quality care and to establish credibility of members of the profession (Bashook, 1985). The quest to measure clinical skills in nursing has led to considerable debate and there is no shortage of information about the problems inherent in this issue (Andrusysyzn, 1989; Bashook, 1985; Benner, 1982; Hepworth, 1989; Krumme, 1975; Scott, 1982; Wood, 1982).

A recurring theme in the above mentioned literature is the need for assessment instruments that are objective, reliable and valid. If we bear in mind that an objective measure is one that can be independently checked by other people (Polit & Hungler, 1985), to be reliable means the ability to measure consistently (Powers & Knapp, 1990), and that to be valid it measures what it purports to measure (Powers & Knapp, 1991), it would seem that these factors should be fundamental to any useful instrument.

Our initial interest in the topic of student assessment arose out of the need to find a more useful assessment instrument than was currently in use in our work, and a wide range of literature was consulted. In doing so it became apparent that, whilst a great deal was written on the topic of assessment of clinical skills, there was little information about assessment instruments which were known to be objective, reliable and valid.

It is particularly important to consider such matters seriously at present as the changes engendered by implementing Project 2000 nursing courses will necessitate

Vivien E. Coates and Mary Chambers: 'Evaluation of Tools to Assess Clinical Competence' in *NURSE EDUCATION TODAY* (1992), 12, pp. 122–129. Reprinted by permission of the publisher Churchill Livingstone.

new means of student nurse assessment. When discussing the challenges for nurse teachers embarking on the Project 2000 recommendation to link nurse education to further and higher education Hollingsworth (1989) noted that,

> 'Project 2000 is about reforming nurse education in order for us to establish nursing as discipline which has a leading part to play in the provision of health care. To do this we have to underpin our practice with research findings . . .' (Hollingsworth, 1989, p. 25)

Both the reform of nurse education and basing practice on research are relevant to the subject of student assessment.

This article will consider the extent to which a small sample of published assessment tools are reported to be reliable and valid instruments. The need to base future development of assessment tools on scientific principles will also be discussed.

Method

An integrative literature review

A literature review was undertaken to evaluate the rigour with which a sample of previously published assessment tools had been developed. The purpose of the review was to summarise and synthesise the results of previous studies in order to gain a more general picture than that which might be achieved by considering individual research findings. This task may be considered an integrative review (Ganong, 1987). If the results of previous studies are subjected to statistical manipulation the term used is meta-analysis (Abraham *et al.* 1987) but such techniques were not employed in this research. Organising the review was guided by the work by Ganong who urges that 'integrative reviews should be held to the same standards of clarity, rigour and replication as primary research.' (Ganong, 1987, p. 2)

The sample

Whilst trying to find a suitable alternative assessment schedule for students we conducted a literature review. This involved both a computer search and subsequent retrieval of all references considered relevant. Several books had been consulted, for example Kenworthy and Nicklin (1989) and Bradshaw (1989) but the bulk of the literature comprised journal articles. For this integrated review it was decided to use all the journal articles which we had gathered over the previous years. This meant that we did not include all published articles reporting the development of an assessment instrument. However the selection of material was not biased as the primary intention at the time the search was conducted was simply to identify what alternative schedules were available, not to look critically at the methodology involved in the design. This review is therefore based on a sample of convenience.

Data gathering

The next step was to decide which aspects of instrument development were to be looked for in each of the articles. As we were interested in tools which had scientific credibility it was felt that the instruments needed to be developed through a research process. The factors which were sought in the integrative review therefore were those which are also important in the research process. In each article we checked whether the following were included:

1. A theoretical framework upon which to base the research/instrument design.

2. Identification of the method of assessment, for example profiling.

3. Details of the pilot study, including the size of the sample involved.

4. Information about the method by which the main study was conducted.

5. Length of time the assessment instrument had been in use.

6. Discussion or measurement of reliability and validity.

7. Evaluation of the assessment instrument.

It was also thought useful if an example of at least part at the assessment tool was included.

Discussion of the criteria

The theoretical framework was considered important because it provides the rationale for the research (Abdellah & Levine, 1965). For example when considering the development of clinical skill Benner (1984) works from theory developed by Dreyfus (1982). The theory helped her to interpret the stages nurses may pass through in order to achieve expert status. Similarly Andrusyszn (1989) when discussing the thorny problem of assessment of nursing skills in the affective domain noted the need to refer to theory to support practice and quoted Epstein (1977), 'the affective domain cannot be evaluated without knowing how values are learned and how we teach them' (Epstein, 1977, cited by Andrusyszn, 1989, p. 76).

According to Diers the theoretical background to the study is one of the most critical in the research process, because every other aspect of the process derives from it (Diers, 1979). Batey (1977) surveyed publications from 25 years of the journal *Nursing Research*, and found that 'the majority of the major inadequacies in published studies were in the conceptual phase of the study, rather than in the empirical or methodological phase' (cited by Diers, 1979, p. 63).

The framework can unite previous work and thinking on a subject, and current research can feed into this, so adding to the body of knowledge on a topic. Brink and Wood (1988) note that the 'framework will be tested in the course of the study and will either be supported or refuted by your results, and in this way will add to the literature on the theory you are using' (Brink & Wood, 1988, p. 48).

In this review if the study was to develop an assessment tool involving continuous assessment (CA) we were looking for a theory underlying CA, rather than a description of what it was thought to be. Points 2–7 listed above were deemed important because they would indicate the rigour with which the tool had been designed and tested, and the reported value of it in practice. To help people decide whether they wish to use assessment schedules designed by others it is important that they have access to such information. However, it is appreciated that the criteria sought in the review could have been considered when the authors were developing the assessment instrument but for various reasons were not, or could not, be included in the publication. The primary purpose of authors is often to publicise results rather than give details of the methods used. It should be noted that the authors whose work was included in the review may have only published a small sample of their work in order to publicise their area of research. They may expect to be contacted by those interested in their work and give further details at this stage.

Method of reviewing

A broadsheet containing the criteria to be looked for in each article was drawn up. The authors independently read the literature and marked off whether the criteria were included in the articles. Each set of broadsheets was subsequently compared. As the criteria were mainly objective items there was little disagreement between the two reviewers. If the authors had categorized, or interpreted information differently, the article was reconsidered and usually the most lenient interpretation was taken. For example, if one reviewer thought the evaluation was included whilst the other did not, the view of the former was that which was recorded. In this way each article reviewed was given 'the benefit of the doubt' to meet the sought criteria.

Results

A total of 49 articles concerning clinical assessment of competence were reviewed; of these 13 were about developing an assessment instrument, 11 concerned nursing, 1 medicine and 1 occupational therapy. It was decided that the 11 articles concerning the development of an instrument to assess clinical competence in nursing would be included in the integrated review. These articles are listed in the Appendix.

The results of the integrative review are illustrated below in the Table.

Table 1   The result of the review

Total number of articles reviewed	49
Number of articles which described the development of an assessment tool for nursing (listed in Appendix)	11

Criterion to be identified	Number of articles in which criterion identified n = 11
1. Theoretical framework included	2
2. Method of clinical assessment identified	11
3. Pilot study undertaken	5
4. Main study described	3
5. Length of time in use stated	3
6. Reliability and validity discussed	5
7. Reliability and validity measured	1
8. Whole instrument illustrated	2
9. Part of instrument illustrated	9
10. Evaluation of pilot study included	4
11. Evaluation of overall assessment schedule development and use included	3
12. No evaluation of the assessment tool	4

Discussion

Meeting the criteria

The first of the criteria was the presence of a theoretical framework, and it can be seen from the Table that only 2 of the 11 articles indicated the tools were based on theory. Whilst the authors of the other articles did discuss the type of assessment instrument they wished to develop, they did not link the work to a theoretical framework, for example to theories of learning from education or psychology. As such the basis for the work was not as thoroughly established as it could have been. Bearing in mind the quotation by Batey (1977) cited above, the lack of a sound theoretical base when developing clinical assessment instruments may be one of the reasons there is so much information about the problems inherent in assessment of competence. By involving a theoretical framework, and a scientific process of development, the opportunity for small studies to contribute to knowledge development increases.

Wood (1982) noted the lengthy process of developing evaluation tools

'The entire process for the development of a form usually took a minimum of two years . . . The costs are high and the results are disappointing.' (Wood, 1982, p. 17)

If the work considered in her review had been linked to theory it could also have been contributing to the development of a body of nursing knowledge, as suggested above by Brink and Wood (1988).

In addition to theory development, but relevant to it, is the need for a definition of terminology. This applies to aspects of nursing competence. For example, what do we mean by 'competent to teach patients? Also, if a grading system is to be used, definition of 'adequate' or 'proficient' grades is required. These issues are more thoroughly discussed by Krumme (1975), and with specific reference to psychiatry by Thompson (1989).

Benner also noted that progress in the development of assessment instruments has been hindered by 'the lack of adequate pre-existing definition of competency' (Benner, 1982, p. 303). Whilst arbitrarily defined terms are used, the objectivity of the assessment procedure will be undermined through lack of standardisation. The other criteria regarding the methods involved in developing the assessment instrument were also often not documented (Table 1–points 3, 4, 6, 7, 11). Information about how the study was undertaken is important 'so that any researcher wishing to replicate it would be able to do so from the information given' (Stephenson, 1985, p. 104).

Despite the accepted need for reliable and valid instruments, as noted above, it appeared from the available published information, that only one article in the review included details of these factors. The need for reliability of assessment tools was obvious to Donabedian over 20 years ago. She wrote

'The reliability or repeatability of judgements using any given method of assessment . . . should be part and parcel of the development of that method.' (Donabedian, 1969, cited by Krumme, 1975, p. 768)

Krumme goes on to say that 'It is difficult to understand the neglect of the pioneers in nursing audit to test and document the reliability of their instruments' (Krumme, 1975, p. 768).

Four articles included an evaluation of the pilot study, but only three studies contained an overall evaluation of the instrument, whilst four did not contain any information of this nature at all. Lack of information may discourage others in nursing from using these tools, which could be of potential value to them. In this way researchers may make similar mistakes as they are denied the opportunity of learning from the experience of those who have previously undertaken similar work.

Only three articles mentioned the length of time the assessment instrument had been in use. This information is also important as nurse teachers may want to know whether an instrument has 'stood the test of time' before considering whether it would be suitable for their own needs. Two articles illustrated the entire schedule, a further seven gave a partial example, whilst two articles did not illustrate any aspect of the assessment schedule. Without an example it may be difficult for others to visualise the instrument in question.

Skills and resources needed for instrument design

The development of assessment instruments is likely to be endemic in nursing circles in the United Kingdom at present. As new curricula are being developed for Project 2000 courses there is widespread realisation that previous methods of assessment will no longer be useful and new schedules will be required (Hepworth, 1989). There is a danger that nurses throughout the UK will be working hard to develop new assessment tools, but working in isolation and perhaps independently covering similar ground.

The results indicate that in the past instrument design may have been undertaken without following a scientific process, and this has led to inadequately tested tools. Nurses must be involved in instrument design as they appreciate the skills the students must master. If necessary, nurses must be given the opportunity to gain any additional skills as are required to undertake instrument design. Time, and resources, to gain any necessary skills therefore need to be allowed for when initially planning and budgeting for the development of assessment instruments. Woods (1982) also notes the importance of allowing adequate time to complete the project, and realistically suggests it may take 2 years to design and test a clinical assessment instrument. Perhaps in the past it has been expected that nurses can design tools much more rapidly than this, and as a result they could not be fully tested.

Replication and implementation of research

From this small integrative review it can be seen that there are few articles about the development of an assessment tool that could be used as a basis to replicate studies. The need for more replication of studies in nursing is acknowledged (MacGuire, 1990) and this is an area in which such work may be particularly important. Another often mentioned subject, akin to the need to replicate studies, is that of the need to implement research findings (Hunt, 1987; MacGuire, 1990).

While discussing the problem of non-implementation of research findings Bergman (1988) raises the following points:

1.   On what basis do practitioners accept or reject research findings?

2.   Do they use research to introduce change?

3.   Have research findings had an impact on nursing practice?

This review indicates that in the case of clinical assessment it would be difficult to know how practitioners could decide whether to accept an assessment tool. Also, the review indicates that practitioners would find it difficult to use the published literature to introduce change, that the research is not sufficiently developed in many cases to warrant introduction, and thus has not had an opportunity to have a positive impact on practice. The volume of literature lamenting the problems associated with this issue may be a result of the lack of thorough research in this area.

While the purpose of the review was not to rate one study against another, but was to gain a general impression of the scientific development of a sample of instruments, it would appear that the most thoroughly reported and tested schedules from the information in the articles were those of Dunn (1986), Ross et al. (1988) and Scott (1984). These articles may serve as valuable examples to others considering assessment design although the type of assessment may not be what they have in mind.

Limitations of the review

It must be remembered that the review comprised only a small part of the total literature available on the subject of clinical assessment. As such the findings can only indicate trends in the articles reviewed above. There may well be articles containing research based development of clinical assessment tools which were not mentioned here. While the literature review was not exhaustive, it was the result of a reasonably wide search. We noted above that the time and energy required of nursing staff who have to attempt to develop new assessment schedules is costly (Woods, 1982). In these days of ever increasing workloads it is likely that few people detailed to develop an assessment schedule will have either the time, or the opportunity to undertake an extensive search and thorough review. In which case the scope of this review may be representative of that which is available to most nursing staff undertaking this task.

Another limitation to the review could arise from adopting the stance that nursing competence must be measured. It should be noted that this belief is not universally held. Over 10 years ago Sheahan wrote of his concerns about a lack of valid measurement in nursing education but concluded, 'Those concerned with nursing education should measure but should not confine themselves to measurement' (Sheehan, 1979, p. 56). Benner also warned that it is premature to place too much faith in assessment of certain competencies. She feels there is a danger that we may be 'carried along by a technological, measurement-orientated age . . .' (Benner, 1982, p. 303).

Similarly Andrusyszyn (1989) addresses the problems in trying to assess competencies in the affective domain, and notes 'the subjectivity associated with clinical evaluation of the affective domain renders it difficult to measure and grade. Although the mechanisms discussed are useful tools with which to provide insight into students' attitudes and values, they may not provide hard data that can be measured for the purpose of assigning a grade.'

Whilst we have focused on the need for measurement of nursing skills, and stressed the need for a scientific basis for the assessment instruments used, we acknowledge that areas of nursing care cannot be ignored because there is not currently an acceptable method of assessing them.

Lest it be thought that we have been unduly critical of our colleagues it should be noted that we have included our own effort at developing a clinical assessment schedule (Coates & Chambers, 1990), and in the course of the review noted that it also fell short of many of the criteria listed in the Table.

Conclusion

The purpose of this review was to draw attention to the need for more rigorously designed and tested instruments of clinical assessment. A small number of articles were reviewed and illustrated that many of the stages considered to be fundamental to the research process (Diers, 1979) were often not mentioned. It is particularly timely to consider such issues at present as Project 2000 courses are being rapidly developed, and the students participating in them will soon need to be assessed.

Whilst it is accepted that objectivity, reliability and validity are difficult to identity and measure it is suggested that clinical assessment cannot be adequately undertaken until the instruments used are known to possess these properties. Nurses who are involved in instrument development must have suitable skills to undertake the task, and must be allowed sufficient resources to formulate and test assessment instruments thoroughly.

References

Abdellah F G, Levine E (1965) *Better patient care through nursing research*. Macmillan, New York.

Abraham I L, Shultz S, Polis N, Vines S W, Smith M C (1987) Research on research: meta-analysis of nursing and health research. In: M C Cahoon (ed) *Recent Advances in Nursing*. Churchill Livingstone, Edinburgh.

Andrusyszyn M A (1989) Clinical evaluation of the affective domain. *Nurse Education Today* 9: 75–81.

Bashoook P G (1985) Clinical assessment: a state of the art review. *Diabetes Educator* 11, Suppl: 30–36.

Benner P (1982) Issues in competency-based testing. *Nursing Outlook* 30, 5: 303–309.

Benner P (1984) *From novice to expert*. Addison Wesley, Menlo Park.

Bergman R (1988) Omissions in nursing research: another look. *International Nursing Review* 35, 6: 165–168.

Bradshaw P L (Ed) (1989) *Teaching and assessment in clinical practice*. Prentice Hall, London.

Brink P J, Wood M J (1988) *Basic steps in planning nursing research from question to proposal.* Jones & Bartlett, Boston.

Coates V E, Chambers M (1990) Developing a system of student nurses profiling through action research. *Nurse Education Today* 10: 83–91.

Diers D (1979) *Research in nursing practice.* J B Lippincott, Philadelphia.

Dreyfus S E (1982) Formal models vs human situational understanding: inherent limitations on the modelling of business expertise. *Office Technology and People* 1: 133–165.

Dunn D M (1986) Assessing the development of clinical nursing skills. *Nurse Education Today* 6: 28–35.

Ganong L A (1987) Integrative reviews of nursing research. *Research in Nursing and Health* 10: 1–11.

Hepworth S (1989) Professional judgement and nurse education. *Nurse Education Today* 9: 408–412.

Hollingsworth S (1989) Securing nursing as a credible profession: the challenge for nurse teachers. *Nursing Standard* 36 (3): 25–32.

Hunt M (1987) The process of translating research findings into nursing practice. *Journal of Advanced Nursing* 12: 101–110.

Krumme U (1975) The case for criterion-referenced measurement. *Nursing Outlook* 23, 12: 764–770.

Kenworthy N, Nicklin P (1989) *Teaching and assessing in nursing practice.* Scutari Press, London.

MacGuire M (1990) Putting nursing research findings into practice: research utilization as an aspect of the management of change. *Journal of Advanced Nursing* 15: 614–620.

Polit D F, Hungler B P (1985) *Essentials of nursing research methods and applications.* J B Lippincott, Philadelphia.

Powers B A, Knapp T A (1990) *A dictionary of nursing theory and research.* Sage, London.

Ross M, Carroll G, Knight J Chamberlain M *et al.* (1988) Using the OSCE to measure clinical skills performance in nursing. *Journal of Advanced Nursing* 13: 45–56.

Scott B (1982) Competency based learning: a literature review. *International Journal of Nursing Studies* 19, 3: 119–124.

Scott B (1984) A Competency based learning model for critical care nursing. *International Journal of Nursing Studies* 21, 1: 9–17.

Sheahan J (1979) Measurement in nursing education. *Journal of Advanced Nursing* 4, 1: 47–56.

Stephenson P M (1985) Reading a research report. *Intensive Care Nursing* 1: 102–106.

Thompson C (1989) *The instruments of psychiatric research.* Wiley, Chichester.

Wood V (1982) Evaluation of student nurse clinical performance — a continuing performance. *International Nursing Review* 29, 1: 11–18.

Appendix

Articles included in the review

Coates V E, Chambers M (1990) Developing a system of student nurse profiling through action research. *Nurse Education Today* 10: 83–91.

Darbyshire P, Stewart B, Jamieson L, Tongue C (1990) A new approach to students' clinical assessment being implemented in Glasgow. *Nursing Times* 86, 27: 73–75.

Dunn D M (1986) Assessing the development of clinical nursing skills. *Nurse Education Today* 6: 28–35.

France M (1988) Dawn of a new age: assessment and evaluation. *Senior Nurse* 8, 12: 25–27.

Ross M, Carroll G, Knight J, Chamberlain M *et al.* (1988) Using the OSCE to measure clinical skills performance in nursing. *Journal of Advanced Nursing* 13: 45–56.

Scott B (1984) A competency based learning model for critical care nursing. *International Journal of Nursing Studies* 21, 1: 9–17.

Shearer M (1989) Progressing nicely. *Nursing Times* 85, 3: 60–61.

Skelton G (1987) Student profiling. *Nursing Times* 83, 5: 62–63.

Sweeney J (1988) Student profiling as a basis for continuous assessment of clinical progress during a registered mental nurse course. *Nurse Education Today* 9: 254–263.

White E (1989) A scheme for continuous practical assessment. *Senior Nurse* 10, 3: 27–29.

Yeun F, Pircombe J, Martin M (1987) Student competence profile: the Wollongong approach. *International Nursing Review* 34, 4: 107–109.

39.   Evaluation

How can we tell . . . ?
Alan Rogers

The need for evaluation

Like earlier sections of this book, this chapter is intended to raise questions rather than to propose firm answers. The approach to evaluation here is a practical one; the intention is to make conscious what most of us do much of the time as part of the process of teaching. It is often assumed that the need for and the means of evaluation are self-evident, but if it were, teachers would be better at doing it and would be able to see themselves doing it, more often and more effectively. Evaluation is one of the more difficult skills required of the teacher, and we need to work at it consciously. There are different possible strategies involved, and our task is to choose between them, to decide for ourselves our own preferred way of working.

Along with this should go a willingness to change what we (and our student participants) are doing. There is no point in evaluating the teaching–learning situation if we are unwilling to change course. Evaluation will be effective only if we are prepared to alter or even scrap our existing programme when we detect something wrong and begin again.

A distinction also needs to be drawn between evaluation and assessment. *Assessment* is the collection of data on which we base our evaluation. It is descriptive and objective; if anyone else were to do it, they would come up with much the same findings. *Evaluation* on the other hand is a process of making personalised judgements, decisions about achievements, about expectations, about the effectiveness and value of what we are doing. It involves notions of 'good' and 'bad' teaching and learning, of worth. It is based on our own ideology.

Why evaluate?

Evaluation is necessary for at least three reasons:

- To improve our performance as teachers. Questions of quality, of accountability, of protecting our 'customers', of being effective are important not just for the providers and organisers but also for our student participants and for ourselves. We must believe in what we are doing and that we are doing it well, in order to do it well.

- To plan new strategies, make choices, establish priorities; to determine where we are in the teaching–learning process at present and what to do next; to identify helps and hindrances and decide what to do about them.

Alan Rogers: 'Evaluation: How can we tell . . .?' from *TEACHING ADULTS* (Open University Press, 1996; 2nd edn), pp. 220–233.

- To learn: to assess how much progress has been made, in which direction and how much farther there is to go. Evaluation is an essential part of learning.

Two main forms of evaluation have been identified by writers on this subject: *formative* — the ongoing evaluation that is inherent in the learning process itself and leads to learning changes; and *summative* — evaluation that takes place at different times, particularly at the end of the programme of learning, to see how far we have got. But these are not in fact two distinct processes, only one. If a summative evaluation undertaken at the end of a course (a teacher's report, for instance) is used to plan new programmes and new approaches, then it becomes a formative one. It is the way evaluation is used that distinguishes it. If it looks only backwards and reviews what has been done, it is summative; if in addition it looks forward to, and influences, new procedures, it is formative. The latter is more productive; evaluation judgements should lead to change. But there is also a time for the former.

Who evaluates?

We can also distinguish between *external* and occasional evaluation, practised by the organiser of the programme or some inspector or external validating body, and *internal*, more regular evaluation, practised by the teacher in the course of the teaching programme.

The *organiser* will be assessing how the programme objectives are being met. Are we getting in our groups the right kind of student-learners, the ones the programme is primarily intended for, those we feel to be in most need? Are they learning the right things? Are the courses meeting their needs and intentions? Are the programmes on offer reflecting the selectivity-, competitiveness- and competency-based criteria of the existing educational system, or are they offering a different (non-selective, non-competitive and effort-based) ethos? In addition, at a time of static or dwindling resources, the providers' concern will be with matters of quality control. They need to determine whether the resources they have at their disposal are being used most effectively and, in certain circumstances, to establish priorities. To do all this, they will need criteria to determine whether some courses are better than others and to plan accordingly.

The *teachers* also evaluate their work in order to plan. They are concerned with whether they are being effective as teachers; whether the objectives they have set are the right ones and at the right level, as well as whether they are being met. They need to assess progress, match between intentions (objectives) and outcomes (the results of the teaching–learning process), to measure change, appraise efforts, identify new needs and assess strengths and weaknesses. They will wish to learn whether the short-term goals and the tasks they have laid before the group have been achieved and whether they are of the kind that will contribute towards the desired learning changes. They need to test whether the learners are ready to move on to the next stage or not. They will want to see clearly the *intended* programme of learning, the *implemented* programme (which may be different from what was intended for various reasons) and whether that again differs from the *received* programme.

Both organiser and teacher, then, evaluate for much the same reason, for their own learning and to plan changes. But teachers also build evaluation into the teaching–learning process for the learners' sake. They use evaluation for (extrinsic) motivation (although not all of the participants need this). What is more, an ongoing programme of evaluation is a necessary part of the learning process and becomes part of the work of the whole group.

So thirdly the *learners* themselves evaluate in the course of learning. Evaluation is an essential tool for developing new skills, knowledge and understanding. Hitting a tennis ball against a line on a wall in a practice session brings about no learning changes by itself (though it may strengthen the muscles). What is needed is a series of judgements: 'That was too high'; modification; 'That was too low'; modification; 'That was about right'; repetition; 'That was good'; once more; and so on. Only by such an evaluative process will learning changes take place. Trial-and-error learning particularly is based on evaluation, but most other kinds of learning also rely on this process for effective changes. The learners then engage in formative evaluation in order to learn. They will also pursue summative self-evaluation for motivation: assessing their own progress and performance, rekindling their enthusiasm for the learning goals in the light of their achievements (what is called ipsative evaluation).

It is likely — though not inevitable and probably not desirable — that the evaluation by the teacher and by the outside body (usually organiser) will not be the same, for their objectives differ to a certain degree (even though those of the organiser are subsumed in those of the teacher). It is also likely — and almost certainly undesirable — that the evaluation by the teacher and by the learner will be different. A hierarchy of evaluation thus emerges and should be developed more consciously, the organisers and inspectors (where they exist) should encourage the teachers to evaluate, and they in their turn should encourage the student participants to engage in evaluation. Since evaluation is largely a skill, the teachers need to teach the learners how to evaluate; they should demonstrate the process. Evaluation is one of those exercises that need to be practised jointly between teacher and student participant rather than be taught by exhortation.

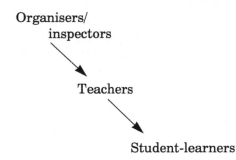

Evaluate what?

There are many different tools of evaluation. One of the more useful ones which may be used for any formative evaluation of adult learning programmes is the appropriately named SWOT approach: to assess the *strengths* and the *weaknesses* of the programme or class and to assess the *opportunities* which it opens and which may or may not have been taken up, also the *threats* which will hamper the effectiveness of the programme and which need to be addressed if the goals of the learning programme are to be achieved. This approach has specific advantages in that it encourages us to look beyond the normal assessment of strengths and weaknesses to explore other possibilities and the risks faced in the programme.

In evaluating our adult education activities, there is one overriding concern — whether the learners are learning or not. That must be the eventual standard by which our programmes need to be judged. In order to assess this, we may look at three main elements: goal achievement, teaching processes, and student attainments.

1. Goal achievement

The learning objectives need to be submitted to evaluation in two main ways: Are they the right ones? How far are they being met? We need to identify clearly the intentions of the programme of learning and to submit these to some form of judgement. Perhaps we take for granted that the objectives of our courses — to learn a craft or other skill, to study literature and so on are the right ones, self-justifying. But these assumptions need to be examined in depth. Is the learning primarily concerned with personal growth, or with socialisation and social change, or with vocational advancement? Whose goals are they, ours or those of the student participants? We also need to assess how far these intentions are being achieved, whether the programme of learning is proving effective. Throughout, we must ask whether the student participants are learning in a particular area, even when this learning is seen as a means of achieving some goal that lies behind the learning. Even if the goal is to pass an examination or to create a work of art for oneself, the means to the satisfactory attainment of these goals is student learning.

2. Teaching processes

The entire process by which the teacher creates the learning opportunity (planning skills as well as powers of exposition) needs to be evaluated. Once again the main concern is with the learner rather than the teacher; the purpose of effective teaching is student learning. The question is less whether we are teaching well than whether the student has been well motivated. There is not much point, as we have remarked before, in the teacher teaching if the learner isn't learning. Evaluation of our own teaching thus includes the process of feedback.

3. Student-learner attainments

At the heart of the evaluation process there lies the question of student learning. Are the learners learning? How much and what are they learning? What form of learning are they engaged in: is it product or process, to handle tools or to produce a table to a set standard? What is the quality and level of their learning? How well is the material learned? Have their skills of learning increased during the programme? These and many other similar questions occur in the process of thinking about the evaluation of our work as teachers of adults.

One of the issues here lies with the concept of progress in learning. If ignorance is seen to be deprivation, then progress will be seen in terms of acquisition — of new skills, knowledge, understanding and attitudes. 'Progress' is usually viewed as advancement along a straight line of development. But there is not always a straight line of progress in learning.

An essential part of this evaluation will be with the attitudinal development of the student participants — with how much additional confidence, how much increased motivation have arisen from the teaching–learning programme. This aspect is often omitted from the evaluation process which concentrates more on increased knowledge and more highly developed skills; but the assurance and enhanced self-image of the students, their willingness to continue to study, their increased interest are all outcomes which need to be evaluated.

And finally we will need to look for the unexpected outcomes, the impact of our teaching–learning programmes. Some of this may have to be done some time after the course has finished — what is sometimes called *post hoc* or postscript evaluation. Experience indicates that at times, whereas the learning objectives of a programme may have been achieved, the longer-term impact of one or other course could be negative (Rogers, 1992).

Evaluation methods

Exercise

Before starting this section, look at the course which you are taking as your case study and try to determine how you plan to evaluate it — what indicators will you look for. I suggest that you write them down here:

How to evaluate?

Student learning is the main focus of our process of evaluation. But there is no single right way of evaluating this; we have to decide for ourselves how to do it. Obviously we need to ask a series of questions, and determining what some of these should be is relatively simple. It is more difficult to come to some agreement on the criteria by which to judge the answers.

Over the years, organisers and providers have used a number of criteria to assess the effectiveness of their programmes and to establish the relative merits of their courses. Some argue (on *a priori* grounds) that longer courses are better than shorter ones (by no means always true) or that those taught by well-qualified teachers are better than those taught by less well-qualified staff (again not always true). They thus judge their programmes in terms of the numbers of longer courses or by the qualifications of the teachers used.

1. Satisfaction indicators

Others rely more heavily on satisfaction indicators such as

- indicated demand — requests from prospective student participants, individually or through organisations, on which the programme is built and which are taken to indicate that it must be meeting needs;

- effective demand — the numbers of student-learners attracted to particular classes; the size of the group is sometimes taken as a means of assessing the value of a course;

- follow-on — whether an extension of the learning situation is requested and taken up; a course is deemed successful if the learners request more of the same;

- follow-up — whether the learners continue to study on their own or pass into new programmes, whether they practise their new skills, read more, etc.;

- attendance figures — in terms of both regularity of attendance and low numbers of drop-outs;

- verbal or written comments by the student participants — both approval and complaints, indicating the learners' sense of success or dissatisfaction.

Teachers, too, often use such popularity or satisfaction indicators to help evaluate their work. But we need to examine them more closely to see whether such popularity signals truly indicate that effective learning is taking place.

2. Contextual preconditions

Among the factors that contribute towards the effectiveness of the learning process are those relating to the context within which the teaching takes place. These too are the concern of evaluation by both organiser and teacher. Since part of the task of evaluation is the identification of the good and bad influences that affect the results of our teaching, we need to consider carefully the *setting* (the room, furniture, temperature, lighting, teaching aids) to see whether it is conducive to the student participants' learning and to remedy any hindrances it contains. The *climate* also needs examination, both that of the institution within which the course is set and that of the learning group itself. There is little hope of creating effective learning changes in the direction of greater self-confidence and self-determination if the whole ethos of the institution is opposed to this or if the class denies the learner any opportunity to exercise such qualities. Overt and covert pressures for or against the goals are important elements in the process of teaching adults, and need evaluation.

3. Criteria from teaching

These two elements in the evaluative process, satisfaction indicators and signs of a conducive context, although valuable, say little about whether the student participants are learning or not. For this, other ranges of criteria can be drawn up, both by organisers concerned with the quality of the programmes they provide and teachers concerned about the effectiveness of their work. These criteria are based on what happens during the teaching–learning experience, and sometimes consist of a description of what happens, moment by moment, an analysis in terms of events and learning episodes. Some attempts have gone beyond this, trying to identify those processes that need to be reinforced and those needing to be corrected or nullified.

1. Some evaluators have looked to the *emotional climate* and *management controls* of the class for their indicators. These are perhaps more properly the preconditions of learning; they do not necessarily indicate whether learning is taking place. However they should contribute to the criteria by which we can assess teaching–learning effectiveness.

2. Another kind of evaluation is based on an analysis of what educational events occur during any teaching session. Thus some have recorded the number of *learning events* taking place and of what kind they are. (One such scheme divides these events into acts of memorisation, acts of divergent and convergent thinking, and acts of evaluative thinking.) Others have concentrated on the logic of teaching and of the language used in teaching; episodes have been listed such as defining, reporting and designating. These techniques however are more readily practised by others than by the teachers themselves; you cannot easily use them on your own group except by watching yourself teach with the use of a video-recorder. (It is well worth doing this, if you can get hold of the equipment; but if not, you can visit other classes and see other teachers at work, and in this case it is valuable to have in mind what you are looking for.)

3. More useful for the practising teacher is the analysis of the number and kinds of *transactions* that take place during any teaching session: transactions between teacher and learner, and between learner and learner. The participation of the student-learner in the work (activities) of the group is seen as one indicator that learning is taking place. If the teacher talks for a long time, only one kind of transaction is taking place; questions on the other hand comprise more transactions. The most frequently cited analysis of these transactions is that by Flanders, which records events every three seconds, but once again teachers usually need to rely on what they can deduce from their own teaching, and sophisticated techniques are probably not appropriate.

4. Others have concentrated on *types of method* used in the class and the involvement of the student participants in their own learning. The use of 'approved' teaching–learning methods such as demonstration or discussion is frequently felt to lead inevitably to learning. But it is not always easy to see how the teacher can test, at the end of each such occasion, how much and what kind of learning has taken place by the use of these methods. A substantial amount of subjective impression will add itself to our evaluation; we will *feel* good about the teaching session. But a reliance on particular teaching methods will not always lead to learning and may introduce an element of artificiality into the experience.

4. Teacher and learner

An analysis of what goes on during the teaching session can tell us about ourselves and about the learners, and may throw light on whether learning is taking place.

The first part of this analysis relates to our *performance* as teacher. Such an analysis will centre upon our subject expertise and skills of presentation and communication. Evidence of preparation, both of the subject-matter and of the modes of teaching; awareness of the student-learners; the clarity with which the goals of learning are defined; the structure of the learning episode — its level, pace of learning, relevance to the learner and to the task in hand — and the clear signposting of each step of the learning process are all capable of assessment. Our personal style of teaching (self-projection, confidence, voice level, powers of organisation, the rapport built up with the learners, the development of interaction and feedback), the methods used, the involvement of the learners in the processes, and the creation of feedback and evaluation procedures can all be recorded on a positive–negative scale. Positive recordings are those which it is believed will produce an occasion conducive to learning. This is perhaps as far as we can go along this line of enquiry.

Secondly the range and nature of *student activity* can be recorded as part of the evaluative process. The nature of the group, the kinds of interaction between members, the range of expectations and intentions they declare and the clarity of their goals, the kind of work they do in each session and between sessions, the questions they ask (as signs that they are grappling with the new material), the involvement of the learners in evaluating themselves — positive recordings in each of these areas are thought to be indicators that learning is taking place. At each stage, judgements need to be made: as to whether the activity in which the participant is engaged really aims 'at the *improvement* and development of knowledge, understanding and skill and not merely at its exercise'. In the end a description of the programme of work is not in itself an adequate means of assessing effectiveness, but a programme in which the learners are active is more likely to lead to learning changes than one in which they are passive recipients of information and instruction.

5. Performance testing

Involvement by the learners in the learning activities does not always reveal the kind of learning taking place, even if it can be relied upon to indicate that some form of learning changes are taking place. We noted [earlier] the two types of learning (inner learning and the behavioural expressions of that learning, the distinction expressed in the terms 'public' and 'private' effects of our teaching) and the discussion as to whether all 'private' outcomes can and should express themselves in behavioural (performance) terms. *Behavioural changes* and performance targets are easier to assess than inner changes in understanding, values and attitudes, and this fact will influence the procedures of assessment and evaluation we adopt. Part of the process of evaluation then is to interpret behavioural patterns and to create a range of performance situations in order to see how the more private learning changes are expressed.

We need to identify or create certain activities (making something, or writing, or speaking, say) that in themselves express the desired learning, in order to assess whether progress is being made and what kind of learning change is being achieved. But once again we need to remind ourselves of a number of caveats:

- These situations should be real ones, not artificial; there is little point in asking adult student-learners to engage in false activities that they will never engage in again once the course is over.

- The primary purpose is to evaluate the hidden depths (expressive objectives) that lie beneath these competency-based activities.

- Outside influences may hinder or prevent the exercise of the desired function. Activities (including words) do not always reflect inner learning changes and they rarely reflect their nature. But they are often the only way we can evaluate the learning changes of others.

6. Examinations

Despite the hesitations of many teachers in adult education, examinations are used with adults to evaluate student learning, and there are signs that their use is increasing. The variety of such so-called objective tests (usually subject based) is also increasing. They range from the very formal (standardised testing) to the very informal: written examinations (unseen, open-book, pre-set or home based), tests, essays (whether structured or subjective; that is, devoted to whatever the learner wishes to write about), practicals, observation of exercises, oral tests, questions, discussion, assignments, projects and so on. They tend to test the end product of the learning, the competencies attained; and their effect on the learning process is usually short-term.

The problems of marking examinations, of norm and criterion referencing (that is, whether each exam is to be marked against a 'normal' distribution pattern of success and failure, say 5 per cent top grade, 20 per cent second, 50 per cent third, etc.; or against an objective standard of competence that is supposed to exist somewhere outside of the examiner) and of whether the learners are thinking for themselves are well known. Their accompaniments — the prejudices of the examiners in relation to particular learners, the problem of extrinsic rewards rather than intrinsic motivation, the increase in competitiveness and selectivity, feelings of anxiety, failure and injustice, the distortion of the curriculum and of the pace of learning, the fact that many exams are set and marked by people unknown to the learners so that the aim comes to be to defeat the examiner rather than to learn — are again well known. They have led to a widespread concern to seek ways to replace élitist and selective examinations with other forms of evaluation; to replace prizes with goals that all may achieve. One of the most significant modern developments is the marathon run, which all may enter and all may win in their own terms because the participants choose their own standard and determine their own attainments; frequently they set themselves against themselves alone and assess their own attainments. Modern processes of evaluation are seeking similar ways of helping student participants to assess their own learning progress.

Nevertheless we may not dismiss such formal methods of evaluation entirely, for they can be formative as well as summative in their nature. Internal tests may be as much a means of new learning as of assessment. Sometimes they are intended to be solely summative, leading to the evaluation of attainment levels and on occasion to the award of certificates of competency. There may be a place for these in some forms of adult education, but a number of factors limit their usefulness:

- The problem of how to evaluate progress made as distinct from levels of attainment. Some adult learners, starting from a base lower than that of others in their group, make more rapid progress but remain well behind the attainment levels of the rest. The way to reward such effort and advances while retaining the prescribed or desired attainment levels is problematic.

- Adult learners not only start at very different points; they also choose different goals for themselves. The ends and intentions of adult learners are not homogeneous.

- There are no age-related criteria for adult learners as there are for many younger people.

7. End product

It remains a fact that the most frequent means of assessment and evaluation in adult education is the quality of the end product, be it a piece of writing, the ability to engage in a series of exercises, a fabricated article or role-play exercise completed to the satisfaction of the teacher, who is for this purpose the assessor. These, as we have seen, are not to be judged solely on their own but according to certain criteria attached to the performance of behavioural objectives: the level, the purpose for which it is being done, the conditions under which the actions are being performed, and so on. Any evaluation will need to include some clarification of these conditions as well as a definition of the activity itself.

The only fully satisfactory mode of assessment as to whether the learners are learning the right things and at the right level is the performance of the student participants after the end of each stage of the learning programme. Do they act in such a way as to reveal increased confidence, in whatever field of learning they are engaged in? Do they exercise the new skills better and/or more often? Do they reveal new understandings and new knowledge in what they say and do? Are they continuing to learn in directions of their own choice? Do they show signs of being satisfied with their own performance in their chosen field or of striving towards further improvement? The ultimate evaluation of the success or failure of our teaching will be seen in the exercise of the new skills, knowledge and understandings and of new attitudes towards themselves and the world around them. It is a question of whether our adult students reveal in their behaviour signs of increased adulthood and maturity, of development of their talents, greater autonomy and a sounder sense of perspective.

This is not easy, especially as most teachers of adults lose contact with their student participants soon after the end of the course or programme. The possibility of delayed learning (we know that it takes time for feelings, creative approaches and understandings to emerge) means that we can never be sure, in the case of seeming failures, that our work will not eventually bear fruit. Nor can we be sure that the learning of those with whom we seem to have been most successful will be permanent. For true evaluation ought to address itself not only to what the learners *can* do but to what they *do* do subsequently.

Does this mean that summative evaluation is impossible for the teacher of adults? The answer must be no. But it does mean

- that formative evaluation is more important in teaching adults than summative;
- that our summative evaluation will always be tentative; we can never know for sure.

Some teachers of adults will find this unsatisfactory; but we will often have to be content to cast our bread upon the waters in the expectation that it will (may?) return to us after many days. Perhaps the most rewarding aspect of the evaluation of adult learning are those signs of satisfaction that so many adults reveal in their relations with their teachers. The student participants are after all the best judges of whether they are getting what they feel they need.

Figure 1   An evaluation schedule: suggested headings

Objectives
- their nature
- the clarity with which they are perceived

Context
- the milieu/setting
- the climate

Teacher
- subject competency
- performance as teacher
- materials used

Student learners
- activities in group
- activities as individual learners

Level of performance
- the finished product

Unexpected outcome
- positive
- negative

Indicators of satisfaction
- whether goals have been/are being attained

Assessment of success or failure
- and reasons

Further reading

Charnley A H, Jones H A (1979) *Concept of Success in Adult Literacy*. Cambridge, Huntington.

Clark N, McCaffrey J (1979) *Demystifying Evaluation*. World Education, New York.

Flanders N A (1970) *Analyzing Teaching Behavior*. Addison-Wesley Pub. Co, Reading, MA.

Guba E, Lincoln E S (1981) *Effective Evaluation*. Jossey, San Francisco, CA.

Rowntree D (1987) *Assessing Students*. Kogan Page, London.

Ruddock R (1981) *Evaluation: A Consideration of Principles and Methods*. Manchester University Press, Manchester.

high degree of positive feeling *generally* about their placement. *In particular,* ┌
seen, they felt very happy with its *value* and its *relevance*. (To see this, look ┌
scores for the two sub-scales which measure value and for the sub-scale w┌
measures relevance. The scores on these particular sub-scales are the nearest of all to
the maximum possible.)

Table 3 **The individual items in the scale and how they are grouped to make up each sub-scale. It should be noted that the items marked with an R are those on which the direction of scoring should be reversed. (This will be understood by looking at Figure 1)**

Item	Sub-scale	Maximum possible score
Valuable (R) Useful Enjoyable Good (R)	Value 1	28
	Value 2	56
Satisfying Interesting (R) Informative Relevant Optimistic Vital	Relevance	28
Large (R) Deep Strong (R) Wide (R)	Breadth	28
Informal (R) Imaginative Active (R) Practical	Liveliness	28
Coherent (R) Consistent Clear (R)	Organisation	21
Stimulating (R) True (R) Fast Easy	Others	–

In contrast, however, the students apparently were not quite so satisfied with the organisation of their placement. This interested us a great deal because our work shows, for other professions, that *organisation* of their placements is one of the things that worries many students on professional training courses. Accordingly, because our work is part of a major Research & Development (R & D) project, this is something which particularly takes our attention from the research point of view.

From this point of view, Table 4 is of particular interest. In it, we have split up the results for the two classes of students which helped us in our study. By doing this, it can be seen that it was the students on the third-year (hospital) placement who had given low ratings to the organisation of their placement. Indeed, they had given *significantly* lower ratings to the way their placement was organised than did the fourth-year students. This result, of course, is explicable in terms of the different ways in which hospital and community placements are typically handled. In the former, the student nurse may have numerous different supervisors. In the latter, by contrast, greater continuity of supervision is often provided because only one midwife or health visitor is primarily responsible for the student.

Table 4   **Mean scores on sub-scales across the different classes: 3rd year students on hospital placement versus 4th year students on community placement**

	Maximum possible score	3rd year/ Hospital (N = 18)	4th year/ Community (N = 22)	F*	P*
Value 1	28	24.7	25.1	0.12	.73
Value 2	56	48.4	49.8	0.43	.52
Breadth	28	18.9	18.8	0.01	.93
Liveliness	28	19.6	21.0	1.41	.24
Organisation	21	13.6	16.0	6.60	.01*
Relevance	28	23.4	24.4	0.83	.37
Total	175	132.4	139.2	1.25	.27

* F – Fisher's F statistic, produced by Analysis of Variance (ANOVA).
    A significantly large F value would imply the two samples have different mean scores.
P – Probability that there is no difference between the sample means.
(This table shows that there was only one statistically significant difference between results from students on the different placements, viz. on organisation.)

(Having seen, from Table 4, that the organisation of hospital placements had been felt as something of a difficulty by the students on them, we further wondered whether a difference also arose, *within* the hospital placements themselves, between medical and surgical placements. Having explored this ourselves purely for interest, we give these further analyses in Table 5. But do read Table 5 merely for interest, and with caution, since the numbers of students involved here are too small to draw worthwhile conclusions.)

Table 5   **Mean scores on sub-scales across the two types of (3rd year students')**
hospital placement

	Maximum possible score	Medical (N = 8)	Surgical* (N = 9)	F	P
Value 1	28	24.3	25.0	0.17	.69
Value 2	56	46.5	49.7	0.77	.39
Breadth	28	17.8	19.7	0.65	.43
Liveliness	28	18.5	20.2	0.84	.38
Organisation	21	12.6	14.6	1.46	.25
Relevance	28	21.9	24.3	2.15	.16
Total	175	125.3	137.3	1.43	.25

* (One student was excluded from this analysis having completed a combined medical and surgical placement.)

The students on surgical placements evaluate them more positively than those on medical placements but not significantly so given the smallness of the sample.

Some implications and suggestions for further work

We have shown, then, from the results we obtained, that Hoste has given us a very interesting, helpful and inexpensive way to find out how nurse students feel about their placements. An exercise of the kind we did can be done as a 'one-off' event. Alternatively, such an exercise could be repeated over several years, so that nurse teachers can see, through their *students'* eyes, which aspects of their placements are usually strong and which aspects may need strengthening. (It so happened in the case of this particular study that student satisfaction with placement was very high. Results of this kind, of course, are pleasing to the people responsible. But even less pleasing results would be equally *useful*, obviously.)

For the work we have described we used the Hoste scale in its classic form, just as it stands. But in our newest work (which is based in Edinburgh and is the largest such project in the UK) we are exploring various expansions and adaptations of the Hoste scale. We are interested, for example, in which adjectives would strike a particularly strong chord with *students themselves*, and which we might therefore incorporate in a new version of the scale. (These adjectives would tell us a lot about what is important about a placement from a student's point of view.) Therefore, with this in mind, we asked our nurse students if they would suggest to us the adjectives which *they* felt should be used in the scale. The students' suggestions to us make fascinating reading and included such descriptions as: stressful/safe; stretching/pedestrian; exhausting/therapeutic. We ourselves are taking this aspect of our work further for other professions and in other parts of Britain. It is certainly an aspect which nurse teachers themselves could take forward with the help of their students. It would, we think, yield enormous benefits to nursing education.

Summary and discussion

This paper has described a general scale for measuring student feelings about their courses. This scale can be used in many different ways but our own work concentrates particularly on its use for measuring student satisfaction with professional placements of various kinds. Our interest in the field of nurse education led us to take the scale into that field. This had not been done before. This novel step has proved fascinating and informative to us as researchers and has also shown that the scale can easily be used for course appraisal and development by nurse teachers themselves.

In addition, the particular students in this study, when they were asked to contribute their own adjectives for describing placement, showed us that students themselves have new and interesting suggestions to make. Such suggestions could easily be incorporated into the original scale so that it would become more 'tailor-made' for nursing placements of various kinds.

Even without such further development, however, the scale as it stands is well validated and worth using. It can certainly give to nurse teachers the kind of honest and useful information they want to help them with their work.

Acknowledgements

We are grateful to CNAA for funding this work which is part of the CNAA-funded placement project. (The opinions expressed in the paper are our own, however.) And we are, of course, particularly grateful to the nurse teachers and students who helped us in this work.

References

Cameron-Jones M (1980) Follow-up note: The usefulness of Hoste's course appraisal scales. *Brit. J. In-service Education* 7: 49–52.

Hoste R (1977a) Semantic differential course appraisal scales. College Curriculum Project, University of Leeds and N.F.E.R. mimeo.

Hoste R (1977b) Evaluating an in-service course in reading. *Brit. J. In-service Education* 4: 84–89.

Hoste R (1981) Course appraisal using semantic differential scales. *Education Studies* 7, 3: 151–161.

Osgood C E, Suci G J, Tannenbaum P H (1957) *The measurements of meaning.* University of Illinois Press, Urbana, Illinois.

United Kingdom Central Council for Nursing, Midwifery and Health Visiting (1986) *Project 2000. A New Preparation for Practice,* UKCC, London.

Warr P B, Knapper C (1968) *The perceptions of people and events.* John Wiley & Sons, New York.

Wheeler H H (1988) Evaluating study modules in basic nurse education programmes. *Nurse Education Today* 8: 77–84.

Whittington D, Boore J (1988) Competence in nursing. In: R Ellis (ed) (1988) *Professional competence and quality assurance in the caring professions.* Croom Helm, London.

Continuing Professional Development in Nursing: A Guide for Practitioners and Educators

edited by F.M. Quinn

The aim of this book is to provide practitioners and educators in nursing, midwifery and health visiting with a comprehensive guide to issues and approaches in CPD, utilising a range of contributors from both within and outside the nursing professions who possess acknowledged expertise in the field of CPD. The book covers a wide spectrum of CPD issues and approaches, and the practical 'how to do it' focus is balanced by a sound underpinning of analysis and discussion.

£18.00   Paperback   0 7487 3337

Orders to:

Stanley Thornes (Publishers) Ltd, Ellenborough House,
Wellington Street, Cheltenham, Gloucester, GL50 1YW
Tel: 01242 228383   Fax: 01242 221914

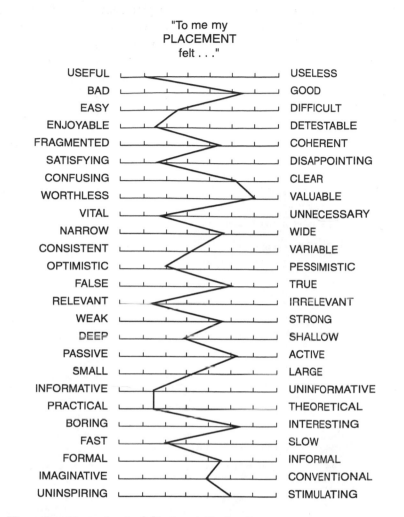

Figure 1   How the 40 students felt about their placements

The details of our own study

For our own study we were given access to two classes of nurse students who had just returned from placement. The third-year class of 18 students had been on hospital placement. The fourth-year class of 22 students had been on community placement.

Both classes of students rated their placement on the scale in the way we have described above (the actual words we gave them were those we show in Figure 1, i.e. 'To me my placement felt . . .'). We combined the replies of both classes to make the profile we have pictured in Figure 1. This figure shows in a graphic way that the students felt very positively indeed about their placements.

When the same results are given in their numerical form, for the various sub-scales, in Table 2, it can be seen clearly again from the *total* score that the students expressed a in. You explain to students either verbally or in writing that on each line they should put a tick in the space which best represents their feeling about the placement. A tick close to an adjective shows strong feeling but a tick at or near to the middle of the line shows undecidedness. Once the sheets are gathered in from the students you can easily score the responses (scoring them as 7 to 1, or 1 to 7 in cases where the 'good-bad' adjectives are reversed) and so can produce from a class a quick impression of their feelings. If you do not have time to calculate sub-scale scores, you can get one useful general measure of your students' feelings merely by adding up the simple total. (The higher the total, the more positive your students' feelings.) This simple total is a helpful statistic just by itself and can be added up even by a clerical assistant, provided that he/she remembers that the direction of scoring for some adjectives must be reversed! (see Table 3, which shows the ones which are reversed and which also explains how to combine the scores on the various separate adjectives in order to make up the six different sub-scale scores if you wish to do this.)

Table 1   Sub-scales in the Hoste scale

Sub-scale	Maximum/minimum scores	Examples of adjectives. One example is given here for each sub-scale. (For example, the student's view of a placement as *informative vs. uninformative* contributes to his/her score on the *Relevance* sub-scale.)
Value 1	28/4	Valuable vs. worthless
Value 2	56/8	Satisfying vs. disappointing
Breadth	28/4	Wide vs. narrow
Liveliness	28/4	Imaginative vs. conventional
Organisation	21/3	Clear vs. confusing
Relevance	28/4	Informative vs. uninformative

Table 2   How the 40 students felt about their placement (Mean scores on the six sub-scales)

	Mean	Maximum possible scores
Value 1	24.9	28
Value 2	49.2	56
Breadth	18.9	28
Liveliness	20.4	28
Organisation	14.9	21
Relevance	24.0	28
Total	136.2	175

One result of this general trend as far as nursing is concerned is that nurse teachers need better methods of discovering just how satisfactory, fruitful and motivating placements are in the eyes of everyone involved, including, and very importantly, in the eyes of the students themselves. This paper describes how to use one method for getting information of this kind. The method is very simple and quick to use. It gives helpful information. And it is ripe for further development by nurse teachers in the future.

The method tells you how students *themselves feel*, in general, and in particular ways, about the placements they have. The method was first developed in the 1970s by Roland Hoste — not in the field of nurse education but in the field of teacher education.

The Hoste scale — some background information and illustration

In the late 1970s Roland Hoste produced and published his scale which could be used for discovering how students felt about courses of *teacher* training. By extension this scale can be used in any other kind of course (Hoste, 1977a; Hoste, 1977b; Cameron-Jones, 1980; Hoste, 1981), a development which Hoste himself suggested and which we ourselves successfully tried out. The scale is a semantic differential scale which presents the person whose views are sought with the name of the thing to be rated (e.g. 'This year's Physiology course') and a list of bi-polar adjectives with which to rate it (e.g. Interesting vs Boring).

Semantic differential scales were first produced in the 1950s (Osgood *et al.* 1957) and were validated in the 1960s (Warr & Knapper, 1968). Hoste's development in the 1970s was notable for applying such scales to *courses*, particularly to their 'theoretical' components (i.e. the parts of a course done in the students' college, rather than the placement part of the course). Our own work in the 1980s took the step of using those scales with students to appraise their *placements*. At first our work was done in the field of *teacher* education. The present paper is the first to move this work into the field of *nurse* education.

Hoste's full scale gives a set of bi-polar adjectives which you can group into six sub-scales. (Two sub-scales measure value; one measures breadth and depth; one measures liveliness; one measures organisation: and one measures relevance.) Each sub-scale is made of a sub-set of the total set of bi-polar adjectives. People using the scale may be particularly interested in the scores on the particular sub-scales, or they may just want to add the scores on all the adjectives to give one total general score.

Examples of the adjectives used in each of the particular sub-scales are given in Table 1. In Figure 1 the whole scale itself is reproduced with, drawn on to it, a 'profile' made by combining all the results we are reporting in this paper. These same results, presented as sub-scale scores, are shown in Table 2, again as an example.

It can be seen from the tables and from the figure that the scale gives very interesting and usable results. The scale also has the merit of being very easy to use and score. Thus, if you want to discover how a whole class of nurse students feel about any part of their course, you give one copy of this scale, with an appropriate heading at the top, to every student in the class. The students will take about 10 minutes or less to fill it

40.   Pleased with Your Placements?

Margot Cameron-Jones and Paul O'Hara

This paper describes a technique for measuring nurse students' feelings about their placements. The method is a semantic differential scale. The scale is robust and we have researched it over a long period with various professions who include placement in their training. It has not been used in nurse education before, but will be a very useful resource indeed to nurse teachers who want to know how their students feel about their placements. The scale gives a general picture of how students feel about a placement generally; it will also show you, more specifically, how students feel about the value, relevance, breadth, liveliness and organisation of their placement. The paper describes how to administer the scale and how to score the results. It also gives some results in graphic (profiled) form, as well as in tables, in order to demonstrate the method and its possibilities in the field of nursing education.

Introduction

In a previous issue of this journal Wheeler (1988) described a tool which can help nurse teachers to measure their students' achievements 'within theoretical and clinical placement settings'. The educational arguments for seeking such information are clear. Without it, nurse teachers will have great difficulty in making rational decisions about the improvement of their courses in the current period of rapid change, and institutional managers will lack the indicators of institutional performance which they increasingly need in these new times.

However, valid tools with which to obtain this information are hard to come by. In addition they are tremendously time-consuming to develop from scratch. And this is particularly so in the very complex field of clinical placement — an area of professional education in which a large number of professions, not just that of nursing, are becoming more urgently interested than ever before.

Thus many professions, including law, teaching, medicine and engineering, now pay increasing attention to the quality of their student placements. The report, Project 2000 (UKCC, 1986), analyses some of the reasons why placement presents a particularly difficult (as well as rewarding) task for its organisers and participants in the profession of nursing. Precisely the same complexities and concerns are found in placements in other professions and they, like nursing (Whittington & Boore, 1988), are now emphasising the critical role of the practitioners who take part in placement. It is a general professional trend, therefore, to highlight the role of practitioners, not only in developing the knowledge base of the profession but also in influencing students in a direct way through offering analyses, modelling and experience to the students placed with them.

Margot Cameron-Jones and Paul O'Hara: 'Pleased with Your Placements?' in *NURSE EDUCATION TODAY* (1989), 9(5), pp. 314–319. Reprinted by permission of the publisher Churchill Livingstone.

high degree of positive feeling *generally* about their placement. *In particular,* seen, they felt very happy with its *value* and its *relevance*. (To see this, look scores for the two sub-scales which measure value and for the sub-scale w measures relevance. The scores on these particular sub-scales are the nearest of all to the maximum possible.)

Table 3   The individual items in the scale and how they are grouped to make up each sub-scale. It should be noted that the items marked with an R are those on which the direction of scoring should be reversed. (This will be understood by looking at Figure 1)

Item	Sub-scale	Maximum possible score
Valuable (R) Useful Enjoyable Good (R)	Value 1	28
	Value 2	56
Satisfying Interesting (R) Informative Relevant Optimistic Vital	Relevance	28
Large (R) Deep Strong (R) Wide (R)	Breadth	28
Informal (R) Imaginative Active (R) Practical	Liveliness	28
Coherent (R) Consistent Clear (R)	Organisation	21
Stimulating (R) True (R) Fast Easy	Others	–

In contrast, however, the students apparently were not quite so satisfied with the organisation of their placement. This interested us a great deal because our work shows, for other professions, that *organisation* of their placements is one of the things that worries many students on professional training courses. Accordingly, because our work is part of a major Research & Development (R & D) project, this is something which particularly takes our attention from the research point of view.

From this point of view, Table 4 is of particular interest. In it, we have split up the results for the two classes of students which helped us in our study. By doing this, it can be seen that it was the students on the third-year (hospital) placement who had given low ratings to the organisation of their placement. Indeed, they had given *significantly* lower ratings to the way their placement was organised than did the fourth-year students. This result, of course, is explicable in terms of the different ways in which hospital and community placements are typically handled. In the former, the student nurse may have numerous different supervisors. In the latter, by contrast, greater continuity of supervision is often provided because only one midwife or health visitor is primarily responsible for the student.

Table 4   Mean scores on sub-scales across the different classes: 3rd year students on hospital placement versus 4th year students on community placement

	Maximum possible score	3rd year/ Hospital (N = 18)	4th year/ Community (N = 22)	F*	P*
Value 1	28	24.7	25.1	0.12	.73
Value 2	56	48.4	49.8	0.43	.52
Breadth	28	18.9	18.8	0.01	.93
Liveliness	28	19.6	21.0	1.41	.24
Organisation	21	13.6	16.0	6.60	.01*
Relevance	28	23.4	24.4	0.83	.37
Total	175	132.4	139.2	1.25	.27

* F – Fisher's F statistic, produced by Analysis of Variance (ANOVA).
      A significantly large F value would imply the two samples have different mean scores.
P   – Probability that there is no difference between the sample means.
(This table shows that there was only one statistically significant difference between results from students on the different placements, viz. on organisation.)

(Having seen, from Table 4, that the organisation of hospital placements had been felt as something of a difficulty by the students on them, we further wondered whether a difference also arose, *within* the hospital placements themselves, between medical and surgical placements. Having explored this ourselves purely for interest, we give these further analyses in Table 5. But do read Table 5 merely for interest, and with caution, since the numbers of students involved here are too small to draw worthwhile conclusions.)

**Table 5   Mean scores on sub-scales across the two types of (3rd year students')
hospital placement**

	Maximum possible score	Medical (N = 8)	Surgical* (N = 9)	F	P
Value 1	28	24.3	25.0	0.17	.69
Value 2	56	46.5	49.7	0.77	.39
Breadth	28	17.8	19.7	0.65	.43
Liveliness	28	18.5	20.2	0.84	.38
Organisation	21	12.6	14.6	1.46	.25
Relevance	28	21.9	24.3	2.15	.16
Total	175	125.3	137.3	1.43	.25

* (One student was excluded from this analysis having completed a combined medical and surgical placement.)

The students on surgical placements evaluate them more positively than those on medical placements but not significantly so given the smallness of the sample.

Some implications and suggestions for further work

We have shown, then, from the results we obtained, that Hoste has given us a very interesting, helpful and inexpensive way to find out how nurse students feel about their placements. An exercise of the kind we did can be done as a 'one-off' event. Alternatively, such an exercise could be repeated over several years, so that nurse teachers can see, through their *students'* eyes, which aspects of their placements are usually strong and which aspects may need strengthening. (It so happened in the case of this particular study that student satisfaction with placement was very high. Results of this kind, of course, are pleasing to the people responsible. But even less pleasing results would be equally *useful*, obviously.)

For the work we have described we used the Hoste scale in its classic form, just as it stands. But in our newest work (which is based in Edinburgh and is the largest such project in the UK) we are exploring various expansions and adaptations of the Hoste scale. We are interested, for example, in which adjectives would strike a particularly strong chord with *students themselves*, and which we might therefore incorporate in a new version of the scale. (These adjectives would tell us a lot about what is important about a placement from a student's point of view.) Therefore, with this in mind, we asked our nurse students if they would suggest to us the adjectives which *they* felt should be used in the scale. The students' suggestions to us make fascinating reading and included such descriptions as: stressful/safe; stretching/pedestrian; exhausting/therapeutic. We ourselves are taking this aspect of our work further for other professions and in other parts of Britain. It is certainly an aspect which nurse teachers themselves could take forward with the help of their students. It would, we think, yield enormous benefits to nursing education.

Summary and discussion

This paper has described a general scale for measuring student feelings about their courses. This scale can be used in many different ways but our own work concentrates particularly on its use for measuring student satisfaction with professional placements of various kinds. Our interest in the field of nurse education led us to take the scale into that field. This had not been done before. This novel step has proved fascinating and informative to us as researchers and has also shown that the scale can easily be used for course appraisal and development by nurse teachers themselves.

In addition, the particular students in this study, when they were asked to contribute their own adjectives for describing placement, showed us that students themselves have new and interesting suggestions to make. Such suggestions could easily be incorporated into the original scale so that it would become more 'tailor-made' for nursing placements of various kinds.

Even without such further development, however, the scale as it stands is well validated and worth using. It can certainly give to nurse teachers the kind of honest and useful information they want to help them with their work.

Acknowledgements

We are grateful to CNAA for funding this work which is part of the CNAA-funded placement project. (The opinions expressed in the paper are our own, however.) And we are, of course, particularly grateful to the nurse teachers and students who helped us in this work.

References

Cameron-Jones M (1980) Follow-up note: The usefulness of Hoste's course appraisal scales. *Brit. J. In-service Education* 7: 49–52.

Hoste R (1977a) Semantic differential course appraisal scales. College Curriculum Project, University of Leeds and N.F.E.R. mimeo.

Hoste R (1977b) Evaluating an in-service course in reading. *Brit. J. In-service Education* 4: 84–89.

Hoste R (1981) Course appraisal using semantic differential scales. *Education Studies* 7, 3: 151–161.

Osgood C E, Suci G J, Tannenbaum P H (1957) *The measurements of meaning.* University of Illinois Press, Urbana, Illinois.

United Kingdom Central Council for Nursing, Midwifery and Health Visiting (1986) *Project 2000. A New Preparation for Practice,* UKCC, London.

Warr P B, Knapper C (1968) *The perceptions of people and events.* John Wiley & Sons, New York.

Wheeler H H (1988) Evaluating study modules in basic nurse education programmes. *Nurse Education Today* 8: 77–84.

Whittington D, Boore J (1988) Competence in nursing. In: R Ellis (ed) (1988) *Professional competence and quality assurance in the caring professions.* Croom Helm, London.

Continuing Professional Development in Nursing: A Guide for Practitioners and Educators

edited by F.M. Quinn

The aim of this book is to provide practitioners and educators in nursing, midwifery and health visiting with a comprehensive guide to issues and approaches in CPD, utilising a range of contributors from both within and outside the nursing professions who possess acknowledged expertise in the field of CPD. The book covers a wide spectrum of CPD issues and approaches, and the practical 'how to do it' focus is balanced by a sound underpinning of analysis and discussion.

£18.00   Paperback   0 7487 3337

Orders to:

Stanley Thornes (Publishers) Ltd, Ellenborough House,
Wellington Street, Cheltenham, Gloucester, GL50 1YW
Tel: 01242 228383   Fax: 01242 221914